NEW CLINICAL GENETICS

Andrew Read
and Dian Donnai

Scion

Department of Medical Genetics, University of Manchester,
St Mary's Hospital, Manchester, UK

A CIP catalogue record for this book is available from the British Library.

ISBN10 – 1 904842 31 3
ISBN13 – 978 1 904842 31 6

Scion Publishing Limited
Bloxham Mill, Barford Road, Bloxham, Oxfordshire OX15 4FF, UK
www.scionpublishing.com

Important Note from the Publisher

The information contained within this book was obtained by Scion Publishing Limited from sources believed by us to be reliable. However, while every effort has been made to ensure its accuracy, no responsibility for loss or injury whatsoever occasioned to any person acting or refraining from action as a result of information contained herein can be accepted by the authors or publishers.

Readers are reminded that medicine is a constantly evolving science and while the authors and publishers have ensured that all dosages, applications and practices are based on current indications, there may be specific practices which differ between communities. You should always follow the guidelines laid down by the manufacturers of specific products and the relevant authorities in the country in which you are practicing.

Typeset by Phoenix Photosetting, Chatham, Kent, UK
Printed by Ajanta Offset and Packagings Ltd, Delhi, India

Contents

Chapter 4 – How can a patient's DNA be studied?

Chapter 5 – How can we check a patient's DNA for gene mutations?

Chapter 7 – What is epigenetics?

Chapter 8 – How do genes affect our metabolism, drug responses and immune system?

Chapter 9 – How do researchers identify genes for mendelian diseases?

Chapter 10 – Why are some conditions common and others rare?

Chapter 11 – When is screening useful?

Chapter 12 – Is cancer genetic?

Guidance for self-assessment questions

Glossary

Index

Case notes – Summary of cases and their page references

CASE 1   Ashton family   1 7 65 104 150 376

- John – 28-year-old son of Alfred Ashton
- ? Huntington disease
- Other family members with similar symptoms
- Autosomal dominant inheritance shown in pedigree
- Diagnostic test ordered – *Chapter 1*

CASE 2   Brown family   2 8 65 126 151 279 376

- Girl (Joanne) aged 6 months, parents David and Pauline
- ? Cystic fibrosis
- Order molecular test? – *Chapter 1*
- Define mutations in *CFTR* gene – *Chapter 5*
- Universal newborn screening? – *Chapter 11*

CASE 3   Choudhary family   3 9 66 242 260 376

- Girl (Nasreen) aged 8 months, parents Aadnan and Mumtaz
- Deaf
- Parents are first cousins
- Pedigree suggests autosomal recessive deafness – *Chapter 1*

- Boy (Martin) aged 24 months, parents Judith and Robert
- Clumsy and slow to walk
- Family history of muscular dystrophy
- Pedigree shows X-linked recessive inheritance
- Order diagnostic DNA test – *Chapter 1*
- Frameshift mutation in the dystrophin gene – *Chapter 6*
- Screening of all new-born boys? – *Chapter 11*

- Miscarriage
- Very small dysmorphic baby girl (Elizabeth), parents Elmer and Ellen
- Heart problems
- Blood taken for chromosome analysis
- Pedigree suggests autosomal dominant condition with reduced penetrance – *Chapter 1*
- Reciprocal translocation – *Chapter 3*

- Frank, aged 22, with increasingly blurred eyesight
- Family history of visual difficulties
- Pedigree suggests X-linked recessive inheritance but not conclusive
- ? LHON
- Order blood test to check for mutation in mtDNA – *Chapter 1*
- Check mutations by Pyrosequencing – *Chapter 5*
- G3460 mutation in mtDNA – *Chapter 6*

- Girl (Gillian) aged 3 years
- Slow to develop
- ? Chromosome abnormality
- Order tests to check for microdeletion at 22q11 – *Chapter 2*

- Helen – new-born daughter of Henry and Anne (33 years old)
- Down syndrome
- Risk of recurrence if they have more children? – *Chapter 2*

- Isabel – first daughter of Irene and Ian
- Small stature despite tall parents
- ? Turner syndrome – *Chapter 2*
- Diagnosis confirmed by karyotyping – *Chapter 7*

- Marfan syndrome – *Chapter 3*

| CASE 11 | Kavanagh family | 81 | 97 | 152 |

- Healthy first baby boy
- Second child, Celia, pale with low hemoglobin levels
- Sickle cell disease – *Chapter 4*
- Single nucleotide mutation, Glu→Val – *Chapter 6*

| CASE 12 | Lawton family | 82 | 98 | 376 |

- Family history of hemophilia
- Baby boy, Lennox, with cephalohematoma – *Chapter 4*

| CASE 13 | Murphy family | 83 | 100 | 376 |

- Baby girl, Michelle, with dysmorphic features
- ? Unbalanced chromosome abnormality – *Chapter 4*

| CASE 14 | Nicolaides family | 115 | 129 | 153 | 376 |

- ? β-thalassemia carriers
- Check mutations – *Chapter 5*
- p.Gln39X nonsense mutation for Spiros
- c.316–106C>G mutation for Elena – *Chapter 6*

| CASE 15 | O'Reilly family | 141 | 154 | 376 |

- Family history of myopia and hip problems
- Orla has severe myopia, is short, and has hip problems
- ? Stickler syndrome
- Frameshift mutation in *COL2A1* – *Chapter 6*

| CASE 16 | Portillo family | 173 | 183 | 214 | 376 |

- Sickly boy, Pablo
- Family history of similar symptoms
- Blood tests suggest X-linked severe combined immunodeficiency – *Chapter 7*
- Check that bone marrow transplantation is appropriate – *Chapter 8*

| CASE 17 | Qian family | 174 | 185 | 376 |

- Girl, Kai, aged 2 years, showing slow development
- Seizure
- ? Angelman syndrome
- Check for causative mutation with FISH – *Chapter 7*

| CASE 18 | Rogers family | 175 | 185 | 376 |

- Baby boy, Robert, born to older parents
- Floppy at birth; failed to suck
- Genetic tests in pregnancy showed normal male karyotype
- ? Prader–Willi syndrome
- Check for causative mutation with PCR – *Chapter 7*

Abbreviations

ACTH	adrenocorticotrophic hormone
AFP	alpha-fetoprotein
ALAS	amino levulinic acid synthase
ALL	acute lymphocytic leukemia
APP	amyloid precursor protein
ASO	allele-specific oligonucleotide
ASP	affected sib pair
CAH	congenital adrenal hyperplasia
CDK	cyclin-dependent kinase
CGH	comparative genomic hybridization
cM	centiMorgan
dHPLC	denaturing high performance liquid chromatography
DMD	Duchenne muscular dystrophy
DNA	deoxyribonucleic acid
DSH	dyschromatosis symmetrica hereditaria
DTDST	diastrophic dystrophy sulfate transporter
DZ	dizygotic
FAP	familial adenomatous polyposis
FDA	Food and Drug Administration
FH	familial hypercholesterolemia
FISH	fluorescence *in situ* hybridization
GvH	graft versus host
HLA	human leukocyte antigen
HNPCC	hereditary non-polyposis colon cancer
Ig	immunoglobulins
IRT	immunoreactive trypsin
IVF	*in vitro* fertilization
LDL	low density lipoprotein
LHON	Leber hereditary optic neuropathy
MCAD	medium chain acyl-CoA dehydrogenase
MH	malignant hyperthermia
MHC	major histocompatibility complex
ML	mucolipidosis
MLPA	multiplex ligation-dependent probe amplification
MMR	mis-match repair
MODY	maturity-onset diabetes in the young
MSAFP	maternal serum alpha-fetoprotein
MZ	monozygotic
NK	natural killer
NSC	National Screening Committee
NTD	neural tube defect

OLA	oligonucleotide ligation assay
OMIM	Online Mendelian Inheritance in Man
PCR	polymerase chain reaction
PKU	phenylketonuria
PWS	Prader–Willi syndrome
QTL	quantitative trait locus
RB	retinoblastoma
RFLP	restriction fragment length polymorphism
RNA	ribonucleic acid
RSTS	Rubinstein–Taybi syndrome
SNP	single nucleotide polymorphism
SSCP	single strand conformation polymorphism
SUMF	sulfatase modifying factor
T2D	type 2 diabetes
TDT	transmission disequilibrium test
TGFβ	transforming growth factor β
TPMT	thiopurine methyl transferase
TS	tumor suppressor
UPD	uniparental disomy
X-SCID	X-linked severe combined immunodeficiency

Preface

This book is the result of a collaboration between a scientist (Andrew Read) and a clinician (Dian Donnai). As such, it represents the way clinical genetics operates. We have been fortunate to work in an integrated genetics unit where clinicians, counselors, diagnostic scientists and researchers all work closely together and strike sparks off each other. When we both arrived in the Department of Medical Genetics at St Mary's Hospital, Manchester one day in 1977, we were assigned adjacent desks in a corridor, the department having as usual outgrown its accommodation. We were both there because we thought this was the most exciting and dynamic area in all biology and medicine. The ensuing years have more than vindicated that judgement.

Our primary audience for this book is medical students, but we hope it will also be useful to counselors and scientists, and indeed established clinicians, who want an introduction to the place of clinical genetics in medicine and biology. Only a few of today's medical students will specialize in genetics. All, however, need to understand genetic principles and their application since, in the future, genetic knowledge will underpin much of medical practice. We have tried to produce a book that will make learning interesting by focusing on patients and real clinical situations, without losing sight of the strong underlying conceptual framework of genetics. As explained in the section, *How to Use this Book*, we have designed the book so that it can be used either for a case-based course of study, or in a more traditional way focusing on the science.

We have based the content of the book around the curriculum of the American Society of Human Genetics and the *List of Competencies* for undergraduate medical students being developed by the UK NHS Genetics Education Centre. Annotated versions of these two documents, showing the main places in the book where the relevant material can be found, are available to download at http://www.scionpublishing.com/newclinicalgenetics

We are grateful to David Cooper, Susan Hamilton, Lauren Kerzin-Storrar, Helen Middleton-Price, Rehat Perveen and Alison Stewart, who read through various sections and provided ideas and suggestions. Susan Hamilton also provided most of the cytogenetic pictures. We also thank the many colleagues who we pestered for photos or data, for their kindness and forbearance, and the families who generously agreed to our use of their photos. We hope we have duly acknowledged the sources of all our illustrations, but if anybody notices a picture of theirs used without due acknowledgement, they should please contact us. Finally, we would like to thank Jonathan Ray of Scion Publishing Ltd for his good ideas, hard work and unfailing patience, without which this book would never have come to fruition.

Andrew Read and Dian Donnai
August 2006

How to use this book

Each chapter addresses a specific question that students may have about genetics, e.g. How can we study chromosomes? Is cancer genetic? etc. Chapters follow a common structure:

- *Learning points* – summarizing what the chapter should enable the student to achieve. These are chosen to cover the curriculum published by the American Society of Human Genetics and the list of competencies being developed by the UK NHS Genetics Education Centre.
- *Case studies* –all chapters except the last one have this section, which introduces a series of short clinically oriented descriptions of a family and the reasons why they sought genetic counseling or testing. The cases are all fictional and the photographs illustrate the condition rather than the patients described; but they are based on our long experience of dealing with real families.
- *Background* – an explanation of the methods and concepts that are necessary in the next section.
- *Investigations of patients* – using the case studies to illustrate the application of the methods and concepts in realistic scenarios. These form running stories that develop over several chapters.
- *Summary and extension* – summarizes and extends the relevant science.

Students can choose different routes through the material:

| CASE 1 | Ashton family | 1 | 7 | 65 | 104 | 150 | 376 |

- John – 28-year-old son of Alfred Ashton
- ? Huntington disease
- Other family members with similar symptoms
- Autosomal dominant inheritance shown in pedigree
- Diagnostic test ordered

- Those who prefer a problem-based approach would move from the initial *Case studies* to the *Investigations of patients* sections. They should treat the other sections as reference material. The page design includes page references to enable students to follow cases that run through several chapters. For example, the Ashton family case is covered on pages 1, 7, 65, 104, 150 and 376. In addition, the bullets associated with each case serve as reminders as to what has been covered previously

- Students who prefer a more didactic approach can concentrate on the science in the *Background* and *Summary and extension* of sections. The other sections provide illustrations and examples.

Chapters finish with self-assessment questions so that students can check that they have mastered the material, regardless which route they chose to take through it.

The book is not intended as a diagnostic manual and so does not aim to describe all the major mendelian and chromosomal disorders. However, the cases and the *Disease boxes* help to show the range and variety of genetic conditions. For specific information you should refer to the reliable websites listed in the *References* section of relevant chapters. The first place to look should be the OMIM database: http://www.ncbi.nlm.nih.gov/omim – OMIM reference numbers are given throughout the book.

Chapter 1

What can we learn from a family history?

Learning points for this chapter

After working through this chapter you should be able to:

- Take a family history

- Draw a pedigree using correct symbols

- Identify the most likely mode of inheritance, given a straightforward pedigree

- Describe how genes segregate in autosomal dominant, autosomal recessive, X-linked dominant, X-linked recessive, Y-linked and mitochondrial conditions

- Define penetrance and expressivity

- Show appreciation of the human and scientific issues raised by the conditions described

1.1. Case studies

| CASE 1 | Ashton family | **1** | 7 | 65 | 104 | 150 | 376 |

- John – 28-year-old son of Alfred Ashton
- ? Huntington disease
- Other family members with similar symptoms

Alfred Ashton, aged 52, had been getting forgetful and was thought to be depressed following losing his job. He has been seeing a psychiatrist, who noted that Alfred was restless and had some choreiform movements (involuntary jerky movements of his fingers and shoulders and facial grimacing). Alfred had told the psychiatrist that he thought he was developing 'the family disease', though he was vague as to what this was. The psychiatrist suspected that Alfred had Huntington disease (OMIM 143100). His 28-year-old son John has been referred to the genetic clinic by his family doctor at the suggestion of the psychiatrist. John knows nothing about Huntington disease; he is preoccupied with other things, having recently married and bought a house.

Figure 1.1 – Huntington disease.
(a) A patient in the advanced stages of the disease showing involuntary movements of the head and face. Photos courtesy of Professor Peter Harper, Cardiff. (b) Post mortem sections comparing normal brain (left) with brain from Huntington disease patient (right); note the loss of tissue in the Huntington disease brain. Photos courtesy of Dr David Crauford, St Mary's Hospital, Manchester.

CASE 2	Brown family	2	8	65	126	151	279	376

- Girl (Joanne) aged 6 months, parents David and Pauline
- ? Cystic fibrosis

Joanne is the second child born to David and Pauline Brown. Her older brother Jason is now 4 years old and very healthy, in fact his parents have to buy age 6 clothes for him. Joanne, however, is a different matter. She has worried her parents from the start. Although she took her bottle well she was very slow to put on weight and in her first few months seemed constantly to have a cold and a cough. At first Pauline and the doctor put this down to the fact that Jason had just started nursery and had a few colds himself. When she was 5 months old Joanne was really ill and was admitted to hospital with a chest infection. The nurses commented that her bowel motions were very bulky and offensive, and when her weight and height were plotted on the charts they were on lower centiles than they had been at birth and in her first month. The doctors suspected she might have cystic fibrosis (OMIM 219700) and therefore arranged for her to have a sweat test. This confirmed their suspicion (Na^+ level of 87 mmol/l, well above the normal upper limit of 60 mmol/l). The diagnosis came as a complete bombshell to Pauline and David. At their request, Joanne's pediatrician arranged for them to see a geneticist to talk things through.

Figure 1.2 – Cystic fibrosis.
(a) The outlook for cystic fibrosis patients has improved over the years but they still need frequent hospital admissions, physiotherapy and constant medications. (b) Chest X-ray of lungs of cystic fibrosis patient. (c) Erect abdominal film of newborn with meconium ileus showing multiple fluid levels. Photos (a) and (b) courtesy of Dr Tim David, Royal Manchester Children's Hospital.

Box 1.1

The pleiotropic* effects of cystic fibrosis

- **Lung**   Abnormal mucus leading to infection and lung damage
- **Gastrointestinal tract** Meconium ileus
                              Distal intestinal obstruction
                              Rectal prolapse
- **Pancreas**   Exocrine pancreas dysfunction
                              Malabsorption
- **Hepatobiliary tract**   Biliary cirrhosis
                              Gallstones
- **Sweat glands**   Elevated chloride and sodium in sweat
- **Reproductive Tract**   Congenital bilateral absence of vas deferens (CBAVD)
                              Thick cervical secretions

*Pleiotropic = having many effects.

| CASE 3 | Choudhary family | 3 | 9 | 66 | 242 | 260 | 376 |

- Girl (Nasreen) aged 8 months, parents Aadnan and Mumtaz
- Deaf
- Parents are first cousins

Nasreen is the first child born to young parents (Aadnan and Mumtaz Choudhary) who are first cousins. The pregnancy and birth were normal and Nasreen thrived. She smiled, lifted her head and rolled over all at the normal times. She was taken regularly to the routine baby clinic. When she had her hearing test at 8 months she didn't seem to react normally to sound. Her mother hoped it was just because she was sleepy but her audiograms showed that she has profound bilateral hearing loss.

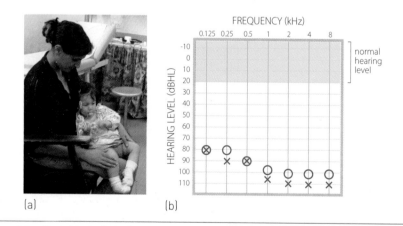

(a)   (b)

Figure 1.3 – Result of a hearing test.
(a) Testing a baby's hearing by checking the auditory brain stem response.
(b) Audiogram showing bilateral severe–profound hearing loss. The horizontal axis shows the frequency and the vertical axis the hearing threshold in decibels. Different symbols are used for readings from the two ears. 0–20 dB is normal hearing; hearing loss is defined as 20–40 dB (mild), 40–70 dB (moderate), 70–95 dB (severe), over 95 db (profound).

| CASE 4 | Davies family | **4** | 10 | 66 | 102 | 151 | 181 | 279 | 376 |

- Boy (Martin) aged 24 months, parents Judith and Robert
- Clumsy and slow to walk
- Family history of muscular dystrophy

Martin is the first son born to Judith and Robert Davies; they already have two daughters Leanne and Kathryn. The girls were very quick with their motor milestones and both were walking just before their first birthdays. Martin seemed slower in many ways and his mum thought it was just that he was a boy. However, when he still wasn't walking at 18 months she asked the doctor at the clinic for advice. The doctor didn't find anything when he examined Martin and arranged for another assessment in 6 months' time. Meanwhile Martin did take his first steps at 20 months but the doctor, at the next appointment, noticed Martin was very clumsy and that when he got up from the floor he had to hold on to a chair or push himself up by propping his hands on his legs. Both the doctor and Judith were very worried at this point because they knew that there was a family history of muscular dystrophy, and although there are many reasons why a little boy might be slow to walk and clumsy, these can also be early signs of that disease. They agreed that Martin needed to be referred to a neurologst, and Judith and Robert needed to see a geneticist.

(a) (b) (c)

Figure 1.4 – Duchenne muscular dystrophy.
(a) Affected boys stand up by bracing their arms against their legs (Gower's maneuver) because their proximal leg muscles are weak. (b) and (c) Muscle histology (Gomori trichrome stain). Normal muscle (b) shows a regular architecture of cells with dystrophin (brown stain) on all the outer membranes. (c) Shows muscle from a 10-year-old affected boy. Note the disorganization, invasion by fibrous tissue and complete absence of dystrophin. Histology photos courtesy of Dr Richard Charlton, Newcastle upon Tyne.

| CASE 5 | Elliot family | **4** | 11 | 42 | 64 | 376 |

- Miscarriage
- Very small dysmorphic baby girl (Elizabeth), parents Elmer and Ellen
- Heart problems

Elmer and Ellen decided they wanted to start a family soon after they came back from their honeymoon in Jamaica where Elmer's parents were born. It wasn't long before Ellen became pregnant but 8 weeks after her last period she started bleeding and after that the pregnancy test was negative. The next pregnancy 5 months later seemed to go well at first but at 30 weeks' gestation a scan showed the baby to be small. This didn't worry the couple since Ellen was petite herself.

Figure 1.5 – A baby with multiple congenital abnormalities and dysmorphic features.

However, when Elizabeth was born at 37 weeks' gestation it was clear that all was not well. Elizabeth was overall a small baby (her length and weight were on the 3rd centiles) but her head circumference was significantly below the 3rd centile. She needed tube feeding and seemed to get breathless very easily. A heart murmur was detected and an echocardiogram showed she had a ventricular septal defect and a narrowing of her aortic valve. The pediatrician asked the geneticist to see Elizabeth and her parents and advise which investigations might be helpful. Ellen told the geneticist her sister had had two early miscarriages and her aunt who lives in Trinidad had a baby who died with a congenital heart defect and a stillborn baby before she had two healthy children.

CASE 6	Fletcher family	5	12	67	131	152	376

- Frank, aged 22, with increasingly blurred eyesight
- Family history of visual difficulties

Frank was an electrician who, at 22 years old, had just finished his college course. He enjoyed going out with his friends and he tended to drink quite a lot of alcohol at weekends. He had always had good eyesight but one week he noticed that his vision was blurred and the colours of the wires he was working on seemed paler than usual. When this didn't improve he went to the optician who noticed changes in Frank's retina and made an urgent referral to the Eye Hospital. There they found he had disk swelling (pseudoedema of the nerve fiber layer), and increased tortuosity of the retinal vessels. Gradually over the next few months his central vision became much worse and he had to give up his job. His mother, Freda, was a healthy woman but her only brother had been registered blind since 28 years of age with what she remembered to be optic atrophy. Her sister Doreen also has serious visual difficulties which came on when she was around 45 years old. The ophthalmologist referred Frank to the genetic clinic because of this family history.

(a) (b) (c)

Figure 1.6 – Leber hereditary optic neuropathy.
(a) Optic disc 3 weeks after patient noted reduction in vision; note hyperemia of disc with blurred margins. (b) Retina of uncle; vision lost several years previously. Note pallor of disc particularly temporally corresponding to optic atrophy. (c) Normal retina. Photos courtesy of Mr Graeme Black, St Mary's Hospital, Manchester.

1.2. **Background**

The first thing to do with any of these patients is to take a family history. Even when the referral letter gives a family history, it is important for the geneticist to go carefully through, following the protocol in *Box 1.2*. The family history can give important clues about the genetic diagnosis; it also forms a necessary background for genetic diagnosis and counseling.

Box 1.2

How to take a family history and draw a pedigree

Take a special pedigree proforma or a sheet of blank paper and rule four lines across the long dimension. Start with the **consultand** (the person who is referred to the clinic) in the middle of the next-to-bottom line. Draw in the appropriate symbol (see below) and note his or her name, date of birth and any relevant clinical features. Next record details of the spouse(s) or partners, if any, then proceed systematically through their children, parents, and brothers and sisters (sibs). For each sib record their partners and children. Next ask about the sibs of each parent and their partners and children. Finally document all four grandparents and their sibs. Unless there is some reason to do so, it should not be necessary to go beyond that. Be careful to ask systematically about each person, and for each person note their name, date of birth, if dead the date and cause of death, and any relevant clinical information. Ask about miscarriages or reproductive problems and, if appropriate, about the place of origin of each person. Even if the consultands are convinced that they know which side of the family is the source of the problem, it is wise to collect full details of both sides – family myths can be very misleading. Some institutions use computerized systems that take you through a series of questions similar to those above, and draw the pedigree for you.

Build up the pedigree as you go along, keeping each generation on one horizontal line. List sibs in the order of their birth if this can be done without too many lines crossing on the drawing. If the pedigree is at all complicated you will probably need to re-draw it neatly later. You can use the pedigrees in this chapter as models. The appropriate symbols to use are:

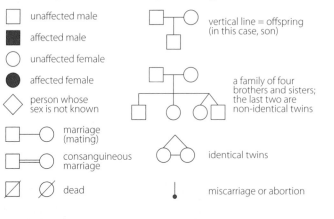

- □ unaffected male
- ■ affected male
- ○ unaffected female
- ● affected female
- ◇ person whose sex is not known
- □—○ marriage (mating)
- □═○ consanguineous marriage
- ⬚ ⊘ dead

- vertical line = offspring (in this case, son)
- a family of four brothers and sisters; the last two are non-identical twins
- identical twins
- ⬙ miscarriage or abortion

1.3. **Investigations of patients**

In each of our cases the initial investigation was to construct a detailed pedigree. The pedigrees below illustrate some of the typical features of autosomal dominant (Huntington disease), autosomal recessive (cystic fibrosis and Nasreen's deafness) and X-linked recessive (Martin's muscular dystrophy) conditions. The final two pedigrees (for the Elliot and Fletcher families) raise issues of interpretation that will be considered towards the end of this chapter.

| CASE 1 | Ashton family | 1 | **7** | 65 | 104 | 150 | 376 |

- John – 28-year-old son of Alfred Ashton
- ? Huntington disease
- Other family members with similar symptoms
- Autosomal dominant inheritance shown in pedigree
- Diagnostic test ordered

John's mother comes to the clinic with John to help construct a family tree. As well as John, she has a daughter who has two young sons. Alfred Ashton's father Frederick (John's grandfather) was killed in an industrial accident aged 38 years but Alfred's mother is alive and well at 77 years. Alfred's paternal grandmother became demented in her 50s and needed institutional care, as did one of her two brothers and her only sister. Although the family have lost touch with the extended family, since they became aware of the diagnosis in John's father they have heard that other people in the family have Huntington disease. They are very worried about Alfred's sister who lives in Australia and who has been demonstrating jerky movements like her brother.

This pedigree shows autosomal dominant inheritance. The child of somebody affected by Huntington disease has a 1 in 2 chance of having inherited the Huntington disease gene. If they do inherit the gene, they will inevitably develop Huntington disease unless they die of something else first, like Alfred's father did. The disease may develop at any age from childhood to 70+, but most usually when the person is in their 40s.

Severe late-onset genetic conditions like Huntington disease cause agonizing dilemmas for at-risk people. John has just got married and bought a house. His wife and he are thinking of starting a family. Although he shows no symptoms of the disease, if he does carry the Huntington disease gene he will inevitably develop this severe disease later in his life, and any child he has would be at 1 in 2 risk. A DNA test is available that could tell John definitively whether or not he carries the mutation. Deciding whether or not to take the test will be one of the biggest decisions of his life. In the UK about 70% of people in this situation

Figure 1.7 – Pedigree of John Ashton's family.
This is shown as it might be recorded in the clinic but because the cases and families in this book are fictional, all subsequent pedigrees show only information that is relevant to following the case and understanding the genetics.

opt, after full counseling, not to take the test. Genetic counselors must always respect a patient's right *not* to know, in this or any other situation, if that is their choice. Before embarking on this whole process, it is crucial to confirm that the family disease really is Huntington disease and not either an unrelated neurodegenerative condition or one of the rare autosomal dominant diseases that can resemble Huntington disease. In this case the psychiatrist is confident of the diagnosis for Alfred, but a test of Alfred's DNA (see *Chapter 4* for a description of type of test) is used to make sure. Note that testing somebody who is already ill constitutes a **diagnostic test** which is not as ethically sensitive as a **predictive test** on a healthy person like John, although a positive result in Alfred would confirm the poor prognosis.

| CASE 2 | Brown family | 2 | **8** | 65 | 126 | 151 | 279 | 376 |

- Girl (Joanne) aged 6 months, parents David and Pauline
- ? Cystic fibrosis
- Order molecular test?

The pedigree shows that there is no family history of cystic fibrosis or other evident genetic problems. "How can it be genetic, when nobody in either family has ever had it?" Pauline asked. In fact this pedigree is typical of the way autosomal recessive diseases present in societies where consanguinity is not common. The affected child is usually the only affected case born to a non-consanguineous couple with no relevant family history. Thus the pedigree gives no clue that the condition is genetic. Identifying the cause usually starts with making a clinical diagnosis. Sometimes the condition is so unmistakable, and the genetics so unambiguous, that a clinical diagnosis provides an adequate degree of certainty. More often the clinical diagnosis is really a hypothesis, more or less plausible. Ideally it would be confirmed by a molecular test demonstrating a mutation.

In most cases of cystic fibrosis the clinical history and a positive sweat test (showing characteristically raised sodium) make the diagnosis fairly secure. Genetically, cystic fibrosis is always autosomal recessive, and always caused by mutations in the *CFTR* gene on chromosome 7 (see *Chapter 3*). A molecular test to demonstrate the mutation is needed for advising relatives about their carrier status, for prenatal testing, and to confirm the diagnosis in atypical cases.

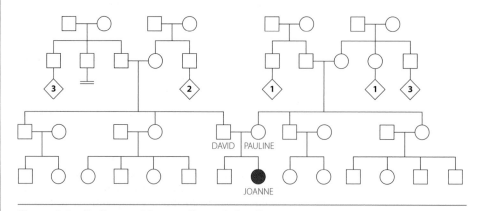

Figure 1.8 – Pedigree of Joanne Brown's family.
Note the complete absence of any family history of cystic fibrosis. Autosomal recessive conditions commonly present as a single isolated case.

| CASE 3 | Choudhary family | 3 | **9** | 66 | 242 | 260 | 376 |

- Girl (Nasreen) aged 8 months, parents Aadnan and Mumtaz
- Deaf
- Parents are first cousins
- Pedigree suggests autosomal recessive deafness

The clinic visit turned out to be a family affair because Aadnan's sister Benazir and Mumtaz's brother Waleed also asked to come, together with Aadnan, Mumtaz and Nasreen. Waleed was deaf, but was skilled at lip-reading, and with careful attention to seating and lighting he was able to play his full part in the consultation. The pedigree revealed an extensive family with several consanguineous marriages. In the UK pedigrees of this type are most often seen in people originating from the Middle East or the Indian subcontinent. Aadnan and Mumtaz are first cousins (see *Box 1.3*). Mumtaz's parents (who are also first cousins) have four children in addition to Mumtaz. Two boys, Waleed and his brother Mohammed, are deaf and attend a college for deaf students where they are doing well academically. Aadnan and Mumtaz want to know the risk of deafness in any children they might have in the future. Mumtaz has had two miscarriages, and she fears that she will never have healthy children.

Congenital deafness can be due to environmental factors such as maternal rubella or birth trauma. The geneticist had checked Mumtaz's notes to make sure there was no evidence of such problems, but she noted the need to check with Mumtaz's mother and her family doctor that there was no evidence of such factors with Waleed or Mohammed. The pedigree is most simply interpreted as showing autosomal recessive deafness. About two-thirds of congenital deafness has such a cause. If this interpretation is correct, then each subsequent child of Aadnan and Mumtaz has a 1 in 4 risk of being deaf. The extensive inbreeding is an additional pointer to a recessive condition. Although consanguineous marriage roughly doubles the risk of abnormal children (depending on the degree of consanguinity - see *Chapter 10*), the increase is only from 2% to 4%. In other words, the chance of a healthy child is only reduced from 98% to 96%. In many traditional societies there are good social reasons to marry a relative rather than a stranger. Mumtaz's two miscarriages are very unlikely to be related to the deafness. They might

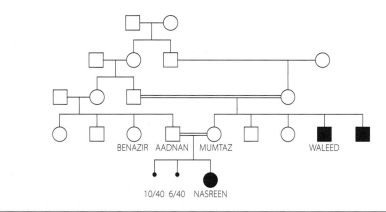

Figure 1.9 – Pedigree of Nasreen Choudhary's family.
Note the use of double marriage lines to highlight consanguineous marriages. Two early miscarriages are indicated. In a real family you would mark the dates of birth of Aadnan's and Mumtaz's sibs, because arranging them in birth order would probably make it difficult to draw a clear pedigree.

be evidence of another, much more severe recessive condition in the family, but there are many non-genetic causes of miscarriage. The geneticist reassured Mumtaz that two early miscarriages is quite a common history that usually has no sinister import.

The presence of Waleed and Benazir at the clinic visit was explained by the fact that they have been introduced and a wedding is planned. Benazir was worried that if a child of theirs was deaf, it might relate exclusively to Waleed and she would be cut out of the family circle. Waleed, however, took a much more relaxed view. The geneticist had to be sensitive to the undercurrents and careful not to try to impose her own views. Consanguineous marriage within a family with a known recessive condition does carry specific risks. In *Chapter 10* we will see how the geneticist calculated the risk for Waleed and Benazir. However, that calculation would only be valid if Waleed's and Nasreen's deafness was confirmed to be autosomal recessive. The family were keen to know if a DNA test was available to confirm the interpretation. This is discussed in *Chapter 3*.

Relationships

Sibs means brothers or sisters, regardless of sex

Cousins: Jack and Jill are **first cousins** if one of Jack's parents is a sib of one of Jill's parents. They are **second cousins** if one of Jack's parents is first cousin of one of Jill's parents.

In some cultures the word 'cousin' is used much more loosely to mean 'kinsman'. For genetic purposes it should be used in the strict sense defined above. More complex relationships such as in the **Choudhary family** (**Case 3**, *Figure 1.9*) are best defined by drawing or describing the pedigree details. We will see in *Chapter 10* how to calculate exact degrees of relationship and inbreeding.

Box 1.3

CASE 4	Davies family	4	**10**	66	102	151	181	279	376

- Boy (Martin) aged 24 months, parents Judith and Robert
- Clumsy and slow to walk
- Family history of muscular dystrophy
- Pedigree shows X-linked recessive inheritance
- Order diagnostic DNA test

The pedigree shows that Judith's aunt (her mother's sister) had had two boys who died in their teens having had a progressive muscle disease. There were no other affected relatives in the family. The pedigree is consistent with X-linked recessive inheritance. If Martin does indeed have the same condition as his two dead relatives, then X-linked inheritance is highly likely, but at this stage this is still not certain.

It was crucial to check the exact diagnosis of these two boys. There are many different degenerative muscle diseases. While these might have roughly similar implications for management of the patient, the implications for the wider family depend critically on a precise genetic diagnosis. The geneticist will request the case notes, paying particular attention to the detailed course of the boys' decline and to any reports of muscle histology. Given the dates of their deaths it is unlikely that any DNA test results would be available. As described in *Chapter 4*, testing Martin's DNA will play a central part in the investigations.

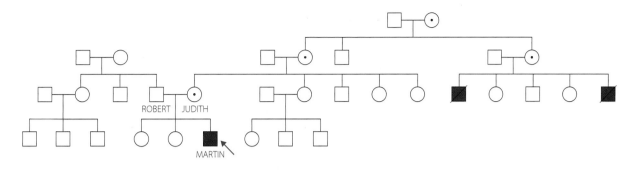

Figure 1.10 – Pedigree of Martin Davies's family.
Assuming this is X-linked muscular dystrophy, the women marked with dots
are **obligate carriers** of the disease gene – that is, they must be carriers
because they have both parents and offspring who are affected or carriers.
Other females (e.g. the sisters of affected boys) may or may not be carriers.

CASE 5	Elliot family	4	**11**	42	64	376

- Miscarriage
- Very small dysmorphic baby girl (Elizabeth), parents Elmer and Ellen
- Heart problems
- Blood taken for chromosome analysis
- Pedigree suggests autosomal dominant condition with reduced penetrance

The family history of miscarriages, stillbirth and liveborn infants with malformations in several generations might suggest an autosomal dominant condition with reduced penetrance (see *Section 1.4* for an explanation of penetrance). However, clinical experience suggests the most likely explanation is a balanced chromosome structural abnormality. The next step is to perform chromosome analysis on the parents and the surviving abnormal child (see *Chapter 2*).

After the birth of a child with malformations or other problems parents experience a whole range of emotions including shock, anxiety, denial and confusion. They often also experience a sense of loss for the normal baby they hoped to have. Naturally other family members have their own responses to the difficult situation and tensions are raised further, particularly if one 'side' blames the other. The role of the pediatric team caring for the baby is to keep the family fully informed about their findings in the baby and about tests and consultations that are being arranged. The roles of the clinical geneticist are to help establish a diagnosis as soon as possible and to convey complex results to the parents in a comprehensible way, and also to explain what they mean for the baby's future. Genetic counseling about recurrence risks and implications for the extended family is often arranged later after urgent clinical management issues have been dealt with.

The clinical geneticist and pediatrician agreed that the most likely explanation for Elizabeth's problems is a chromosomal abnormality. Blood was therefore taken from the baby and both parents for chromosome analysis. The results and implications are discussed in *Chapter 2*. Over several sessions the counselor built up the pedigree shown below. The poor reproductive outcomes (miscarriages or abnormal babies) in this family appear to show an autosomal dominant pattern. As explained below, this is not incompatible with the suspicion that the problems are caused by a chromosomal abnormality.

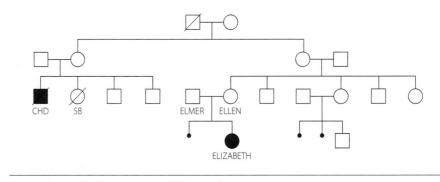

Figure 1.11 – Pedigree of the Elliot family.
This shows the family history of reproductive problems. SB denotes stillbirth and CHD congenital heart disease.

| CASE 6 | Fletcher family | 5 | **12** | 67 | 131 | 152 | 376 |

- Frank, aged 22, with increasingly blurred eyesight
- Family history of visual difficulties
- Pedigree suggests X-linked recessive inheritance but not conclusive
- ? LHON
- Order blood test to check for mutation in mtDNA

Frank attended the genetic clinic with his mother. He was still very shocked after having the diagnosis and poor prognosis explained to him by the ophthalmologist. He hadn't even started to come to terms with the major changes this would bring in his life, including losing his job and not being able to drive. It had, however, begun to occur to him that because of the family history his own children might be at risk. When he came to the clinic he very much wanted to discuss this aspect of things since his girlfriend and he were very worried.

The clinical geneticist first of all drew up a detailed family tree with the help of Frank's mother Freda. Her brother, Derek, was registered blind and had been diagnosed as having optic atrophy. He had first noticed problems like Frank in his 20s; encouragingly he had attended college after his diagnosis and now worked for a large company in their telephone sales department. He had also told Frank about the national organization for people with visual disabilities and about all the help and advice they could offer. Freda's sister Doreen didn't develop any problems until she was in her 40s and her visual deterioration was slower, although still affecting her central vision. At a recent check-up she had been found to have an unusual heart rhythm and had requested Freda to find out in the clinic if that was linked to the eye problems.

The following clues led the geneticist to a hypothesis about the condition in Frank's family:

- the nature of the eye problems
- the rapid progression of symptoms in the affected males
- the later onset and slightly milder disease in Doreen
- Doreen's heart rhythm problems

Based on these observations, the geneticist thought the condition could be Leber hereditary optic neuropathy (LHON). LHON (OMIM 535000) has a wide range of symptoms and ages of onset. It is caused by a mutation in mitochondrial DNA (mtDNA – see *Chapter 3*). The geneticist therefore arranged for blood samples to

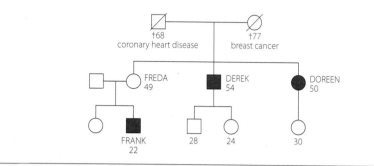

Figure 1.12 – Pedigree of Frank Fletcher.
This pedigree was difficult to interpret. At first sight the geneticist considered X-linked recessive inheritance because of two similarly affected males linked through a normal female. However, Doreen was also affected, which made X-linked inheritance less likely. This nevertheless remained a possibility because sometimes in such families there are 'manifesting female carriers' with milder problems than affected males (see *Chapter 7*). Other types of inheritance such as X-linked dominant and mitochondrial inheritance have to be considered when affected people are linked through the female line.

be taken from Frank and Freda. If this type of inheritance is confirmed then it is good news for any children Frank and his girlfriend may have, since a male does not pass on his mtDNA to his children.

1.4. **Summary and extension**

The art of pedigree interpretation

In laboratory animals like fruit flies or mice, the mode of inheritance of a character can always be established beyond doubt by breeding experiments. With humans we have to take pedigrees as we find them, and they are rarely large enough to define the mode of inheritance unambiguously. For research purposes, collections of pedigrees can be analyzed statistically, using the tools of segregation analysis to work out the most likely mode of inheritance. In the clinic, pedigree interpretation is an art as much as a science. It is more a matter of forming hypotheses for subsequent investigation. The hypothesis might involve any of the following causes:

- a chromosomal abnormality
- an autosomal dominant condition, fully or partially penetrant
- an autosomal recessive condition
- an X-linked condition, dominant or recessive
- a condition caused by a defect in the mitochondrial DNA
- a multifactorial condition
- a non-genetic cause

Case 5 (Elliot family) showed that chromosome abnormalities can give a mendelian pedigree pattern. A mendelian pattern will be seen whenever a phenotype is caused by something at a single fixed chromosomal location – whether that 'something' is a classical gene or a chromosomal abnormality.

Box 1.4 summarizes the features of the main mendelian pedigree patterns. Possible investigations include:

- clinical identification of a syndrome – but bear in mind that some clinically defined syndromes can show more than one mode of inheritance
- karyotyping (see *Chapter 2*)
- analysis of candidate genes for mutations (see *Chapter 5*)
- checking for biochemical abnormalities, including abnormalities of mitochondrial function (see *Chapter 8*)
- checking for skewed X-inactivation (see *Chapter 7*)

Summary of modes of inheritance

Autosomal dominant:
- a vertical pedigree pattern, with multiple generations affected
- each affected person normally has one affected parent
- each child of an affected person has a 1 in 2 chance of being affected
- males and females are equally affected and equally likely to pass the condition on

Autosomal recessive:
- a horizontal pedigree pattern, with one or more sibs affected; often only a single affected case
- parents and children of affected people are normally unaffected
- each subsequent sib of an affected child has a 1 in 4 chance of being affected
- males and females are equally affected
- affected children are sometimes the product of consanguineous marriages. In families with multiple consanguineous marriages, affected individuals may be seen in several generations

X-linked recessive:
- a 'knight's move' pedigree pattern – affected boys may have affected maternal uncles
- parents and children of affected people are normally unaffected. Never transmitted from father to son
- affects mainly males: females can be carriers, and affected males in a pedigree are linked through females, not through unaffected males
- subsequent brothers of affected boys have a 1 in 2 risk of being affected; sisters are not affected but have a 1 in 2 risk of being carriers

X-linked dominant:
- features very similar to autosomal dominant pedigrees, except that all daughters and no sons of an affected father are affected
- condition is often milder and more variable in females than in males

Y-linked:
- a vertical pedigree pattern
- all sons of an affected father are affected
- affects only males

Mitochondrial:
- a vertical pedigree pattern
- children of affected men are never affected
- all children of an affected woman may be affected, but mitochondrial conditions are typically extremely variable even within a family

Box 1.4

To form a hypothesis, individual pedigrees are checked to see what mode of inheritance gives the best fit. The initial hypothesis is based on two questions:

(1) Does the pedigree show that affected people have at least one affected parent? If the answer is yes, the condition is most likely dominant; if no, it is most likely recessive. A dominant condition is manifest in anybody who carries the relevant gene. Barring new mutations, an affected person must have inherited the gene from one parent, who should therefore also be affected.

(2) Are there any gender effects? For example, does the condition affect both sexes, and can it be passed on by a parent of either sex to a child of either sex? If there are no gender effects, the condition is most likely autosomal. Look especially for male-to-male transmission: this is a powerful pointer against X-linked inheritance because a father should never transmit his X chromosome to a son. If there appear to be gender effects, then it may be X-linked, although as explained below, there can be other reasons for a sex bias. Unless the pedigree is exceptionally large, apparent effects may be just random fluctuations.

Having arrived at an initial hypothesis, the next step is to test it by writing in genotypes, as in *Figure 1.13*. Given sufficient coincidences (new mutations, carriers of the disease happening to marry into the family, etc.) almost

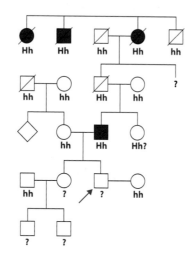

Figure 1.13 – The Huntington disease pedigree of *Figure 1-1* with genotypes written in.

By convention, upper case is used for the allele determining the dominant character and lower case for the allele determining the recessive character. In this example the disease allele is dominant. Note that affected people in this family are heterozygotes. This is the normal situation with human dominant conditions. Homozygotes are usually extremely rare or unknown; when they are recorded, they are often far more seriously affected than heterozygotes. Nevertheless, such a condition is correctly described as dominant (not semi-dominant). Dominance and recessiveness are properties of phenotypes (characters, diseases...) not genes. A character is **dominant** if it is manifest in the heterozygote, and this is the case for Huntington disease. As it happens, Huntington disease is one of the rare human cases where homozygotes are known to exist and to be phenotypically identical to heterozygotes.

any pedigree can be made to fit almost any mode of inheritance. The most likely mode of inheritance is the one that requires the least number of such coincidences – preferably none. If you require any coincidences to make your initial hypothesis fit, then you should see if an alternative hypothesis gives a better fit. Pedigrees in student examination papers should always have one 'right' answer. Real life is not always so kind: many real pedigrees are ambiguous, or do not fit any of the standard mendelian patterns. The condition may be multifactorial, or other evidence may suggest a chromosomal abnormality or a non-genetic cause.

Penetrance and expressivity – pitfalls in interpretation and counseling

Many human conditions show a mainly autosomal dominant pedigree pattern, but occasionally skip a generation: that is, an unaffected person who has an affected parent produces one or more affected children. Thus occasionally a person can carry the relevant gene but not manifest the condition. Such occurrences are described as non-penetrance. The **penetrance** of a character is defined as the proportion of people with the relevant genotype who show the character.

Penetrance is a property of both the gene and the character. Different syndromes show characteristically different penetrances, but different features of a syndrome can also have different penetrances. Penetrance can also be age-related, as with Huntington disease.

Non-penetrance is a pitfall in both pedigree interpretation and counseling. *Figure 1.14* shows an example. Individual III-11 must carry the disease gene despite being unaffected. Before starting a family he might have requested counseling to find out his risk of having a child with the family disease. The counselor would have had to know the penetrance of that particular condition in order to be able to calculate the risk that despite being phenotypically normal, he might be a non-penetrant gene carrier. Fortunately in many cases a molecular test would be available that could give a definitive answer.

Figure 1.14 – Pedigree of an autosomal dominant condition with reduced penetrance. The condition is non-penetrant in individual III-11. Other unaffected individuals in generation IV who have an affected parent might also be non-penetrant gene carriers.

Reduced penetrance is a nuisance for counselors, but there is no mystery about why it happens. The surprise is really that some conditions show 100% penetrance. For such a condition, if you have the relevant gene then you will inevitably manifest the condition, absolutely regardless of all your other genes, your environment and your lifestyle. For many conditions, having the gene means that you are highly likely to manifest the condition, but occasionally a lucky combination of other genes and/or environmental factors will save you.

There is a complete spectrum of characters and genes, from 100% penetrance down to very low penetrance (*Figure 1.15*). For example, in cancer research there is much interest in identifying low-penetrance genes that make a person more likely to develop cancer, but do not in any way make that fate inevitable (see *Chapter 12*). Characters at the high-penetrance end of the spectrum are usefully described as mendelian, while those at the low-penetrance end would be called multifactorial (see *Chapter 13*). There is no hard and fast rule where the changeover occurs. Reduced penetrance must occur with characters showing recessive inheritance, but it would be much less obvious from the pedigree, so in practice incomplete penetrance is largely a problem of dominant conditions.

Figure 1.15 – Continuum of penetrance.
There is a continuum of penetrance from fully penetrant conditions, where other genes and environmental factors have no effect, through to low-penetrance genes that simply play a small part, along with other genetic and environmental factors, in determining a person's susceptibility to a disease. Multiple sclerosis is used as an example of a multifactorial condition where genetic factors play a major part in determining susceptibility, but current research suggests that each individual factor has very low penetrance (see *Chapter 13*).

Genetic conditions often show **variable expression**. That is, the full-blown condition involves a number of features, but many affected people show only some of those features, or may show a certain feature to differing degrees. Type 1 neurofibromatosis (NF1; see *Disease box 1*) is an example of a common autosomal dominant condition that is very variable. We could say that each feature of the syndrome has its own characteristic penetrance, or we could say that the syndrome as a whole shows variable expressivity. Either way, this is a reflection of the fact that genes do not act in isolation, but against a background of innumerable other genes and a variable environment. Each child of somebody with NF1 has a 50% chance of inheriting the disease gene, and this might be checked with a DNA test, but the test cannot tell us how severely a child would be affected.

Type 1 Neurofibromatosis (OMIM 162200)

NF1, also known as von Recklinghausen disease, is an autosomal dominant condition caused by mutations in the *NF1* gene on chromosome 17. The disease affects about 1 person in 3500 and is seen in both sexes and all ethnic groups. Penetrance is complete, in that some feature of the condition can be found in every affected person, but the disease can manifest in many ways and varies greatly in severity.

(a)

(b)

(c)

Mildly affected patients show only café-au-lait skin macules (a), Lisch nodules (hamartomas in the iris) and/or axillary freckling. Dermal neurofibromas (b) are frequent, and they can be numerous and grossly disfiguring (c).

NF1 patients are also liable to develop a variety of benign or malignant tumors, including nerve sheath tumors and gliomas and other tumors in the central nervous system. Occasionally NF1 patients have learning difficulties, short stature or seizures.

Counseling in NF1 can be difficult. Approximately half of all cases represent new mutations (a common observation with clinically severe dominant conditions, see *Chapter 10*). Patients with no family history may not understand the genetic risks, and mildly affected people may not appreciate that their children could be severely affected. Although the *NF1* gene has been cloned, molecular testing for mutations is difficult because the gene is large (59 exons covering 350 kb of genomic DNA, see *Chapter 3*). Even if DNA analysis does characterize the mutation in a family, it cannot predict how severely affected a mutation carrier will be.

NF1 is a prime example of the problems of variable expression in an autosomal dominant disease.

Rarer modes of inheritance

X-linked dominant inheritance

For males, X-linked diseases are neither dominant nor recessive, because dominance and recessiveness are properties of heterozygotes, and males have only a single X chromosome. As explained further in *Chapter 7*, the phenomenon of X-inactivation means that even for heterozygous females, dominance and recessiveness are not as clear-cut for X-linked as for autosomal conditions. Most X-linked diseases seldom affect heterozygous females significantly, and so are described as recessive. Occasional X-linked conditions do commonly affect heterozygotes badly, and so are dominant. An example is X-linked hypophosphatemia (OMIM 307800; an inability of the kidneys to retain phosphate, leading to vitamin D-resistant rickets). At first sight the pedigree pattern (*Figure 1.16*) might well be interpreted as autosomal dominant. Consistent with this interpretation, there is a vertical pedigree pattern and on average 50% of the children of an affected person are affected. However, a male passes his X chromosome to all his daughters but none of his sons. Thus all the daughters but none of the sons of an affected father are affected. Because of X-inactivation, X-linked dominant conditions tend to be milder and more variable in females than in males.

Other causes of sex bias

A sex bias is not a reliable indicator of X-linkage. An autosomal condition may affect just one sex for anatomical or physiological reasons. For example, ovarian cancer may be caused by mutations in the *BRCA2* gene on chromosome 13, but obviously affects only females. Such conditions are called **sex-limited**. Sometimes a condition may be lethal in one sex but not the other. If this happens before birth, the result is a condition seen in only one sex. This is most likely with X-linked dominant conditions where heterozygous females survive but affected males die *in utero*. An example is Rett syndrome (OMIM 312750 – see *Disease Box 7*). Affected males normally miscarry early in pregnancy, so the classical syndrome is only seen in girls. A few affected males do in fact survive to birth, but their phenotype is so different that its cause was not recognized until molecular tests demonstrated that they had mutations in *MECP2*, which is the gene mutated in most cases of Rett syndrome.

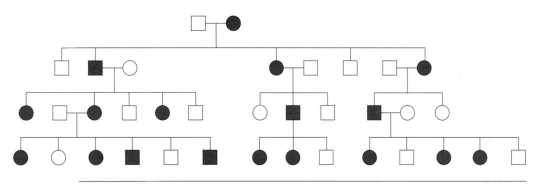

Figure 1.16 – Pedigree of an X-linked dominant condition.
Although heterozygous females are affected, such conditions are usually milder and more variable in females than in males.

Y-linked inheritance

For a condition determined by a gene on the Y chromosome the inheritance pattern would be simple and striking. It would affect only males, and all the sons of an affected man would be affected. However, the Y chromosome carries only about 50 genes, and since females manage perfectly well without any of them, none of these genes can be essential to life or general health. Y-linked genes are important for male sexual function, and abnormalities of the Y chromosome are a common cause of male infertility. Such abnormalities are clinically important, but because the resulting phenotype is infertility, they do not segregate in multi-generation pedigrees.

Mitochondrial inheritance

The problem in the Fletcher family – Case 6 (*Figure 1.12*) illustrates an unusual mode of inheritance. All the previous cases have involved the chromosomal DNA in the cell nucleus. But, as we shall see in *Chapter 3*, mitochondria also contain

DNA. Mutations in the mitochondrial DNA (mtDNA) are responsible for a few diseases, including the Fletcher case. Note four important points:

(1) All the mitochondria of an embryo are derived from the egg, and none from the sperm. This gives rise to a matrilineal pattern of inheritance: mitochondrial mutations are passed on by the mother, but never by the father. Most conditions caused by mutations in mtDNA affect both sexes equally. Leber hereditary optic neuropathy is unusual in that, for unknown reasons, it affects mostly males.

(2) Most of the components and functions of mitochondria are controlled by genes located on the chromosomes in the nucleus (see *Chapter 3*). Most diseases caused by malfunction of mitochondria therefore follow typical mendelian inheritance patterns. Only a very few mitochondrial diseases are caused by mutations in the mtDNA and follow the pattern of inheritance we see in the Fletcher case.

(3) Because each cell contains many mitochondria, people can have a mix of normal and mutant mitochondria in each cell (**heteroplasmy**). The proportion can vary between tissues and in the same tissue over time. This helps explain why diseases caused by mitochondrial mutations typically have low penetrance and extremely variable expressivity.

(4) Ova contain many mitochondria; therefore a heteroplasmic mother can have heteroplasmic children. This is in stark contrast to mosaicism for nuclear abnormalities (chromosomal or single gene), which cannot be inherited (see below and *Chapter 2*)

Some further problems in pedigree interpretation

A condition is not necessarily genetic just because it is **congenital** (present at birth) or **familial** (tending to run in families). Huntington disease is an example of a condition that is genetic but not congenital, while many birth defects (congenital by definition) are caused by environmental teratogens (rubella or thalidomide, for example). Unless a familial condition shows a clear-cut mendelian pedigree pattern or a demonstrable chromosomal abnormality, it can be very difficult to decide what role genes play in its causation. Innumerable behavioral and occasional physical characters can be the result of shared family environment rather than genes. *Chapter 13* describes how these 'nature – nurture' problems can be approached. The converse is also true: a negative family history does not rule out a genetic cause for a problem. This is especially true of autosomal recessive conditions, as illustrated here by the cystic fibrosis case of the Brown family – (Case 2), but it may also be seen with an autosomal dominant or X-linked condition where cases are often the result of new mutations. *Chapter 10* explains why new mutations are frequent with some genetic conditions and rare with others.

Mosaicism

A person whose body contains two or more genetically different cell lines is called a **mosaic**. As explained in *Chapter 2*, the process of mitosis should ensure that every cell in the body carries a complete and identical set of genes. Our discussion so far has tacitly assumed that if a person has a mutation, it is present in every cell of his body. This is true of inherited mutations, but what about freshly arising mutations? Mutations can happen to any cell at any time. Only the descendants of that cell will carry the mutation. Given the number of cells in the human body, and typical mutation rates of genes, it is clear that everybody will have the odd cell or small clone of cells carrying a mutation in almost any gene you care to think of. Normally these odd rogue clones will have absolutely no effect. There are three circumstances in which mosaicism may be clinically important:

(1) if the mutant cells have a tendency to grow and take over – see *Chapter 12*
(2) if the mutation arose sufficiently early in embryonic development that the mutant line makes up a significant part of the whole body. The person may show features of the disease, maybe with a milder phenotype (if the product of the mutated gene is diffusible) or with a patchy distribution reflecting the distribution of mutant cells (if the gene product remains in the cell where it is produced)
(3) if the mutation affects the **germ line** (sperm or egg cells or their progenitors)

Germ-line mosaicism is a major source of uncertainty and confusion in pedigree interpretation and genetic counseling. A person who by all clinical and genetic tests is entirely normal may produce several children with the same dominant or X-linked disease if he or she has a germ-line clone of mutant cells. When a normal couple have a child with a dominant condition, with no previous family history, this is evidently a new mutation. The counselor must remember that one or other parent may be a germ-line mosaic. The risk of recurrence is rarely possible to quantify, because we have no idea what proportion of germ-line cells carry the mutation, but it is not negligible. If a normal couple have two or more affected children, the pedigree pattern (*Figure 1.17*) looks recessive because the parents are unaffected. Misinterpreting the condition as recessive would cause serious errors when the affected children ask about their risk of passing it on. The risk would be very low for a rare recessive condition, but 50% for a dominant condition.

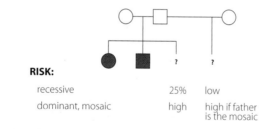

RISK:

recessive	25%	low
dominant, mosaic	high	high if father is the mosaic

Figure 1.17 – A problem in counseling.
A couple with no previous family history of this condition have two affected children. Is this an autosomal recessive condition, or is it autosomal dominant with one of the parents being a germinal mosaic? The risks are very different depending which theory is correct.

1.5. **References**

Useful website

For detailed information on genetic deafness see the Hereditary Hearing Loss Homepage: http://webhost.ua.ac.be/hhh

1.6. **Self-assessment questions**

Each of the following 10 pedigrees shows a rare disease.

(a) Identify the most likely mode of inheritance, chosen from autosomal dominant (fully penetrant), autosomal dominant with about 90% penetrance, autosomal recessive or X-linked recessive

(b) Define the risk that the next child of the arrowed person or people will be affected.

Hints on pedigrees 1–4 are provided in the solutions section at the back of the book.

SAQ 1

SAQ 2

SAQ 3

SAQ 4

SAQ 5

SAQ 6

SAQ 7

SAQ 8

SAQ 9

SAQ 10

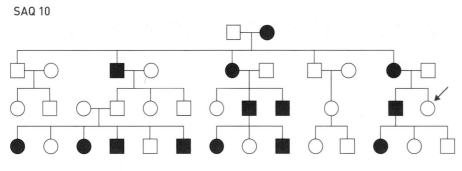

Chapter 2

How can a patient's chromosomes be studied?

Learning points for this chapter

After working through this chapter you should be able to:

- Describe the results of mitosis and meiosis, and how these are achieved
- Identify normal and simple abnormal karyotypes
- Describe human sex determination and the effects of errors
- Describe triploidy, trisomy, reciprocal translocations, robertsonian translocations, paracentric inversions, pericentric inversions, and deletions
- Explain the origins of the main types of numerical and structural chromosome abnormalities
- Work out the main possible reproductive outcomes for carriers of translocations or inversions

2.1. **Case studies**

| **CASE 7** | Green family | **25** | 38 | 68 | 99 | 376 |

- Girl (Gillian) aged 3 years
- Slow to develop
- ? Chromosome abnormality
- Order tests to check for microdeletion at 22q11

Figure 2.1 – Child with 22q11 deletion. Note small mouth, narrow nose and upward slant of her eyes.

Gillian is the second child born to healthy parents. Everything seemed fine at birth although her birth weight was less than her sister's. At her routine neonatal examination the doctor heard a heart murmur and referred her for an echocardiogram. This showed that she had a small hole between the two lower chambers of her heart (a ventricular septal defect - VSD). It was not considered serious and follow-up was recommended. By 3 years of age the murmur had disappeared and a further echocardiogram showed the VSD had closed. However, Gillian's parents were still worried about her since all her developmental milestones had been slower than her sister's. Her speech development had been particularly slow and she was difficult to understand. The pediatrician referred her for speech studies and she was found to have poor movements of her palate. He then asked the opinion of a clinical geneticist. The geneticist noted that Gillian had a very narrow nose, over-folding of the upper part of her ears, and long fingers. He organized a chromosome test and in addition to the routine karyotype requested a molecular test to see if there was a deletion of part of chromosome 22 (22q11).

| CASE 8 | Howard family | **26** | 38 | 68 | 100 | 275 | 376 |

- Helen – new-born daughter of Henry and Anne (33 years old)
- Down syndrome
- Risk of recurrence if they have more children?

Figure 2.2 – A child with Down syndrome.

Pregnancy was a surprise for Helen's parents Anne and Henry who were both 33 years old. They had had a son and daughter when they were in their early 20s. Nevertheless when they got used to the idea they were pleased. At the antenatal clinic they were offered screening tests for Down syndrome but they decided against these since they had had no tests in their previous pregnancies, and anyway, they both agreed they wouldn't really consider a termination of pregnancy. Everything went well in pregnancy and labor started at full term. When Helen was born, Anne thought she looked like her sister but the midwife was worried because she was very hypotonic (floppy), had loose skin at the back of her neck and single creases across her palms. The pediatrician was called and gently told Anne and Henry that he was concerned that Helen might have Down syndrome. He arranged to send a blood sample to the cytogenetics laboratory and requested that the result be sent as soon as possible since by now the parents and grandparents were extremely anxious. The pediatrician and the midwife saw the family several times over the next two days until the result was available. This confirmed that Helen did indeed have Down syndrome. The parents had lots of questions about Helen's future which the pediatrician answered, but he suggested he refer them to the genetic clinic in a few weeks' time to respond to their questions about how Down syndrome occurs and whether, if they were to have more children, there would be a high risk of recurrence.

| CASE 9 | Ingram family | **26** | 41 | 68 | 101 | 182 | 376 |

- Isabel – first daughter of Irene and Ian
- Small stature despite tall parents

Isabel was the first baby born to Irene and Ian who were both quite tall. She had some swelling of her feet for the first few months, and was quite petite, but in general she was a healthy little baby. She developed normally in childhood but was always the smallest in the class. By 10 years of age, her classmates' growth rate had increased and a couple of her friends had even started puberty. Although Irene and Ian were not really worried, the school nurse suggested that Isabel be referred to a pediatrician since her small stature seemed unusual given her parents' height. As part of her initial investigations the pediatrician requested a chromosome analysis.

(a) (b) (c)

Figure 2.3 – Turner syndrome.
(a) Puffy feet, (b) redundant skin at back of neck. (c) Histology of gonads: ovarian cortical stroma devoid of germ cell elements. Photo. (c) courtesy of Dr Godfrey Wilson, Manchester Royal Infirmary.

2.2. **Background**

Why clinicians need to know about chromosomes

Chromosome abnormalities are important in a number of different clinical situations:

- they are a cause of infertility and recurrent miscarriages
- over 50% of embryos that abort spontaneously in the first trimester have a chromosomal abnormality
- about 1 newborn in 200 has multiple congenital abnormalities because of a chromosomal abnormality. Prenatal screening can detect most such abnormalities in time for the pregnancy to be terminated, if the parents so wish
- most chromosomally abnormal babies are born to parents who are entirely normal, but about 1% of people have a subtle chromosomal change that has no effect on their own health, but puts them at high risk of having miscarriages or abnormal babies
- cancer cells typically acquire extensive chromosome abnormalities not present in the normal cells of the patient, and many particular abnormalities have diagnostic and prognostic significance

How are chromosomes studied?

If you want to study chromosomes under the microscope you need dividing cells. As described below, chromosomes are only visible in cells that are in the act of dividing. Taking blood, skin or other samples from a person will yield plenty of cells, but few if any will be dividing. Thus chromosome analysis usually involves taking a sample of non-dividing cells, which are then cultured in the laboratory and persuaded to divide (*Figure 2.4*). Suitable sources are shown in *Box 2.1*. In addition to the methods for studying chromosomes that are described in this chapter, a set of more recent techniques collectively called molecular cytogenetics can be used either to study chromosomes in much finer detail or to check chromosome numbers in non-dividing cells. These are described in *Chapter 4*.

Karyotyping by standard microscopic analysis involves preparing a slide on which a number of dividing cells can be examined, following the protocol of *Figure 2.4*. *Figure 2.10* shows one such cell. The cytogeneticist counts the chromosomes, identifies each one and checks that its structure appears normal. The analysis is typically based on 10 cells, so that if a particular feature is not clear in one cell it can be checked in others. For record-keeping, the chromosomes in one cell are arranged (usually by manipulation of a digital image) into a standard karyogram (often loosely called a karyotype) as in *Figures 2.9* or *2.11*. This is the only method of surveying the entire genome for *any* numerical or structural chromosomal abnormality.

Chromosomes are always prepared from dividing cells, in which the DNA has already been replicated, and therefore under the microscope they are always seen to consist of two identical sister chromatids joined at the centromere. In

Figure 2.4 – Flowchart for processing a blood sample to obtain a standard G-banded chromosome preparation.

Box 2.1

Material for chromosome analysis

- **Peripheral blood lymphocytes** are the commonest material used. 0.5–10 ml of blood is treated with phytohemagglutinin, which stimulates lymphocytes to divide. Cultures are harvested after 48 hours. The protocol is summarized in *Figure 2.4*.

- **Chorionic villi** are used for early prenatal diagnosis. They are usually collected at 10–12 weeks' gestation by transvaginal or transabdominal routes. The procedure carries around a 2% risk of causing a miscarriage. Spontaneously dividing cells are present and can be used for rapid analysis, but results are best confirmed on cultured cells. It is important to dissect out fetal material in order to avoid culturing maternal cells.

- **Amniotic fluid** collected at 14–20 weeks' gestation contains shed fetal cells. These are slow to grow and require around 2 weeks in culture to provide enough dividing cells for analysis.

- **Skin biopsies** are used to look for chromosomal abnormalities that may not be present in blood.

- **Testicular biopsies** are the only way to study male meiosis. In females, meiosis takes place in the fetal ovaries before birth, so there is no way of investigating meiosis clinically in a female patient.

former times the standard preparation protocols made this structure very clear (see inset to *Figure 2.10*). The centromere and sister chromatids are much less obvious in chromosomes prepared according to current protocols, which leave the sister chromatids pressed tightly together. Cytogeneticists rely more on the banding pattern for identifying each individual chromosome and detecting structural aberrations. Banding makes each chromosome stain in a reproducible and characteristic pattern of dark and light bands. The usual method is G-banding. This involves subjecting the chromosomes, spread out on a microscope slide, to a brief digestion with trypsin, followed by staining with Giemsa stain. Other banding methods are sometimes used for particular analyses. R-banding produces a reversed pattern of dark and light bands, useful for checking chromosome ends. Other specialized procedures stain centromeres (C-banding) or the short arms of the acrocentric chromosomes (silver staining).

Chromosomal locations are named according to the Paris Convention as described in *Box 2.2*. Bands are numbered counting outwards from the centromere. *Figure 2.5* shows the standard ideograms and nomenclature of G-banded chromosomes at a resolution of 550 bands. Higher resolutions can be obtained by harvesting the cells well before the chromosomes become maximally contracted at metaphase of cell division (see *Figure 2.6*). In these highly extended chromosomes, bands split into sub-bands and sub-sub-bands, allowing more precise localizations such as 7q11.23 (pronounced '7q one one point two three'). However, longer chromosomes are more likely to be tangled up, making analysis under the microscope at the highest resolutions (1500–2000 bands) very difficult. Abnormalities too small to be seen by standard 550-band analysis are best detected by switching to molecular methods. We will see this process in action as we follow the case of Gillian Green (Case 7).

Box 2.2

Chromosomes and their abnormalities: nomenclature and glossary

Karyotypes are described by the number of chromosomes, the sex chromosome constitution, and any abnormality. Locations on chromosomes are described in relation to the Paris Convention of nomenclature shown in *Figure 2.5*. p means the short arm, q the long arm, t signifies a translocation, del a deletion, dup a duplication, inv an inversion, and der a derivative chromosome, whose structure would then be specified.

- 46,XX – a normal female
- 47,XY,+21 – a male with trisomy 21
- 46,XX,t(1;22)(q25;q13) – a female with a translocation between chromosomes 1 and 22 with breakpoints at 1q25 and 22q13 (the abnormality in **Case 5**, *Figure 2.14*)
- 46,XY,del(2)(q34;q36.2) – a male with a deletion on the long arm of chromosome 2 taking out the material between 2q34 and 2q36.2.

This is enough detail for present purposes. For the full nomenclature, covering every possible abnormality, see Shaffer and Tommerup (2005).

Acrocentric – a chromosome that has its centromere close to one end – chromosomes 13, 14, 15, 21, 22 and Y.

Autosome – any chromosome that is not the X or Y sex chromosome.

Centromere – the position on a chromosome where the sister chromatids are joined, and where the spindle fibers attach during cell division to pull the chromatids apart.

Chromatid – in a dividing cell, a chromosome consists of two identical sister chromatids joined at the centromere. After cell division, and until the DNA is next replicated, a chromosome consists of a single chromatid.

Chromatin – a general term for the DNA–protein complex that makes up chromosomes.

Euchromatin – chromatin with a relatively open structure in which genes can be active; the opposite of heterochromatin.

G-banding – a standard procedure in which chromosomes are treated so that they stain in a characteristic and reproducible pattern of dark and pale bands, as shown in *Figure 2.5*.

Heterochromatin – chromatin that is highly condensed and genetically inactive. Found mainly at centromeres.

Homologous chromosomes – the two no.1s or 2s etc. in a person. Note that unlike sister chromatids, homologous chromosomes are not copies of one another, and they may differ in small ways (minor DNA sequence differences) or sometimes in large ways (because of translocations, etc.).

Inversion – a structural abnormality in which part of a chromosome is in the wrong orientation compared to the rest (see *Figure 2.19*).

Karyotype – a person's chromosome constitution – also used loosely to describe a display of a person's chromosomes, as in *Figure 2.9*, etc.

Metacentric – a chromosome that has its centromere in the middle (e.g. chromosomes 3 and 20).

Monosomy – having one copy of one particular chromosome, but two of all the others (i.e. 45 in total for an autosomal monosomy).

Robertsonian translocation – a special type of translocation in which two acrocentric chromosomes are joined close to their centromeres as in *Figure 2.20*.

Box 2.2 – continued

Sister chromatids – the two chromatids of a chromosome as seen in a dividing cell. Sister chromatids are copies of each other, made during the preceding round of DNA replication.

Submetacentric – a chromosome that has a long arm and a short arm, e.g. most human chromosomes.

Telomere – the special structure at the end of a chromosome arm.

Translocation – a structural abnormality in which two chromosomes swap non-homologous segments.

Triploidy – having three complete sets of chromosomes.

Trisomy – having three copies of one particular chromosome, but two of all the others (i.e. 47 in total).

Chromosome abnormalities

Chromosomal abnormalities can involve having the wrong number of chromosomes, or having one or more structurally abnormal chromosomes. The nature and origin of chromosome abnormalities are discussed in more detail in Section 2.4. Several numerical chromosome abnormalities occur sufficiently frequently to produce syndromes that are recognizable clinically (*Box 2.3*). So, for example, the midwife recognized the characteristic features of Down syndrome in Helen Howard (Case 8). Abnormalities of chromosome structure are usually the result of chromosome breakages. Certain chromosome regions are predisposed to specific breakages which produce recognizable syndromes (*Box 2.4*). An alert clinician would suspect one such syndrome in the case of Gillian Green (Case 7). Most structural abnormalities, however, are one-off events caused by random chromosome breaks. Although these do not produce specific named syndromes, clinicians have learned to suspect a chromosomal abnormality in babies who have multiple congenital abnormalities that are not ascribable to failure of one specific developmental event, or in patients with a combination of mental retardation and dysmorphism. For these reasons it would be appropriate to request chromosome analysis in the case of Elizabeth Elliot (Case 5).

Why do we have chromosomes?

A human cell contains 2 m of DNA. Imagine a typical cell, 10 μm across, expanded to the size of a lecture room 10 m across. The DNA would be represented by 2000 km of string, occupying much of the space in the room. Now replicate the DNA, turning each single strand of string into a double strand like a twin electric flex. And now you must divide the cell. In about an hour a cell succeeds in precisely dividing its replicated DNA, so that each daughter cell gets exactly one copy of every piece of DNA. If you are going to avoid hopeless tangles and confusion in your lecture room full of twin flex, you need to organize it in some very precise way. That is what chromosomes do in a cell.

Figure 2.5 – Nomenclature of cytogenetic bands.
The ideograms show ideal G-banding patterns at 550 band resolution. Major bands are labeled 1, 2, 3, etc., going from centromere to telomere. Major band 11q1 (11q means the long arm of chromosome 11, 11p the short arm) is divided into sub-bands 11q11 – 11q14, and at the highest resolution 11q14 splits into 11q14.1 – 11q14.3. Redrawn from Shaffer and Tommerup (2005) with permission from S. Karger AG, Basel.

Box 2.3

Syndromes due to numerical chromosome abnormalities

Triploidy (69,XXX, XXY or YYY)

Triploidy is common at conception but triploid embryos and fetuses almost never survive to term, and those that do so do not live for long.

Autosomal trisomies

All possible autosomal trisomies can be found among early miscarriages, but only trisomies 13, 18 and 21 generally survive to term. It may be significant that chromosomes 13, 18 and 21 have the lowest density of genes of any chromosomes in our genome. This means that fewer genes are present in abnormal numbers in these trisomies, compared to trisomies of other similar sized chromosomes. How trisomies originate is discussed below.

- +21 Down syndrome – see **Case 8**. The only autosomal trisomy compatible with survival into adult life.

- +18 Edwards syndrome – affected babies normally die in the first year of life. Although they can be externally relatively normal, they have subtle signs, are growth retarded and have many internal malformations. Rare long-term survivors show very little developmental progress.

- +13 Patau syndrome – 50% of affected babies die in the first month, and the rest within the first year. They can have mid-line malformations of the head and face, ranging from mild (closely-spaced eyes, central cleft lip) to very severe (gross malformations of the face with a single central eye and holoprosencephaly – failure of the brain to develop two hemispheres). Polydactyly is another common feature.

Sex chromosome abnormalities

Having wrong numbers of sex chromosomes is much less deleterious than having wrong numbers of autosomes. For the Y chromosome this is because it carries very few genes, and none are essential to life. The X chromosome is different: it carries about 1000 genes including many that are essential to life, but the mechanism of X-inactivation (see *Chapter 7*) greatly reduces the effect of having differing numbers of X chromosomes.

As the examples below show, a person is male if he has a Y chromosome, regardless of the number of X chromosomes. The *SRY* gene on the Y chromosome is believed to be the master switch in sexual differentiation (see *Disease Box 6*).

- 45,X   Turner syndrome – females, pubertal failure, infertile, often short stature, normal intelligence. May have neck webbing, heart defects (coarctation) and horseshoe kidneys.

- 47, XXY Klinefelter syndrome – males, pubertal failure, infertile and often tall with female distribution of body fat. There may be a slightly lowered IQ compared to siblings.

- 47,XXX   females, mostly undiagnosed because they are relatively normal. There may be a slightly lowered IQ compared to siblings.

- 47,XYY   males, tall, possibly mildly reduced intelligence but within the normal range. The great majority of XYY men are living normal lives and are not diagnosed, but there may be a slightly increased risk of behavior problems.

Box 2.4

Recurrent microdeletion syndromes

A number of well-recognized clinical syndromes are caused by **microdeletions** – that is, deletion of a chromosomal segment that is too small to be noticed on a standard chromosome preparation like the one shown in *Figure 2.9*. When an alert clinician suspects a microdeletion on clinical grounds it can be detected and characterized using the molecular cytogenetic techniques described in *Chapter 4*. Some well-defined microdeletion syndromes are listed in the table below.

Syndrome	OMIM number	Location of microdeletion	Comments
Wolf–Hirschhorn	194190	4p16	Low birthweight, mental retardation, fits, typical face
Cri-du-chat	123450	5p15	Mental retardation, typical face, high-pitched cry
Williams–Beuren	194050	7q11.23	See *Disease Box 3*
Angelman	105830	15q11–q13	See *Chapter 7*
Prader–Willi	176270	15q11–q13	See *Chapter 7*
Miller–Dieker	247200	17p13	Lissencephaly, mental retardation, typical face
Smith–Magenis	182290	17p11	Mental retardation, behavioral problems, abnormal sleep patterns
Di George–VCFS	188400	22q11	See **Case 7, Green family**

Many other one-off or recurrent microdeletions have been described. Of those listed in the table, Wolf–Hirschhorn, cri-du-chat and Miller–Dieker syndromes involve deletion of the end of a chromosome arm. These are usually the result of random breakages; the proximal breakpoint varies between different patients but the deletion always encompasses a critical region specific to the syndrome. The other syndromes in the table normally have exactly the same breakpoints in every patient, causing deletion of a specific internal chromosome segment. These usually arise through recombination between misaligned low-copy DNA repeats, as explained in *Disease box 3*.

Centromeres and telomeres

Chromosomes are not simply passive packages of DNA. They are functional cellular organelles, and parts of their function depend on two special structures, centromeres and telomeres.

• A functional chromosome must have one, and only one, centromere. As mentioned previously, the two sister chromatids are joined at the centromere. Importantly, the centromere (or strictly, the kinetochore, a structure located at the centromere) is the attachment point for the spindle fibers that pull the chromosomes apart during cell division (see below).

- Telomeres are special structures at each end of a chromosome. Telomeres contain long arrays of tandemly repeated DNA sequences, $(TTAGGG)_n$. Because of the detailed enzymology of DNA replication, each chromosome end loses around 10–20 repeat units each time a cell divides (see *Figure 12.3*). If the telomere is totally lost the chromosome becomes unstable, normally leading to cell death. Some theories link this process with ordinary aging, but that is controversial. Telomeres have enough repeats to survive the cell divisions that occur within the lifetime of a person, but between generations they need to be renewed. Germ-line cells, and also cancer cells, produce a special enzyme, **telomerase,** that is able to restore telomeres to full length, helping to make such cells immortal.

The behavior of chromosomes during cell division

Preparing to divide

As discussed above, the primary function of chromosomes is to allow cells to distribute their DNA to daughter cells in an orderly fashion.

(a) *Replicating the DNA*. Each chromosome initially contains a single immensely long DNA double helix. When a cell is preparing to divide, during S phase of the cell cycle, the DNA is replicated, but the two copies remain attached to each other. Each chromosome then consists of two identical sister chromatids, each containing a full copy of the DNA double helix and joined together at the centromere. As seen under the microscope, chromosomes always have this structure (even though, as mentioned above, the two sister chromatids are rarely distinct in standard preparations) – but it is important to remember that the normal state of a chromosome in a non-dividing cell is as a single chromatid.

(b) *Condensing the chromosomes*. During the early part of cell division (**prophase**) the chromosomes become much more compact, until they become visible under the microscope.

What is seen next depends on what daughter cell is to be produced. There are two sorts of cell division:

- **Mitosis** is the normal form of cell division, and the form in which chromosomes are almost always studied for clinical purposes. In mitosis the replicated DNA is divided exactly equally between the two daughter cells, so that they are genetically identical.
- **Meiosis** is a specialized form of cell division that is used only to produce gametes (sperm or eggs). Meiosis has two purposes. First, the number of chromosomes must be reduced from 46 to 23, so that when the sperm and egg fuse, the result is a 46 chromosome zygote. Second, meiosis uses two mechanisms, described below, to ensure that every gamete carries a novel and unique combination of the parental genes. As mentioned in *Box 2.1*, clinically meiosis can be studied in males through a testicular biopsy, and this may be part of investigations of male infertility. Female meiosis is virtually impossible to study in humans because most stages take place in the fetus before birth. However, the consequences of errors in meiosis are central to clinical cytogenetics.

PROPHASE
chromatin condenses into chromosomes

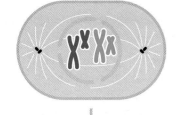

METAPHASE
nuclear envelope disappears
chromosomes align at the equatorial plate

ANAPHASE
sister chromatids separate
centromeres divide

chromatin expands
cytoplasm divides

Figure 2.6 – The stages of mitosis.

Mitosis

In mitosis (*Figure 2.6*), when each chromosome becomes visible it consists of two highly condensed sister chromatids held together at the centromere. At the end of prophase the nuclear membrane dissolves and the chromosomes move to the center of the cell. The positions of the nuclei of the two daughter cells are already marked by radiating arrays of microtubules. These attach to the centromere of each individual chromosome. Each chromosome is held by microtubules radiating from both ends of the cell. The microtubules contract, pulling the chromosomes to lie on the equatorial plane of the cell (**metaphase**). Eventually the centromere of each chromosome splits, so that as the microtubules continue to contract, one chromatid of each chromosome is pulled to each pole of the cell (**anaphase**). Once all the chromatids have arrived at the poles they decondense, nuclear membranes are formed round them, and the cell divides into two daughter cells.

Note the essential feature of mitosis:

- the sister chromatids are copies of each other, and each daughter cell receives one chromatid of each chromosome
- each chromosome behaves independently. Although there are two copies (homologs) of each chromosome, the two do not interact in any way. Look at *Figure 2.10* and note the random arrangement of the chromosomes in the spread. This is a key difference between mitosis and meiosis.

Meiosis

As mentioned above, meiosis is the highly specialized form of cell division that is used only to produce gametes (*Figure 2.7*). Gametes have 23 chromosomes and each gamete is genetically unique. Meiosis consists of two successive cell divisions; meiosis II is similar to mitosis, but meiosis I has special features.

During prophase I the chromosomes condense and become visible, as in mitosis, but in meiosis I the bodies that appear are not 46 separate chromosomes but 23 bivalents (*Figure 2.8*). Each bivalent is a four-stranded structure, consisting of two homologous chromosomes (the two no. 1s, etc.), each of which consists of two sister chromatids. The two sister chromatids of a chromosome are identical, because they are copies of each other, but the two homologs are not identical. You might think of each as a long line of pigeon-holes. Each will have the same set of pigeon-holes, but the content of corresponding pigeon-holes on the two may be different. For example, near the bottom of the long arm of each copy of chromosome 9 there is a locus (a pigeon-hole) for ABO blood group. But one homolog may carry the A gene and the other the O gene. They are not copies of each other.

The pairing of homologs is extraordinarily accurate. When there is a structural abnormality, so that the homologs do not completely match, matching segments pair (unless this involves tying the chromosomes in impossible knots). *Figure 2.17* shows an example of this effect when there is a translocation, and *Figure 2.21* shows what happens when one homolog has an inversion. In male meiosis the X and Y chromosomes also pair. Although most of their sequence is completely different, there is a short region of homology at the tips of the short arms (the **pseudoautosomal region**, see *Section 7.2*) and the X and Y use this to pair end-to-end.

At anaphase I the spindle fibers pull the chromosomes apart. In mitosis the centromere of each individual chromosome splits and the two sister chromatids are pulled apart; but in meiosis I the two homologous chromosomes pull apart, each still consisting of two sister chromatids joined at the centromere. Thus at the end of meiosis I each daughter cell has 23 chromosomes, each of which consists of two sister chromatids. In meiosis II the sister chromatids are pulled apart, just as in mitosis, so that the final product of meiosis is four cells, each containing 23 single-chromatid chromosomes. Case 8 (Howard family) and Case 5 (Elliot family) show examples of what can go wrong at this stage.

Whatever its other merits and demerits, sex has one sole purpose in biology: to produce novel combinations of genes. Partly this is achieved simply by involving two different people in the process of sexual reproduction. But there are two additional mechanisms at work generating yet more novelty, and both of these depend on the way chromosomes behave during meiosis (*Figure 2.7*).

(1) When a person forms a gamete, only one of his two no.1 chromosomes will be picked to go into the gamete. It might be the one he got from his mother or it might be the one he got from his father. With each chromosome we have two choices – we could pick the maternal or the paternal one. Over all 23 chromosomes we have $2 \times 2 \times 2 \times 2 \times ... = 2^{23}$ different ways of picking the one no. 1, one no. 2, etc. that go into a particular gamete; 2^{23} is 8 388 608.

(2) A second mechanism increases the number of possible variations from 8 million to effectively infinity. As previously mentioned, in the early stages of meiosis homologous chromosomes (the two no. 1s, etc.) pair up. But they don't simply stick together (synapse); they exchange segments. This is genetic recombination. The DNA of one homolog is physically cut and joined to the DNA of the homologous chromosome. Not surprisingly, the mechanism of recombination is complicated. It appears to involve cutting the DNA of the two chromosomes at precisely the same position to the nearest single nucleotide, and joining the ends the other way round. Actually that is not exactly how it is done – in reality, after the first cut, the second is made somewhere in the right vicinity, and then DNA is resynthesized around the position of the crossover to get the correct matching sequences. This complicated process requires many enzymes and is still not very well understood.

Regardless of the precise molecular mechanism, the effect is that homologous chromosomes swap segments. Normally there is at least one crossover (point of recombination between synapsed chromosomes) in each arm of each chromosome

Figure 2.7 – The stages of meiosis.
Meiosis is used only for the production of sperm and eggs. It consists of two successive cell divisions, producing four daughter cells (although in oogenesis only one of these develops into a mature oocyte; the others form the polar bodies). Meiosis has two main functions: to reduce the chromosome number in the gamete to 23, and to ensure that every gamete is genetically unique.

(a)

(b)

Figure 2.8 – Examples of chromosomes during meiosis.
(a) Two cells from a testicular biopsy showing chromosomes during prophase
I of male meiosis. Each of the 23 structures is a bivalent, consisting of two
homologous chromosomes, each having two chromatids. Note the end-to-end
pairing of the X and Y chromosomes. (b) A bivalent seen in meiosis in an amphibian,
which has large chromosomes that make the four-stranded structure clear.

pair. On average there are about 60 crossovers in each cell in spermatogenesis,
and about 90 in oogenesis, though the actual number varies considerably between
people and between cells. To a first approximation, crossovers are distributed at
random along each of the 22 pairs of autosomes (although closer investigation
reveals some interesting non-random features). Thus each chromosome in every
sperm or egg that a person produces carries a unique combination of genes
that came from his or her father and mother. This topic is discussed further in
Chapter 9 where we consider how disease genes can be mapped to a particular
chromosomal location, because recombination is the key to genetic mapping.

As a result of these mechanisms, every conceptus is a unique combination of
a unique sperm with a unique egg. The only people who are not genetically
unique are monozygotic twins, whose cells are all derived by mitosis from
a single original conceptus. The fact that monozygotic twins are unique
individuals despite being clones reminds us that genetics is not everything
in life.

2.3. **Investigations of patients**

| CASE 7 | Green family | 25 | **38** | 68 | 99 | 376 |

- Girl (Gillian) aged 3 years
- Slow to develop
- ? Chromosome abnormality
- Order tests to check for microdeletion at 22q11

The combination of slow development, a heart defect, palatal problems and mildly dysmorphic features in Gillian suggested a chromosomal abnormality. Blood was taken for cytogenetic analysis, but the result (*Figure 2.9*) was a normal female karyotype, 46,XX. Because of her particular combination of clinical features the geneticist suspected that Gillian might have the Di George – velo-cardio-facial syndrome (VCFS) which is caused by a microdeletion at chromosome 22q11. As described in *Box 2.4*, the Di George–VCFS deletion is too small to be visible under the microscope. He therefore requested a molecular test. The test and its result are described in *Chapter 4*.

Figure 2.9 – **Gillian Green's karyotype.**
The result (at this resolution) shows a normal female karyotype, 46,XX.

| CASE 8 | Howard family | 26 | **38** | 68 | 100 | 275 | 376 |

- Helen – new-born daughter of Henry and Anne (33 years old)
- Down syndrome
- Risk of recurrence if they have more children?

The clinical diagnosis of Down syndrome in Helen was confirmed by karyotyping. A 2 ml blood sample was taken and, as shown in *Figure 2.4*, the cells were cultured, harvested after 48 hours, spread on a microscope slide and stained by G-banding. The cytogeneticist analysed 10 cells by eye down the microscope (one of the cells is shown in *Figure 2.10*), and for record purposes she used an image analyzer program to arrange chromosomes from one cell into a standard karyotype (*Figure 2.11*). Her report gave the karyotype as 47,XX,+21, confirming that Helen had typical Down syndrome, trisomy 21. An additional reason for checking Helen's karyotype is discussed below in *Section 2.4*.

As expected, the pedigree showed nothing noteworthy (no previous abnormal babies or recurrent miscarriages) in either Anne's or Henry's family, and it is not

Figure 2.10 – 47,XX,+21 spread.
There are three copies of chromosome 21. Note that homologous chromosomes (the two no. 1s etc.) behave entirely independently in mitosis. The preparation method used here leaves the two sister chromatids of each chromosome tightly pressed together, so that the position of the centromere is not obvious to the eye. This makes the banding pattern easier for the cytogeneticist to recognize. The inset shows some chromosomes that have been handled differently, to make the structure of sister chromatids joined at the centromere more obvious.

illustrated here. Their first question was why it had happened, and why to them? The counselor explained that it was a one-off accident in meiosis (see *Figure 2.12*). Either the two paired chromosomes 21 (in the first meiotic division), or the two sister chromatids of the one copy of 21 in the second division, had

Figure 2.11 – Karyotype showing trisomy 21 (47,XX,+21).

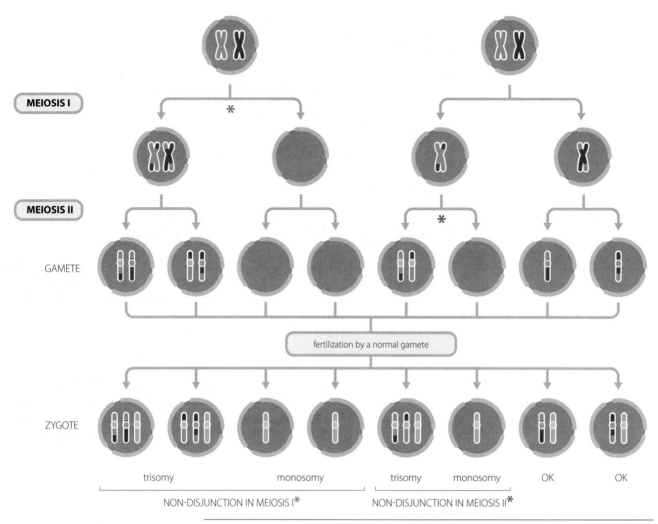

Figure 2.12 – The effects of non-disjunction in meiosis.
The non-disjunction involves only the single pair of chromosomes (meiosis I) or the single chromosome (meiosis II) shown; all the other chromosomes (not shown) disjoin and segregate normally.

failed to disjoin at anaphase and segregate into separate daughter cells. They had both ended up in the same daughter cell, producing an egg or sperm with 24 chromosomes, including two copies of no. 21.

Anne asked if it was always the woman's fault, as she had heard that said. No; in the first place these things are nobody's fault, and secondly, in principle the non-disjunction could happen at either division of meiosis in either parent, though DNA marker studies showed that 70% of cases were due to non-disjunction in the first meiotic division in the mother. This might possibly be a reflection of the extremely long duration of that stage in women, from before birth until whenever the relevant egg ovulated. In men, meiosis goes on continuously in the testes from puberty to old age. The individual risk rises sharply with the age of the mother (*Table 2.1*) but because most babies are born to younger women, most Down syndrome babies are also born to younger mothers. This led to the discussion of population screening that is summarized in *Chapter 11*.

Table 2.1 – **Risk of Down syndrome vs. maternal age**

Age (years)	20	30	34	36	38	40	42	45
Risk	1 in 1500	1 in 900	1 in 500	1 in 300	1 in 200	1 in 100	1 in 60	1 in 30

With the exception of Turner syndrome (45,X), all the numerical abnormalities listed in *Box 2.3* show a similar age dependence.

Later, Anne and Henry requested an appointment to discuss options for prenatal diagnosis in any subsequent pregnancy. This led to the discussion and intervention described in *Chapter 4*.

| CASE 9 | Ingram family | 26 | **41** | 68 | 101 | 182 | 376 |

- Isabel – first daughter of Irene and Ian
- Small stature despite tall parents
- ? Turner syndrome

As described earlier, although Isabel had a few mildly abnormal features at birth, she only came to medical attention because she was small compared to her parents' heights and her peer group. Her phenotype and history of swollen hands and feet were strongly suggestive of Turner syndrome. Chromosome analysis confirmed this (*Figure 2.13*). This is the only human monosomy that is not lethal early in development. Because males survive with only one X chromosome, maybe it is not surprising that Turner syndrome is not always lethal. But in fact it is lethal in over 90% of cases. Fetuses with Turner syndrome can be grossly distended with fluid and the great majority abort spontaneously. The survivors are often born with puffy (edematous) hands and feet and with redundant skin on the neck, which represent the remains of presumably milder fetal edema.

Figure 2.13 – **Karyotype of Isabel Ingram.**
Although Isabel will never be able to have children normally, treatment with estrogens can allow her to develop normal secondary sex characteristics and greatly assist her personal and social life. Modern reproductive technology has allowed some Turner syndrome patients to bear children using donor eggs. Treatment with growth hormone can result in improved growth and final height.

Unlike all the trisomies, the risk of Turner syndrome does not increase with maternal age. The mechanism is different. Rather than non-disjunction, Turner syndrome is the result of anaphase lag, in which one of the sex chromosomes moves too slowly to the pole of a daughter cell during cell division, and ends up outside the nucleus, whereupon it is broken down. It can arise during gametogenesis or after conception during an early mitotic division. Many Turner women are mosaics (see *Section 1.4*, and below), and they can be either 45,X / 46,XX or 45,X / 46,XY mosaics. Where there is XY tissue in the gonad, it has a propensity to become malignant, and therefore the gonads are best surgically removed.

| CASE 5 | Elliot family | 4 | 11 | **42** | 64 | 376 |

- Miscarriage
- Very small dysmorphic baby girl (Elizabeth), parents Elmer and Ellen
- Heart problems
- Blood taken for chromosome analysis
- Pedigree suggests autosomal dominant condition with reduced penetrance

Previously it had been found that baby Elizabeth suffered from multiple congenital abnormalities (*Figure 1.5*). This suggested she had a chromosomal imbalance, but did not allow the geneticist to guess which chromosomes might be involved. Ellen had had one previous miscarriage, not in itself remarkable, but it was noted that her sister had also had two miscarriages. Further enquiries revealed a family history of reproductive problems – the pedigree is shown in *Figure 1.11*. Blood was taken from the baby and both parents for chromosome analysis. The results showed:

- Elmer – normal male karyotype, 46,XY
- Ellen – a balanced translocation between chromosomes 1 and 22 (*Figure 2.14*)
- Elizabeth – an unbalanced segregation product (*Figure 2.15*)

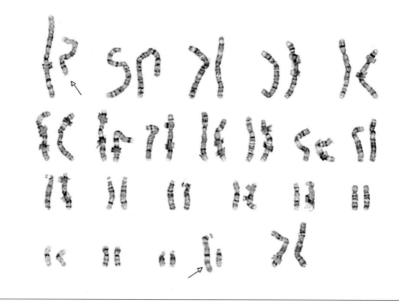

Figure 2.14 – G-banded karyotype of Ellen's chromosomes.
There is a balanced translocation. Chromosomes 1 and 22 have exchanged segments (arrows). The translocation is described as 46,XX,t(1:22)(q25:q13).

Figure 2.15 – G-banded karyotype of baby Elizabeth.
She has inherited Ellen's normal chromosome 1 but her translocated chromosome 22 (arrow). She is trisomic for the portion of chromosome 1 distal to 1q25, the translocation breakpoint, and monosomic for chromosome 22 distal to 22q13.

When they learned these results, the parents, as well as being very distressed and wanting to know the implications for Elizabeth, were keen to understand exactly what had happened and why. An explanation of the cytogenetics was given using language familiar to the family and explaining technical terms.

Ellen was a constitutional carrier of a balanced translocation – that is, it was present in every cell of her body (see below for a discussion of balanced vs. unbalanced abnormalities). The translocation had been present in the fertilized egg from which Ellen developed, and the pedigree suggested it was already present in one of Ellen's maternal grandparents. At some time in that person or a more distant ancestor, chromosomes 1 and 22 had undergone breakages. Chromosome breaks are common events, but cells have machinery to repair them so that most go unnoticed. In this case, two simultaneous breaks had generated four broken ends, and by bad luck the repair machinery had joined those up the wrong way round (*Figure 2.16*). Alternatively, maybe the translocation had been produced by the machinery responsible for genetic recombination during meiosis activating inappropriately and cutting and joining non-matching chromosomes in a germ-line cell. Because each derivative chromosome nevertheless had a single centromere, mitosis proceeded with no problems, and because no genetic material was extra or missing, there was no phenotypic effect.

Although Ellen's cells could go through mitosis with no problems, meiosis was a different matter. In the first division of meiosis, homologous (matching) chromosomal segments pair (*Figure 2.7*). In this case, pairing would produce a cross-shaped structure containing four whole chromosomes – a tetravalent. When spindle fibers attached to the four centromeres and pulled them

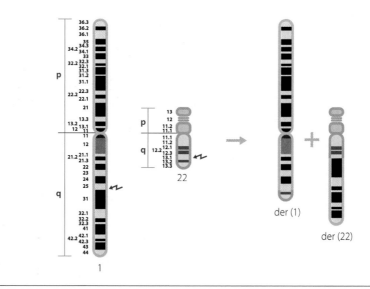

Figure 2.16 – How the 1;22 translocation in Ellen Elliot originated.
Chromosomes 1 and 22 broke at the positions indicated by the arrows, and the cell's DNA repair machinery rejoined the ends to form the two derivative chromosomes as shown. The derivative chromosomes are labeled der(1) and der(22).

apart, they could segregate in various ways (*Figure 2.17*). She could produce entirely normal gametes, gametes carrying the balanced translocation, or various unbalanced forms, one of which had produced Elizabeth. The baby had partial trisomy of chromosome 1 and simultaneously partial monosomy of chromosome 22. The resulting genetic imbalance was the cause of her abnormalities.

There was a risk of problems in future pregnancies, which could take various forms depending on the way the translocated chromosomes segregated. The result could be another child with the same problems as baby Elizabeth, or a different segregation pattern could result in a child with a different set of multiple abnormalities; maybe the result would be severe enough to cause a miscarriage; or of course they could hope to be lucky and have a normal baby. All these various outcomes could be seen in other family members on the pedigree (*Figure 1.11*). The risk was substantial, but it was not easily quantifiable for several reasons:

- we can't predict the exact probability that the translocated chromosomes would segregate in each of the various possible ways
- with some possible unbalanced outcomes a conceptus might abort so early that it would not be recognized as a problem
- it is uncertain whether other less fatally unbalanced karyotypes would result in a miscarriage or a live-born abnormal baby

If it had been Elmer who carried the translocation the risk would be lower, because abnormal sperm are less likely to win the race to fertilize the egg. If Elmer and Ellen wished, it would be possible in future pregnancies to check prenatally and offer termination where the fetus had one of the unbalanced karyotypes. The ways this might be done are discussed in *Chapter 14*.

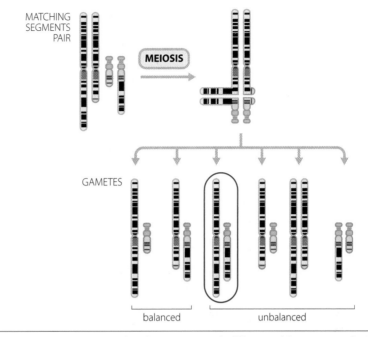

Figure 2.17 – Possible ways the chromosomes in Ellen could segregate in the first meiotic division.
During prophase I matching chromosome segments pair, resulting in a cross-shaped tetravalent containing the normal and translocated copies of chromosomes 1 and 22. At anaphase I they pull apart, and the diagram shows various ways this could happen. The gamete that gave rise to Baby Elliot is circled. Other more complex segregation patterns (3:1 segregation) are also possible.

Months later, once Elmer and Ellen had begun to cope with Elizabeth's health problems, and had absorbed the information about the translocation and their own risks for future children, the question of family risk was discussed. The family history suggested that Ellen's aunt and sister could well be carrying the same balanced translocation, as might her younger sister, who was not yet married. The counselor explained that they needed to be made aware of the risk, preferably by Elmer and Ellen having a word with them to raise the subject. The counselor offered to see the relatives to explain the situation and the options available, including genetic testing. In the genetic clinic it is important to deal with each branch of a family separately, unless family members indicate otherwise. Confidentiality should be maintained and information about one family member only given to another with permission.

2.4. Summary and extension

What are chromosomes?

Chromosomes are packages of DNA. Each chromosome contains a single immensely long DNA double helix, packaged by a diverse set of proteins. Chief among these are four types of histones H2A, H2B, H3 and H4, but there are also many other proteins. Chromatin is the generic name for the resulting DNA–protein complex. The basic structure of chromatin is a string of beads

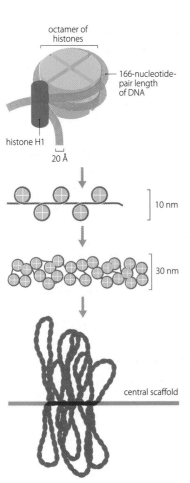

Figure 2.18 – Packaging DNA into a chromosome.
If you stretched out the DNA in one of the chromosomes in *Figure 2.9*, it would be 10 000 times the length of the chromosome. The DNA in chromosomes exists as a DNA–protein complex called chromatin. The most basic component of chromatin is the nucleosome, consisting of approximately 170 bp of double–stranded DNA wrapped round an octamer of histone proteins. This 'string of beads' is coiled up into a 30 nm fiber then hung in loops from the protein scaffold of the chromosome.

(*Figure 2.18*). The string is DNA and the beads are called nucleosomes. A nucleosome has a roughly spherical core made up of eight histone molecules, with the DNA wrapped round it for 1.75 turns, and a ninth histone molecule on the outside. The chromatin forms large loops, anchored at their bases to a protein scaffold that forms the backbone of a chromosome.

Above this basic structure, chromatin exists in several alternative configurations, depending on what that particular stretch of DNA and that particular cell are doing. Most of the time the string of beads is coiled into an extended 30 nm fiber. The nucleosomes can be loosely or tightly packed, depending whether or not the genes in that stretch of DNA are being expressed (see *Chapter 3* for a description of transcription). When cells are dividing the chromatin is much more tightly packaged. At this time the chromosomes can be seen under the light microscope (*Figures 2.10* and *2.11*). Chromosomes are equally present in non-dividing cells but cannot be seen under the microscope because the 30 nm chromatin fibers are so thin.

Numerical and structural chromosome abnormalities

Chromosome abnormalities can be **numerical** (wrong number of chromosomes, e.g. Helen Howard (*Figure 2.11*), Isabel Ingram (*Figure 2.13*) and the examples in *Box 2.3*) or **structural**, when one or more chromosomes contain the wrong DNA, as with Ellen Elliot (*Figure 2.14*).

Numerical abnormalities
These are of two types:

- **Errors of ploidy** are errors where there are the wrong number of complete sets of chromosomes. Normal cells are **diploid** ($2n$ = 46 chromosomes). Gametes are **haploid** (n = 23). Occasionally two sperm fertilize one egg, producing a triploid ($3n$ = 69). Triploids can also be produced if the whole meiotic process fails, resulting in a diploid gamete that then fertilizes a normal haploid gamete. As mentioned in *Box 2.3*, triploidy in humans is a common error at conception, but triploids virtually never survive to term. Tetraploidy results when a cell replicates its DNA but then does not divide. Tetraploidy and higher degrees of ploidy (polyploidy) may be seen in individual cells, but not in a whole person.
- **Aneuploidy.** All the above abnormalities involve cells with complete sets of chromosomes, which are called **euploid**. **Aneuploid** cells have just one or more single chromosomes extra or missing. Cells or people with one chromosome extra or missing are trisomic or monosomic for that chromosome. Tetrasomy and nullisomy are also possible. The reasons why aneuploidy causes clinical problems are discussed in *Chapter 7*.

Structural abnormalities
These include:

- **Reciprocal translocations.** These arise when any two chromosomes swap non-homologous segments (see *Figure 2.16*). A carrier of a balanced reciprocal translocation is at risk of producing offspring with trisomy of one of the translocated segments and, at the same time, monosomy of the other (*Figure 2.17*). This was the problem in Case 5 (Elliot family).

- **Robertsonian translocations.** These involve a translocation between two acrocentric chromosomes (13, 14, 15, 21, 22) with the breakpoints in the proximal short arm, just above the centromere (*Figure 2.20*). A carrier of a Robertsonian translocation is at risk of producing a conceptus with either complete trisomy or complete monosomy for one of the chromosomes involved. For example, somebody carrying a Robertsonian translocation involving chromosome 21 is at risk of producing a child with trisomy 21. About 3–4% of Down syndrome cases are due to such translocations. Phenotypically such a child will be indistinguishable from any other child with Down syndrome, but the recurrence risk is much higher. That is an additional reason why Helen Howard (Case 8) was karyotyped, even though there was little doubt about the diagnosis of Down syndrome.

- **Deletions** can be interstitial or terminal, though a chromosome must always have telomeres, so any stable terminal deletion must have somehow acquired a telomere. Ring chromosomes (see *Figure 2.19*) are a special type of terminal deletion. Deletions generally have severe effects, and large deletions are lethal.

- **Duplications** normally have less severe effects than the corresponding deletions.

- **Inversions** can be of any size. If they involve the centromere (pericentric inversions) they change the overall chromosome shape; if not (paracentric inversions) they can only be detected by careful examination of the banding pattern.

Balanced and unbalanced abnormalities

- A chromosomal abnormality is described as **balanced** if there is no material extra or missing: the DNA is just divided into packages incorrectly. Provided each chromosome has a single centromere and proper telomeres, a balanced abnormality does not interfere with the ability of a cell to go through mitosis. Thus a fertilized egg with a balanced abnormality should be able to develop into a normal adult. Ellen Elliot (*Figure 2.15*) is an example of a person who has a balanced chromosomal abnormality but is phenotypically normal. Robertsonian translocations are regarded as balanced even though two acrocentric short arms have been lost (*Figure 2.20*) because they have no effect on the phenotype of a carrier, and the short arms of the remaining acrocentric chromosomes supply all the functions of the missing two.

- If there is pathogenic extra or missing material the abnormality is **unbalanced**. The word 'pathogenic' is used here because recent research has overturned the older view that there is a fixed correct amount of chromosomal material for humans. Certain DNA segments are frequently absent or duplicated in normal people (so-called large scale

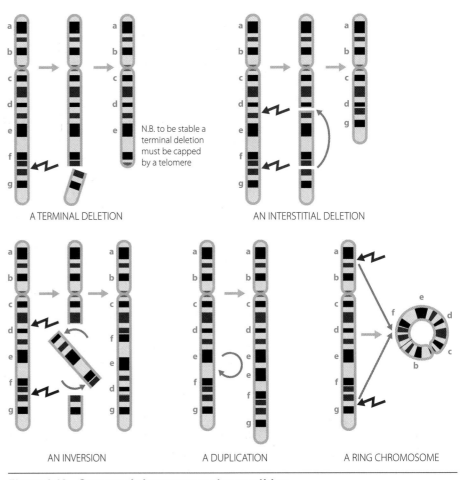

Figure 2.19 – Structural chromosome abnormalities.
These can arise either through mis-repair of chromosome breaks or through inappropriate function of the genetic recombination machinery. See *Figures 2.16* and *2.20* for translocations.

copy number polymorphisms). One would not describe these variants as unbalanced. Nevertheless, much of our DNA does have to be present in the correct quantity and Helen Howard (*Figure 2.11*) and Elizabeth Elliot (*Figure 2.15*) exemplify the problems of unbalanced chromosomal abnormalities.

Balanced abnormalities become important in meiosis when homologous chromosomes pair up. Things can go wrong in two ways.

• Translocated chromosomes have segments derived from more than one original chromosome. During prophase of meiosis I they will pair with multiple partners, forming trivalents or quadrivalents instead of bivalents (associations of two homologs). These are liable to segregate incorrectly at anaphase (*Figure 2.17*)

• Chromosomes with inversions pair with a single partner forming a looped structure (*Figure 2.21*), but if a crossover occurs within the loop the recombinant chromosomes are abnormal (see also *SAQ 4*).

Figure 2.20 – A Robertsonian translocation.
The inset shows how this common type of chromosome abnormality arises. The short arms of all the acrocentric chromosomes (13, 14, 15, 21, 22) contain similar DNA. Inappropriate recombination between two non-homologous chromosomes produces the fusion chromosome, which functions as a normal single chromosome in mitosis. The small acentric fragment comprising the two distal short arms is lost.

Although balanced abnormalities do not normally affect a person's phenotype, there are exceptions.

- One or more of the breakpoints may slice through a gene. This will prevent that gene from working, which may or may not matter to the individual. Case 12 (Lawton family) in *Chapter 4* is an example where it did matter.
- Sometimes, as described in *Chapter 3*, a breakpoint does not disrupt a gene itself, but separates a gene from a control element located some way away on the same DNA strand. Again, this may prevent the gene from working.
- Occasionally, when a misplaced recombination or DNA repair joins together segments from different chromosomes, the join creates a novel gene out of parts of two genes that were located near the breakpoints on the different chromosomes. Such chimeric genes are important in cancer (*Chapter 12*).
- Finally, balanced X-autosome translocations cause special problems because of X-inactivation. This is discussed in *Chapter 7.*

Constitutional and mosaic abnormalities

Chromosomal abnormalities can be:

- **constitutional** (present in every cell)
- **mosaic** (present only in some cells)

Figure 2.21 – During meiosis I matching chromosome segments pair. If one chromosome has an inversion compared to its homolog, they usually form a looped structure.

Mosaicism has already been discussed in *Chapter 1* and in connection with Case 9 (Ingram family, Turner syndrome). It is always the result of post-zygotic events, when a person or embryo consists of more than one cell. Because mosaicism depends on post-zygotic events, the recurrence risk for the parent of a mosaic child is negligibly low; however, if mosaicism in a person extends to the germ line, the risks for his or her children may be substantial. These considerations introduce some uncertainty into genetic counseling, because whether or not a chromosomal abnormality has been detected, it is impossible ever to formally exclude mosaicism (you can't examine every cell of a person) and the chromosomes of the germ line can only be studied through their effects in a person's children.

People can be mosaic for either a single gene disorder or a chromosome abnormality, but historically, discussion of clinically relevant mosaicism has focused on chromosomal mosaicism. This is because techniques for studying chromosomes have been available for 40 years, while studying mosaicism for point mutations requires molecular tests that have only recently become available. Cytogeneticists look at many cells when analyzing a patient's chromosomes, and so they often note mosaicism. Any chromosomal abnormality (except triploidy) that can arise in constitutional form through a meiotic error can also arise in mosaic form through a mitotic error. Thus, for example, mosaic Down syndrome is well known. The phenotype will lie somewhere along the spectrum between normal and full Down syndrome, but exactly where along the spectrum is unpredictable because it depends on the proportion of trisomic cells in different tissues and organs. In addition, many abnormalities that would be lethal if present in constitutional form can survive in mosaics. For example, a patient may have mosaic trisomy 8, but is unlikely to have full constitutional trisomy 8.

Sometimes mosaicism is present only in some tissues – for example, mosaic 12p tetrasomy (four copies of the short arm of chromosome 12; the two extra copies are in the form of a small additional metacentric chromosome) causes Pallister–Killian syndrome (OMIM 601803), where affected individuals have a characteristic appearance and pattern of malformations. But the abnormal cells are seen only in skin and not in the standard blood samples – it is likely that in the blood, which has a rapid cell turnover, abnormal cells are at a disadvantage and the normal cell lines come to predominate. Tissue-limited mosaicism can be a particular problem in prenatal diagnosis. The procedure of chorion villus biopsy (*Chapter 14*) provides the cytogeneticist with a sample of the placenta for analysis. Although the placenta is a fetal tissue, if it shows mosaicism there is great uncertainty whether this might be confined to the placenta or whether the fetus itself might also be mosaic, which could have implications for the pregnancy.

Alpha-thalassemia / mental retardation syndrome: a chromatin disease

Alpha-thalassemia (OMIM 301040) is the result of a deficiency of the α-globin component of hemoglobin. A complete deficiency causes lethal fetal hydrops, while a partial deficiency causes HbH disease with microcytosis and hemolysis. Alpha-thalassemia affects millions of people in malarial regions worldwide, especially in south-east Asia. It is caused by deletions, or sometimes point mutations, of the α-globin genes on chromosome 16p. The association with malaria is discussed in *Chapter 10*. Among indigenous populations of non-malarial regions it is exceedingly rare.

During the 1980s a number of cases were reported of native Northern Europeans who had α-thalassemia (HbH disease) and mental retardation. Mental retardation is not a normal feature of thalassemia. On investigation, several of these individuals proved to have large deletions of chromosome 16p that took out the α-globin gene, and presumably other genes whose loss would explain the mental retardation (see OMIM 141750). However, other affected cases did not have any identifiable abnormality of chromosome 16. Moreover these patients were always male, sometimes had affected male relatives in a pattern suggestive of X-linked inheritance, and had a characteristic facial appearance (see photograph). The HbH disease, though present, was often atypically mild, and only detectable on laboratory testing. Affected people often had other features including male to female sex reversal. Genetic mapping and positional cloning (as described in *Chapter 9*) eventually led to the identification of mutations in a gene called *ATRX* on the X chromosome at Xq13.

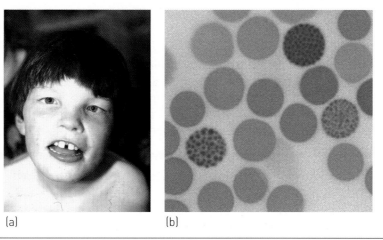

(a)   (b)

(a) A patient with ATRX. Reproduced from *J. Med. Genet.* 1991; **28**: 742–745 with permission from the BMJ Publishing Group. (b) Lymphocytes from an ATRX patient showing characteristic inclusions. Photo. courtesy of Dr Richard Gibbon, Oxford.

How could mutations in an X-chromosome gene result in α-thalassemia, together with a whole range of other features? On the evidence of its amino acid sequence, the ATRX protein is a member of a large family of proteins, the SWI2/SNF family, that regulate gene expression and chromosome behavior through effects on the structure of chromatin. As explained earlier, DNA is packaged by being wrapped round an octamer of histone proteins to form nucleosomes. The string of nucleosomes is then subject to further levels of packaging, under the control of numerous other proteins. There are two basic configurations of chromatin:

- heterochromatin is tightly packed and genes in heterochromatin are not expressed

- euchromatin is more open and variable; genes in euchromatic regions of chromosomes may or may not be expressed

ATRX is a helicase, that is, a protein that can unwind DNA double helices. It is believed to form part of large multiprotein complexes that control the local structure of chromatin. This in turn controls the expression of the genes in the packaged DNA. ATRX is particularly associated with centromeres, which have the repressive heterochromatic structure. Other local regions of chromatin can also form these repressive structures, shutting off expression of the genes in the region in response to signals about the metabolic state of the cell. ATRX is probably involved in establishing or maintaining repressive chromatin structures.

ATRX is an example of a **chromatin disease**. Other examples include ICF syndrome (see OMIM 242860) and Rett syndrome (see *Disease Box 7*). These diseases have mutations in genes encoding proteins that control the structure of chromatin, and hence have effects on the expression of a potentially large number of genes. With our present state of knowledge, it is not possible to predict which genes would be affected by a given defect, or what clinical phenotypes would result. However, these diseases give us a window into an important function of chromosomes. They show us that chromosomes are more than just vehicles for partitioning the genome between daughter cells during mitosis and meiosis. Through local variations in chromatin structure, chromosomes provide a dynamic environment for regulating the way genes are expressed.

Chromatin has a highly dynamic structure. Chromatin remodeling complexes, of which the ATRX protein is a component, constantly shuffle nucleosomes along the DNA, exposing sites for selective modification of the DNA and histones. Active and inactive chromatin are marked by different patterns of DNA methylation (see figure) and by a variety of modifications of the histones, including acetylation, methylation and phosphorylation of specific residues.

2.5. **References**

Gardner RJM and Sutherland GR (1996) *Chromosome Abnormalities and Genetic Counseling*, 2nd edition OUP, Oxford. *Gives an in-depth treatment of the material covered in this chapter.*

Shaffer LG and Tommerup N, eds (2005) *ISCN 2005, An International System for Human Cytogenetic Nomenclature.* S. Karger AG, Basel.

More detail on mitosis and meiosis can be found in any cell biology textbook.

Useful websites

A useful web resource is the Online Biology Book by MJ Farabee (see the chapters on mitosis and meiosis):
http://www.emc.maricopa.edu/faculty/farabee/BIOBK/BioBookTOC.html

The website of Hironao Numabe at Tokyo Medical University contains many (English language) graphics and animations relevant to this chapter: http://www.tokyo-med.ac.jp/genet/index-e.htm

2.6. **Self-assessment questions**

(1) Which meiotic divisions in which parent could, by non-disjunction, potentially produce a child with:
   (a) 45,X [*guidance provided for this one*]
   (b) 47,XXY
   (c) 47,XYY

(2) Draw the tetravalent and possible gametes and conceptuses from the following translocations.
   (a) t(2;4)(q22;q32) [*guidance provided for this one*]
   (b) t(5;10)(p14;p13)
   (c) t(7;9)(q32;p21)

(3) Using the diagrams of tetravalents that you drew for the previous question, put in a crossover between the translocated and normal chromosomes in each of the paired segments. Work out the consequences. (*This is not done just to give you a headache – there is normally at least one crossover per chromosome arm during meiosis.*)

(4) Consider the carrier of a balanced Robertsonian 14:21 translocation whose karyotype is shown in *Figure 2.20*. During meiosis the translocation chromosome will form a trivalent with the normal chromosomes 14 and 21. Draw the possible ways this can segregate when a gamete is formed, and describe the consequences of each of these for any conceptus.

(5) Work out the possible gametes, conceptuses and live-born babies that a carrier of a balanced Robertsonian 21:21 translocation married to a chromosomally normal person could have.

(6) Considering the inversion heterozygote shown in *Figure 2.21*, work out the consequences of a crossover occurring either within the inversion loop or outside it. Is it different if the centromere lies within the inverted segment (a pericentric inversion) rather than outside it as in the figure (a paracentric inversion)?

Chapter 3

How do genes work?

Learning points for this chapter

After working through this chapter you should be able to:

- Name the bases, sugars and nucleosides that form normal DNA and RNA, and sketch a DNA double helix, marking in base pairs and the 5′ and 3′ ends
- Draw a diagram showing the principles (but not the detailed enzymology) of DNA replication, of transcription, of splicing of the transcript and of the way an mRNA sequence specifies the amino acid sequence of a polypeptide
- Describe the general features of the nuclear and mitochondrial genomes
- Sketch a typical human gene structure, showing exons, introns, the promoter, the start and stop codons, the 5′ and 3′ untranslated regions and splice sites
- Describe in outline the role of the promoter, transcription factors and chromatin structure in determining gene expression

3.1. Case studies

| CASE 10 | Johnson family | **55** | 64 | 376 |

- Marfan syndrome

Figure 3.1 – Pedigree of James Johnson

James first came to the genetic clinic when he was 14 years old. His father, Henry, and several other relatives had been known to the genetics department for many years. They were originally referred by an eye specialist who had noted that Henry had dislocated lenses and was rather tall. The ophthalmologist was alarmed to find out that Henry's brother, aged 45 years, had died suddenly of aortic rupture and that his mother had died unexpectedly at a similar age. The diagnosis of Marfan syndrome was made and Henry was counseled that his own offspring would have a 50% risk of inheriting this dominant genetic condition. At that time the gene responsible for the syndrome had not been identified, and diagnosis rested on well-defined clinical criteria. These included a positive family history and involvement of the systems that are typically affected in Marfan syndrome (mainly the skeletal, ocular, and cardiovascular systems). Years later, when James came to the clinic, the doctor carefully checked for the clinical features of Marfan syndrome using the Ghent criteria (De Paepe *et al.*, 1996). An echocardiogram showed early dilatation of the ascending aorta, and James was very tall for his age. The doctor concluded that these features and the positive family history left no room for doubt. By this time the gene involved in Marfan syndrome had been identified, but on clinical criteria alone it was obvious that James was affected.

(a)　　　　　　　　　　　　　　　　　　　　　(b)

Figure 3.2 – Marfan syndrome.
(a) Arachnodactyly (long fingers). (b) Dislocated lens.

3.2. **Background**

How genes work is the subject of two famous hypotheses. Neither of them is wholly true, but both are nevertheless useful tools for thinking about genes.

- In the 1940s Beadle and Tatum proposed that the job of each gene was to specify one particular enzyme (the **one gene – one enzyme hypothesis**). It is not completely true because many genes specify non-enzymic proteins, and some specify functional RNA molecules rather than proteins – but in the form of 'one gene – one polypeptide' it remains a useful first tool for thinking about what genes do.
- Some years later, Francis Crick defined the essential function of DNA in the 'Central Dogma' of molecular biology (**Figure 3.3**). Genes are functional units of the DNA, and the usual function of a gene is to specify the structure of a protein. There are thought to be about 24 000 protein-coding genes in the human genome, though this is only a provisional estimate. The Central Dogma is useful but not absolutely true. Occasionally the flow of information from DNA to RNA is reversed, when a special enzyme (reverse transcriptase) makes a DNA copy of an RNA molecule. This is a critical part of the life cycle of RNA viruses, but is not

Figure 3.3 – The Central Dogma of molecular biology.
The arrows don't mean that DNA is turned into RNA, etc; they mean the information contained in DNA is transferred to an RNA molecule, which in turn transmits its information to a protein. In other words, genes consist of DNA, but exert their effects through proteins. DNA also specifies the information in other DNA molecules (DNA replication).

part of the mainstream metabolism of a human cell. More importantly, RNA has many functions apart from specifying the amino acid sequence of proteins. Ribosomal RNA and transfer RNA are the best-known examples of such functional RNAs, but there are many others.

A full account of the structure and function of genes would take a whole book. All the processes involved are vastly complicated and involve innumerable proteins and other molecules to effect and control them. Fortunately most of the detail is irrelevant to clinical practice. For clinicians, while there is no limit to the level of detail that it would be desirable to understand, the amount that is essential is much more manageable. The basic essential topics are explained below and in *Boxes 3.2* and *3.3* and are:

- the general structure of nucleic acids as chains of A, G, C and T (or U) units
- the double helix
- 3′ and 5′ ends of DNA
- the exon-intron structure of genes
- splicing of the primary transcript
- the genetic code

If you are interested in finding out more, many excellent textbooks cover these topics in more detail. Additionally there are several websites that provide freely accessible course material (see *Section 3.5 References*).

Structure of nucleic acids

Nucleic acids (DNA and RNA) are made of subunits called **nucleotides** linked together into long chains. Each nucleotide comprises three modules: a base, a sugar and a phosphate. DNA chains are made of only four types of nucleotide. The sugar is always deoxyribose and the base can be adenine (A), guanine (G), cytosine (C) or thymine (T). The chemical formulae are given in the last section of this chapter, but it is not necessary to know them in order to use this book. RNA is also made up of four types of nucleotide. Here the sugar is always ribose, the bases are A, G and C as in DNA but instead of T, RNA has uracil (U).

DNA, as famously described by Crick and Watson in 1953, normally exists as two polynucleotide chains wrapped round each other – the double helix. Its crucial feature is that the two chains will only fit together correctly if opposite every A in one chain is a T in the other, and opposite every G is a C. Base-pairing, A with T and G with C, explains how DNA is able to be replicated (*Figure 3.4*). This mechanism enables the genetic information in the mother cell to be copied and passed during mitosis to both daughter cells, as described in Chapter 2. RNA does not normally exist as double helices. This is not because of any feature intrinsic to the chemical structure of RNA, but because normal cells do not contain complementary strands of most RNA molecules, nor any enzyme that would construct an RNA strand using an RNA template. Cells use DNA and RNA to do different jobs, and they use the chemical differences between them as recognition signals for targeting enzymes to DNA or RNA as appropriate.

adenine A C cytosine

thymine T G guanine

Figure 3.4 – Principle of DNA replication.
Each strand of the double helix serves as a template for synthesis of an exact replica of the other strand. A similar mechanism is used to make an RNA copy of one strand of the double helix when a gene is transcribed (U in RNA pairs with A in DNA). This diagram shows the principle and the result of DNA replication; the actual molecular events are much more complicated. In particular, this diagram ignores the fact that nucleic acid chains can only grow in the 5′ → 3′ direction (see *Box 3.2* and *Chapter* 4).

The human genome comprises around 3 x 10^9 bp of DNA (see *Box 3.1* for an explanation of the units). A normal diploid cell contains two copies of the genome (two copies of chromosome 1, two copies of chromosome 2, etc.). As described in *Chapter 2*, each chromosome contains a single immensely long double helix of DNA, packaged by histones and other proteins into chromatin. Chromosome 21, the smallest, contains 47 Mb of DNA, chromosome 1, the largest, 245 Mb. In addition to this nuclear genome, mitochondria have their own little genome, comprising a single circular DNA molecule 16 569 bp long.

A note on units

The size of a piece of DNA is measured in nucleotides (nt), base pairs (bp), kilobases (kb or kbp = 1000 bp) or megabases (Mb or Mbp = 1 000 000 bp). Because DNA is virtually always double-stranded, the distinction between bases and base pairs is often ignored when talking about the size of a piece of DNA. Thus a DNA double helix comprising one million base pairs can be described as either 1 Mbp or 1 Mb – it is not 2 Mb.

Box 3.1

The structure of genes: exons and introns

Most genes of humans and other higher organisms are organized in a strange and unexpected way. The DNA sequence that will ultimately specify the amino acid sequence of a protein is split into segments (**exons**) interrupted by non-coding sequences (**introns** or intervening sequences). The number and size of introns varies without any evident logic. The average human gene has nine exons averaging 145 bp each and the introns average 3365 bp each, but the range is very wide – see *Table 3.1* in *Section 3.4*.

Box 3.2

5′ and 3′ ends

To understand clinical genetics it is not crucial to know a lot about the chemical structure of DNA, but there is one non-obvious feature that does matter. Writing a DNA sequence as a string of letters like AGTTGCACG obscures one important point: the two ends are not chemically identical. Looking at the chemical formula of the sugar–phosphate backbone (see figure below), successive deoxyribose units are linked through the carbon atoms labeled 5′ ("5 prime") and 3′. The uppermost deoxyribose has its 5′ carbon free, while the lowermost has its 3′ carbon free. Biochemically this difference is crucial. Enzymes that act on the 5′ end of DNA will not act on the 3′ end, and *vice versa*. This has several important consequences.

* The two chains in a DNA double helix are anti-parallel. If a double helix is drawn vertically one chain will have its 5′ end at the top, and the other will have its 3′ end at the top. The same is true of the DNA–RNA double helices that are temporary intermediates when a gene is transcribed.

* All DNA replication proceeds in the 5′→3′ direction. That is, all the enzymes that string nucleotides together (DNA polymerases) can only add nucleotides to the 3′ end of a polynucleotide. This will turn out to be crucial when we consider the polymerase chain reaction in *Chapter 4*. The same is true of the RNA polymerases that synthesize RNA.

* It is a universal convention that DNA or RNA sequences are written in the 5′ to 3′ direction. The sequence AGTTGCACG means 5′–AGTTGCACG–3′. It is just as wrong to write a sequence 3′ to 5′ as it is to write English from right to left. If for any reason you need to write a sequence in the 3′ to 5′ direction, it is essential to label the ends to make this clear.

* Only one strand of the DNA of a gene is transcribed. This is called the **template strand**. Suppose part of this sequence reads 5′–AGTTGCACG–3′. The RNA transcript is complementary to this, with A wherever the template strand has T, G where the template has C, etc. (see *Figure 3.5a*). Writing it in the conventional 5′→3′ direction, its sequence would be CGUGCAACU (remember the strands are anti-parallel and RNA uses U in place of T). Even with very short sequences like these, their relationship is not immediately obvious. To avoid this problem, by convention we write the DNA sequence of a gene not as the template strand but as its complementary strand – CGTGCAACT in this case. This strand is called the **sense strand**. The RNA sequence is just the same as the sense strand, except for replacing T with U.

* Sequences lying 5′ of a gene or sequence of interest (on the sense strand) are often referred to as **upstream**; those 3′ are **downstream**.

A single strand of DNA showing the 5′ and 3′ ends. The carbon atoms of the deoxyribose sugars are numbered 1′, 2′ etc. The prime (′) is to distinguish them from the carbon atoms of the bases, which have their own numbering scheme (not shown here). The phosphate groups carry a negative charge – this is the basis for separating nucleic acids by electrophoresis (see *Box 4.1*).

Splicing of the primary transcript

When a cell needs to make a particular protein it first makes an RNA copy of one strand of the DNA of just the relevant gene (*Figure 3.5a*). Transcription is a very dynamic process, involving only scattered small segments of the genome at any one time, but varying according to the needs of the cell. The way this works is described in a little more detail in the final section of this chapter. The entire sequence of exons and introns is transcribed to make the **primary transcript**. Within the cell nucleus this is then processed by physically cutting out the introns and splicing together the exons (*Figure 3.5b*). The RNA of the introns is broken down and appears to have no useful purpose. Splicing is accomplished within the cell nucleus by a large multimolecular machine called the spliceosome, which is a complex of proteins and small RNA molecules. We can safely ignore most of the complicated molecular details, but we do need to consider how introns are recognized.

Almost all human introns start with GU (GT in the DNA of the sense strand – this is called the donor splice site) and end with AG (the acceptor splice site). By themselves these signals would not be sufficient to define splice sites – there are innumerable GU and AG dinucleotides within exons or introns that are not used as splice sites. To be recognized as a splice site the GU or AG must be embedded in a broader **consensus sequence**. A functional splice site has a suitable combination of short sequence motifs that bind proteins or small RNA molecules in the spliceosome. These individual motifs are only loosely defined, making splice sites very hard to predict by analysis of DNA or RNA sequences.

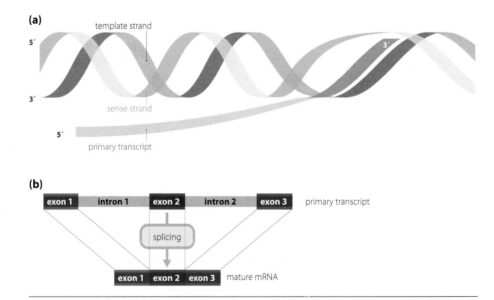

Figure 3.5 – Summary of transcription.
(a) The DNA double helix unwinds locally to allow RNA polymerase to assemble the primary transcript, and rewinds after the polymerase has moved on along the chain. The transcript is made using the template strand; its sequence is complementary to the template strand and identical to the sense strand. (b) The primary transcript is processed by cutting out introns and splicing exons together to form the mature messenger RNA (mRNA).

This is frustrating for clinical geneticists because, as we will see later, sequence variants affecting the efficiency of splice sites are major causes of diseases.

Translation and the genetic code

The mature mRNAs, now comprising just exon sequences, are exported to the cytoplasm where they engage with a ribosome. Ribosomes are yet another large multimolecular machine including many different proteins and several species of non-coding RNA. Again, more details of the mechanism of protein synthesis can be found in textbooks or the recommended websites; for present purposes we need note only the following (see also *Figure 3.6*):

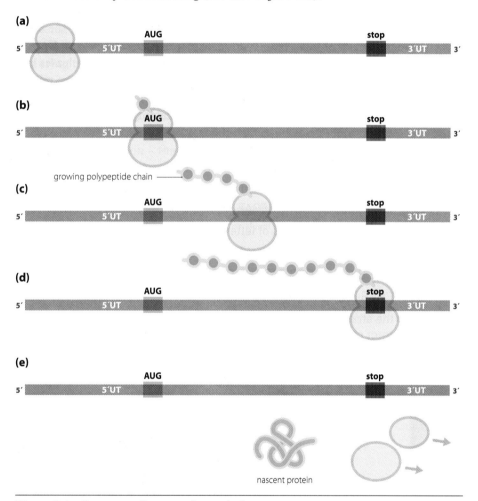

Figure 3.6 – Summary diagram of translation.
(a) A ribosome attaches at the 5′ end of the mRNA. (b) It moves along the 5′ untranslated sequence until it encounters the AUG initiation codon. At this point it picks up the first amino acid. (c) The ribosome moves along the mRNA, picking up amino acids according to the codons of the mRNA and incorporating them into the growing polypeptide chain. (d) When it reaches a stop codon, translation of the message is complete. (e) At this point the ribosome falls off the mRNA and dissociates into its two subunits, and the polypeptide is released. The mature functional protein must be correctly folded, perhaps chemically modified, and transported to the appropriate intracellular or extracellular location.

DOMAINS AND GLYCOSYLATION/BINDING SITES

◀ N-terminus   ◆ Hybrid   ■ Pro   ● Sugar attachment sites

▶ C-terminus   ⬭ TB   ▨ EGF   ● MAGP-1

(a) The large fibrillin protein is organized into more than 50 structural domains.
(b) An isolated microfibril has a string of beads structure under the electron microscope. Reproduced from Kielty *et al.*, (2005) *Advances in Protein Chemistry*, **70**: 405–436 with permission from Elsevier.

Box 3.4 – continued

3.3. **Investigations of patients**

Many of the cases described so far in the book will require DNA investigations. Here we describe how each case fits into the picture of gene structure developed in the previous section. First, however, we will note two cases where no DNA-level tests will be used.

| CASE 5 | Elliot family | 4 | 11 | 42 | **64** | 376 |

• Reciprocal translocation

The chromosome analysis tells us all we need to know in this family. DNA testing is not relevant.

| CASE 10 | Johnson family | 55 | **64** | 376 |

• Marfan syndrome

James didn't have a gene test when he first attended the clinic because his diagnosis was obvious on clinical grounds. For most genetic disorders molecular tests were only introduced into clinical practice in the 1990s. For many years diagnoses for most disorders relied on family history, clinical signs and symptoms and on investigations such as X-rays. There is a great deal of information available about Marfan syndrome because it is a relatively common genetic condition, and formal diagnostic guidelines have been assembled as knowledge increases (Ghent criteria, see De Paepe *et al.*, 1996). However, even for disorders where a diagnosis is usually possible on clinical grounds alone, there may be a need for molecular testing. This might be for use in prenatal testing, or where a person does not quite fulfil the diagnostic criteria but there remains considerable suspicion.

For the remaining cases, DNA tests are required.

| CASE 1 | Ashton family | 1 | 7 | **65** | 104 | 150 | 376 |

- John – 28-year-old son of Alfred Ashton
- ? Huntington disease
- Other family members with similar symptoms
- Autosomal dominant inheritance shown in pedigree
- Diagnostic test ordered

Huntington disease is caused by a change to the coding sequence of a gene on chromosome 4, position 4p16. The Huntington disease gene *HD* has 67 exons, covers 169 kb of genomic DNA (*Figure 3.7*) and encodes a 3141 amino acid protein called huntingtin. Huntington disease patients always have a sequence change in exactly the same place in the gene. Part of exon 1 encodes a run of glutamines in the huntingtin protein. Every patient with Huntington disease has an expansion of this sequence, so that the encoded protein contains a much longer run of glutamines. How this makes the patient ill is discussed in *Disease Box 4*. The DNA test needs to check the size of the sequence encoding this polyglutamine run.

Figure 3.7 – Structure of the Huntington disease gene.
Short vertical bars represent the exons. Human Genome Project data as displayed by GENATLAS (http://www.dsi.univ-paris5.fr/genatlas/).

| CASE 2 | Brown family | 2 | 8 | **65** | 126 | 151 | 279 | 376 |

- Girl (Joanne) aged 6 months, parents David and Pauline
- ? Cystic fibrosis
- Order molecular test?

As mentioned previously, cystic fibrosis is always caused by mutations in the *CFTR* gene on chromosome 7. The disease is recessive, so if Joanne has cystic fibrosis both copies of her *CFTR* gene must be mutated. *CFTR* is quite a large gene, with 27 exons spread over 188 kb of chromosome 7 at position 7q31.2 (*Figure 3.8*). Unlike in Huntington disease, mutations may be anywhere in the gene. Different patients with cystic fibrosis may have different mutations – over 1000 different mutations are described in the Human Gene Mutation Database. Joanne's two mutations might be the same or different. All the mutations are changes to a single nucleotide or a small number of adjacent nucleotides. Scanning both copies of the gene for any such change will be a challenge.

Figure 3.8 – Structure of the *CFTR* gene.
An alternative graphical display of Human Genome Project data, as displayed by the ENSEMBL genome browser. Some closely spaced exons appear as a single bar. The arrow shows the 5′→3′ direction of the sense strand.

| CASE 3 | Choudhary family | 3 | 9 | **66** | 242 | 260 | 376 |

- Girl (Nasreen) aged 8 months, parents Aadnan and Mumtaz
- Deaf
- Parents are first cousins
- Pedigree suggests autosomal recessive deafness

The problem with deafness is that, even when the cause is genetic, mutations in over 50 different genes can cause it. The reason for this diversity is not hard to understand. Our sense of hearing uses a wonderfully complex and subtle mechanism to convert air pressure waves reaching the ear into nerve impulses. Naturally the mechanism involves many components, encoded by many different genes. If any one of these fails, the whole mechanism may fail. It is not practical to start testing genes until we know which gene to test. This is normally an insuperable problem – as described in *Chapter 9*, the usual approach is to check for one particular mutation in one particular gene that is a relatively common cause of the problem. If this test is negative a normal diagnostic DNA laboratory would not be able to justify the expense of looking through a whole long list of genes. However, Nasreen's unusually large family and affected uncles means that it might be possible to narrow down the list of candidate genes using linkage analysis. This investigation is pursued in *Chapter 9*.

| CASE 4 | Davies family | 4 | 10 | **66** | 102 | 151 | 181 | 279 | 376 |

- Boy (Martin) aged 24 months, parents Judith and Robert
- Clumsy and slow to walk
- Family history of muscular dystrophy
- Pedigree shows X-linked recessive inheritance
- Order diagnostic DNA test

Duchenne muscular dystrophy is X-linked, so the causative gene must be located on the X chromosome. It is in the proximal short arm, at Xp21, and encodes a protein, dystrophin, that is essential for making muscle cells robust enough to withstand mechanical stresses over many years. The dystrophin gene (*DMD*) is one of the most remarkable in the human genome. It is huge, covering over 2 million base pairs of DNA – 99.3% of this comprises introns; after they are spliced out of the primary transcript the 79 exons make a 13 kb mature mRNA. Two-thirds of cases are caused by partial deletions of the gene. Because almost all the genomic sequence is intronic, the deletion breakpoints almost always fall in introns, so their effect on the mature mRNA is to remove one or more contiguous exons (*Figure 3.9*). Searching for mutations anywhere in this vast gene would be a major challenge. The initial test is therefore to check the genomic DNA for missing exons, concentrating on those exons that are most commonly deleted. Missing exons are obvious in DNA from an affected boy; in a carrier woman they are masked by her normal X chromosome, which of course has all exons intact.

Figure 3.9 – A deletion of part of the dystrophin gene.
This figure shows a 500 kb region containing exons 41–50. These exons are all 100–200 bp long, and so if drawn to scale each exon would be represented by a line occupying less than 0.05% of the width of the figure. Random deletion breakpoints therefore almost always fall in introns. Their effect is to remove one or more complete exons from the mature mRNA. The deletion shown removes exons 45–47 from the mature mRNA, while leaving all the other exons intact.

| CASE 6 | Fletcher family | 5 | 12 | **67** | 131 | 152 | 376 |

- Frank, aged 22, with increasingly blurred eyesight
- Family history of visual difficulties
- Pedigree suggests X-linked recessive inheritance but not conclusive
- ? LHON
- Order blood test to check for mutation in mtDNA

The pedigree and clinical phenotype suggested a diagnosis of Leber hereditary optic neuropathy (LHON). This is caused by mutations in the DNA of the mitochondria, rather than the DNA of the chromosomes in the cell nucleus.

The small mitochondrial genome (*Figure 3.10b*) is markedly different from the nuclear genome. In many ways it is much more similar to bacterial genomes – an observation consistent with the belief that mitochondria evolved from bacteria that lived in a symbiotic relationship inside some ancestral cell. The mitochondrial genome is circular and compact. Though only 16 569 bp long, it contains 37 genes. Like bacterial genomes, the genes are tightly packed together with very little intergenic DNA – a marked contrast to the nuclear genome which averages only eight genes per megabase. Mitochondrial genes have no introns – another point of resemblance to bacterial genes. However, mitochondria are very far from being independent micro-organisms. Most mitochondrial functions depend on proteins encoded by nuclear genes that are transported to the mitochondrion after being synthesized. Importantly, this means that diseases caused by mitochondrial dysfunction are not necessarily caused by mutations in the mitochondrial DNA. LHON is one of the few diseases caused by mutations in the mitochondrial DNA.

The DNA extracted from a clinical sample includes the mitochondrial as well as the nuclear DNA. The diagnosis in Frank Fletcher will be confirmed if his DNA sample can be shown to have one of the mitochondrial DNA mutations characteristic of LHON (see *Chapter 5*).

Figure 3.10 – (a) A cell showing the nucleus and mitochondria. (b) The mitochondrial genome. The 13 protein-coding genes are labeled and the locations of the three common LHON mutations shown. The other 24 mitochondrial genes encode functional RNAs: the two ribosomal RNAs (red segments) and 22 transfer RNAs (small genes indicated by unlabeled thin lines).

| CASE 7 | Green family | 25 | 38 | **68** | 99 | 376 |

- Girl (Gillian) aged 3 years
- Slow to develop
- ? Chromosome abnormality
- Order tests to check for microdeletion at 22q11

Gillian's combination of learning difficulties and mild dysmorphism suggested a chromosomal abnormality, and her clinical features resembled those of patients with an interstitial deletion of chromosome 22 at position 22q11. Under the microscope her karyotype appeared normal (*Figure 2.9*) but a deletion of less than 3–5 Mbp of DNA would not have been visible. Given an average density of genes across the whole human genome of about eight per Mb of DNA (24 000 genes spread over 3000 Mbp of genomic DNA), a deletion that is too small to see under the microscope can still affect a dozen or more genes. Checking the diagnosis requires a test able to see deletion of a region of DNA that is small in cytogenetic terms but still very large in molecular terms. This will require a different technique from the previous cases.

| CASE 8 | Howard family | 26 | 38 | **68** | 100 | 275 | 376 |

- Helen – new-born daughter of Henry and Anne (33 years old)
- Down syndrome
- Risk of recurrence if they have more children?

The clinical features and chromosome analysis (*Figures 2.2* and *2.11*) establish the diagnosis. Many couples request prenatal testing for Down syndrome, either because, like Helen's mother, they have had an affected child, or because of the increased risk when the woman is older. As will be explained in *Chapter 14*, it takes 2 weeks from obtaining fetal cells to get them dividing well enough for conventional cytogenetic analysis. The waiting can be very stressful for the patient. To avoid this, a DNA test is increasingly used that allows immediate analysis of the non-dividing cells.

| CASE 9 | Ingram family | 26 | 41 | **68** | 101 | 182 | 376 |

- Isabel – first daughter of Irene and Ian
- Small stature despite tall parents
- ? Turner syndrome

Clinical features and chromosome analysis (*Figures 2.3* and *2.13*) establish the diagnosis. As explained in *Chapter 2*, Isabel may have started life as a 46,XY conceptus and lost the Y chromosome in one of the early mitotic divisions. If any of the cells in her streak gonads retains a Y, these cells can give rise to a malignant gonadoblastoma. Therefore it is important to check for the presence of Y-chromosome DNA sequences. If any are found, then gonadectomy is usually recommended.

3.4. **Summary and extension**

Some chemistry

For reference, *Box 3.5* gives the chemical structures of the bases A, G, C, T and U, and *Box 3.6* shows the 20 amino acids that are used to make proteins.

Box 3.5

Chemical formulae of A, G, C, T and U.

The formulae and names show the bases, and indicate how each base is attached to a sugar (ribose in RNA, deoxyribose in DNA). Bases are classified into purines (A, G) and pyrimidines (C, T, U). See *Figure 5.2* for a formula of a complete nucleotide.

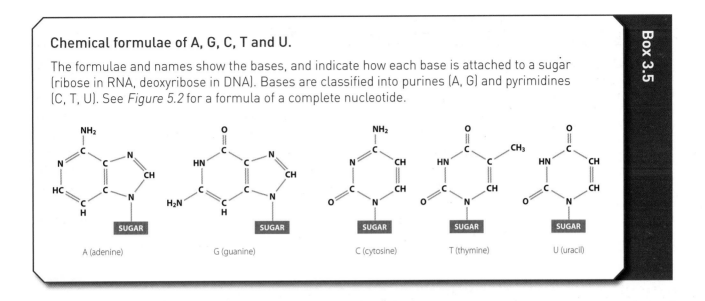

A (adenine)   G (guanine)   C (cytosine)   T (thymine)   U (uracil)

Genes are much bigger than you think

A gene, defined as a functioning DNA unit, is much larger than just its protein-coding sequence.

- The exons of a gene include the 5′ and 3′ untranslated sequences, which are important for the stability of the mRNA. These average 200 and 800 nt, respectively, in human genes.
- The primary transcript is derived from intronic and exonic DNA sequence. These are often considerably larger than the exons. *Table 3.1* gives a few examples.
- Sequences upstream of the transcription start site (the **promoter**) are necessary for the gene to be expressed. See below for a description of what promoters do. Promoter sequences are close to the transcription start site, usually within a hundred or so base pairs, though other more distant sequences often affect the activity of a promoter.
- Expression of some genes or gene clusters is known to be controlled by short sequence elements tens or even hundreds of kilobases away. The existence of such distant control elements is another reason why genes occupy stretches of DNA far longer than their coding sequence. At present we have no way of systematically identifying these **locus control regions**. They are discovered by chance when a small deletion or a chromosomal breakpoint some way away from a gene abolishes expression of the gene, even though the coding sequence is intact. It is interesting that genes crucial in controlling early development are often located in 'gene deserts', megabase-sized regions containing no other genes. It is likely that such regions contain long-range control elements. The intervening DNA probably loops out, so that these elements actually lie physically close to the gene they control, and proteins bound to them can interact directly with proteins bound to the gene promoter.

Box 3.6

Structure of proteins

(a) Chemical formula of a polypeptide. The amino acids differ according to the nature of the side chain, labeled R_1, R_2, R_3, here. A real protein would probably contain several hundred amino acid residues. (b) Chemical formulae of the side chains (R groups) of the 20 amino acids used to make up proteins. The three letter and single letter abbreviated names of each amino acid are shown.

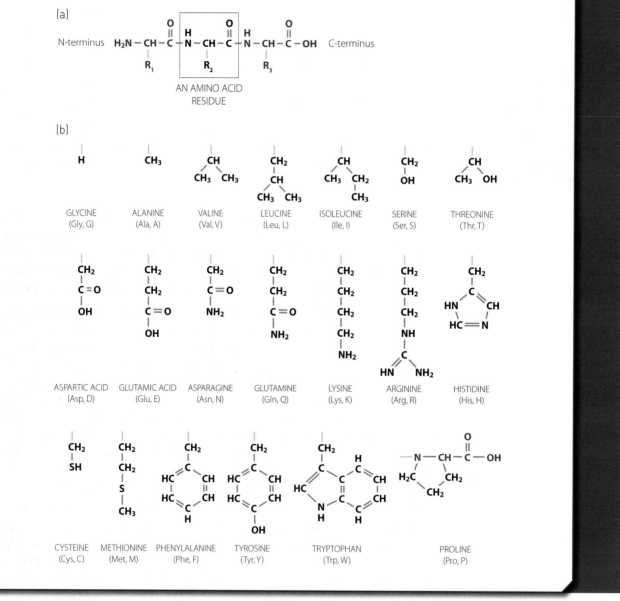

Switching genes on and off – transcription and its controls

All the cells of our body contain an identical set of genes – that is the purpose of mitosis. So how do they become so very different from each other – brain cells, liver cells, skin cells, muscle cells, etc? The answer is that they express

Table 3.1 – **Structures of some human genes**

Gene	Size in genome (kb)	No. of exons	Average exon size (bp)	Average intron size (bp)	Exons as % of primary transcript
Interferon A6 (*IFNA6*)	0.57	1	570	–	100%
Insulin (*INS*)	1.4	3	154	483	32%
Class 1 HLA (*HLA-A*)	2.7	7	160	269	41%
Collagen VII (*COL7A1*)	51	118	78	358	18%
Phenylalanine hydroxylase (*PAH*)	78	13	206	6264	3.4%
CFTR (cystic fibrosis)	188	27	227	7022	3.2%
Dystrophin (*DMD*)	2090	79	178	26615	0.7%

The number and size of introns varies very widely between genes. You can look at the size and exon–intron structure of any gene using the ENSEMBL genome browser as explained in *Box 3.7*.

different subsets of their repertoire of genes. Additionally, an individual cell will switch genes on or off depending on its current needs. A major way of switching genes on or off is to switch transcription on or off. Switching also occurs at the level of translation, but at present it is less clear how generally important this is, and the mechanisms used are only beginning to be explored.

Selectivity is the key to transcription. Although the DNA of a chromosome is a single huge molecule, the RNAs produced by transcription are a diverse collection of much smaller molecules. Only selected small segments of the DNA are transcribed, and choosing them appropriately is crucial to the life of the cell. Partly this is controlled by the way the DNA is packaged. As explained in *Chapter 2* (*Section 2.4* and *Disease Box 2*), DNA is packaged by histones and other proteins into chromatin. Chromatin has two basic configurations, heterochromatin which is tightly packed and represses gene expression, and euchromatin which is more open and variable. Genes in euchromatic regions of chromosomes may or may not be expressed. The local chromatin structure, determined by chromatin remodeling complexes of proteins such as ATRX (*Disease Box 2*) provides a permissive or repressive environment for transcription.

Transcription only begins when a large multiprotein initiation complex has been assembled at an appropriate place on the DNA. The promoter of a gene is defined by a number of different short (typically 4–8 nt) sequence motifs that each bind specific proteins. These DNA-binding proteins are called **transcription factors**. They in turn bind other proteins, and so build up a complex including the RNA polymerase that does the actual transcription. Each individual DNA–protein interaction is weak, but once several different transcription factors are loosely bound, protein–protein interactions between them glue the complex together. Some of the proteins of the initiation complex are present all the time in every cell, but others (themselves the products of genes that are highly regulated) occur only in certain cells, or only when the cell responds to certain signals. By acting in different combinations, a limited (though large) number of transcription factors can achieve flexible control over the expression of a much greater number of genes.

Once started, transcription proceeds until some loosely defined stop signal is reached. The end result (the primary transcript) is a single-stranded RNA molecule, typically 1–100 kb long, corresponding precisely in sequence to the sense strand of the DNA (*Figure 3.5*).

One gene often encodes more than one protein

Contrary to the one gene – one enzyme hypothesis, very often a single gene can encode several different proteins (*Figure 3.11*). The main mechanism for this is **alternative splicing**. Often there is more than one way of splicing the primary transcript. Certain exons may be variably incorporated or skipped in the mature mRNA, giving rise to **splice isoforms**. Sometimes there are two alternative splice

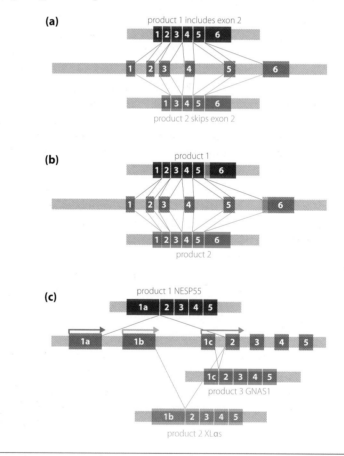

Figure 3.11 – **How one gene can encode more than one protein.**
(a) Exons may be variably incorporated into the mature mRNA or skipped. (b) An exon may have two alternative splice sites. (c) A gene may have two or more alternative promoters and first exons (this example shows the *GNAS1* gene, which encodes three differently named proteins). Any of these mechanisms may result in use of an alternative reading frame for the downstream parts of the gene. About half of all human genes use one or more of these mechanisms to encode more than one protein.

sites marking the beginning or end of an exon. A gene may also have several alternative promoters and first exons (the dystrophin gene has eight). All these variables mean that one gene can encode more than one protein. The average number of transcripts per locus in genes examined by the ENCODE project (see *Chapter 6*) is 5.4. Probably some of this variability is just noise in the system, where the cell is bad at recognizing the one correct signal – but in many cases it is functional, with both products having distinct functions. Mutations that affect the balance of splice isoforms can be clinically significant, but hard to recognize in the DNA sequence.

The Human Genome Project

The first 'big science' project in biology was launched in 1990 and culminated triumphantly with the publication of the "finished" human genome sequence in 2004. The key publications (International Human Genome Sequencing Consortium, 2001, 2004) do not of course print out all 3 000 000 000 As, Gs, Cs and Ts – those are in computer databases – but they describe the methods used and key features of the genome. The 2004 paper is quite brief, but the blockbuster 2001 paper ranks with *The Origin of Species* and Watson and Crick's 1953 paper describing the double helix, as one of the seminal milestones in biology.

The finished sequence was obtained by piecing together literally millions of short runs of sequence, derived from several different anonymous donors. Thus it does not represent the sequence of any one person. Indeed, probably nobody has exactly this sequence. But just as we are all recognizably human despite our individual differences in appearance, so we all have recognizably human genomes despite individual variants. A major interest now is in defining how the sequence varies between individuals.

The raw sequence is held in a freely accessible public database. To access it you use a genome browser program. There are several of these that are freely available on the internet as a public service. Widely used ones include the SANTA CRUZ and ENSEMBL browsers. For example, you can use ENSEMBL to view the intron–exon structure and DNA sequence of any gene whose name you know. Here is how to do so:

1. go to http://www.ensembl.org/Homo_sapiens/index.html
2. fill in the search boxes to get ENSEMBL to look for a gene with the appropriate name e.g. *CFTR*
3. if you have got the name right, this will produce a list that may contain a number of items. Check carefully to get the right one (for *CFTR* this is ENSEMBL Gene: ENSG00000001626)
4. having selected the correct gene, you will see one or more transcripts listed, each with options to view *transcript information*, *exon information* or *protein information*: viewing *exon information* gives you the structure and sequence of your gene. *Figure 1* shows another example of how the browser can present information (the actual screen display contains much more data than this figure, which has been heavily edited in the interests of clarity).

The human genome sequence is a stunning achievement – but it is important to understand its limitations. In fact, by itself, the raw sequence does not tell us very much. It needs to be annotated to identify the genes and other functional elements contained in the sequence. Genome browsers like ENSEMBL bring together not just the raw sequence but huge amounts of annotation data – for example, in defining the genes shown in *Figure 1*. Annotating the sequence is now a major occupation of scientists the world over. They use a combination of laboratory experiments and computer analysis of the sequence. Comparison of the human

Box 3.7

- In addition to these high copy-number repeats, there are many low copy-number repeats that have arisen by recent duplication events. There are many traces of sequences, including gene sequences, being duplicated and then the copies diverging by accumulation of mutations. Often when genes are duplicated, only one copy stays functional, the other becoming a non-functional **pseudogene**. See Case 19 (*Chapter 8*) for an example.
- After accounting for all these categories, we are left with a large amount of intergenic DNA with unique (single-copy) sequence that is not conserved between humans and other mammals, and that has no known function.

How much of the so-called 'junk DNA' really is junk, and how much has some function, as yet undiscovered, is a matter of much debate. Overall, the human genome appears chaotic. Evidently there has been no selective pressure for a tidy genome. The contrast with the elegance and efficiency of most of our anatomy and physiology is very striking. It is fascinating to speculate on how and why all this has evolved.

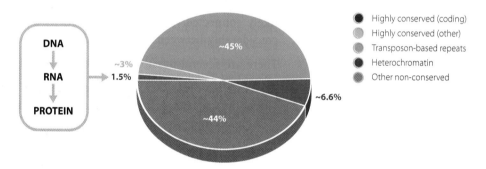

Figure 3.12 – What does all our DNA do?
About 1.5% does what the Central Dogma says DNA does. A further ~3% is conserved between humans and mice, implying that it has some sequence-dependent function. At least some of the heterochromatin functions as the centromeres of chromosomes. About half of the rest of our DNA is made up of many copies of transposable elements that have spread within the genome like an infection. Data from the Draft Human Genome Sequence (2001).

A hidden RNA world?

Recently many non-translated RNAs have been discovered that, at least in some cases, exert major controls over gene expression or chromatin structure. These raise many unanswered questions. Up to 50% of our genome gets transcribed, at least in some cells and at some time. Known genes can account for only a minority of this. Does most of this activity represent noise in the system, accidental transcription of non-functional sequences because the cell is not very good at recognizing genes? Or is there a whole world of functional RNA species waiting to be discovered? We don't know.

Williams–Beuren syndrome (OMIM 194050)

Children with Williams–Beuren syndrome (WBS) are recognized by their combination of learning difficulties, small size and characteristic face with full lips and cheeks and short nose (*Figure 1*). Many have a heart problem, supravalvular aortic stenosis (SVAS), which may require surgery, and some suffer from infantile hypercalcemia, which worsens their failure to thrive and may lead to kidney damage, but which tends to resolve spontaneously. WBS occurs sporadically; there is almost never any family history. About 1 in 20 000 births is affected in both sexes and all ethnic groups.

WBS is interesting both for its mechanism of origin and for its cognitive and behavioral phenotype. The mechanism of origin relates directly to the presence of low copy number repeats, as described above. A crucial clue to the cause of WBS came from a family in which several members had SVAS, but not WBS. The affected people all carried a balanced chromosomal translocation t(6;7)(p21.1;q11.23). The breakpoint on chromosome 7 disrupted the elastin gene. As mentioned in *Box 3.4*, elastin, together with fibrillin, is a major component of the elastic microfibrils that give skin and arterial walls their elasticity. SVAS is a consequence of a relative deficiency of elastin. Reasoning that people with WBS must also have a deficiency of elastin, researchers examined the relevant region of chromosome 7 in WBS patients and identified a microdeletion. All WBS patients have this deletion, on one of their copies of chromosome 7. It is now known that the deletion takes out 1.4 Mb of DNA, including the elastin gene. Although the deletion is too small to be seen by conventional cytogenetics, this WBS-critical region includes at least 24 genes.

Figure 1 – **Williams–Beuren syndrome.**

The WBS deletion is a recurrent one, almost always arising *de novo* in each new case. The reason why the same pathogenic deletion occurs over and over again is that the deleted region is flanked by low copy repeats. Over a 300–500 kb region the DNA either side of the WBS critical region shows greater than 98% sequence homology. When the two copies of chromosome 7 pair during meiosis, occasionally these repeats mispair. If there is then a crossover within the mispaired repeats, the result is to generate one chromosome carrying the WBS deletion and another carrying a duplication of the region (*Figure 2*).

Figure 2 – **Generation of a deletion and the reciprocal duplication by recombination between mispaired repeats flanking the WBS critical region.**
Low-copy repeats are a common feature of the human genome, and recombination between mispaired repeats is a frequent cause of duplications or deletions of various sizes that cause a large number of different human syndromes.

Disease box 3 – *continued*

A particular fascination of WBS comes from the cognitive and behavioral phenotype that affected individuals display. Although WBS children have a global IQ similar to children with Down syndrome (usually in the range 40–85), their pattern of abilities and deficiencies is strikingly different. They have relatively good verbal skills which contrast with their poor spatial skills. Asked to draw an object or copy a diagram, a WBS child will crudely reproduce the details but fail to integrate them into any overall picture (*Figure 3*). On the other hand, they can be very eloquent verbally. They also have characteristic behavior and personality traits. They manifest anxiety in unfamiliar situations but may be inappropriately friendly to strangers.

WBS allows us to see how changes in a small number of defined genes lead to rather constant effects on speech development, cognition and personality. Many researchers hope that this syndrome will give us clues to the more general genetic determinants of normal speech acquisition, cognition and behavior.

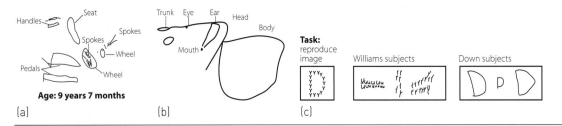

Figure 3 – Drawings by people with WBS.
(a) A bicycle and (b) an elephant. In each case the drawing consists of disconnected parts (labeled by the tester), not integrated into a whole. (c) Children with WBS and children with Down syndrome matched for age and IQ were asked to copy the diagram on the left. Again, note how the WBS children see the details but not the overall design. Illustrations reproduced with permission from Dr Ursula Bellugi, The Salk Institute for Biological Studies.

3.5. References

De Paepe A *et al*. (1996) Revised diagnostic criteria for the Marfan syndrome. *Am. J. Med. Genet.* **62**: 417–426. *Ghent criteria for diagnosing Marfan syndrome.*

International Human Genome Sequencing Consortium (2001). Initial sequencing and analysis of the human genome. *Nature*, **409**: 860–921.

International Human Genome Sequencing Consortium (2004). Finishing the euchromatic sequence of the human genome. *Nature*, **431**: 931–945.

General background

NCBI Science primer – http://www.ncbi.nlm.nih.gov/About/primer/

The Online Biology Book produced by MJ Farabee – http://www.emc.maricopa.edu/faculty/farabee/BIOBK/BioBookTOC.html
Chapters 14–19 are good background reading for *Chapters 3–6* of this book

More detail of DNA structure and function can be found in any reasonably recent genetics or cell biology textbook, such as:

- Strachan T and Read AP (2004) *Human Molecular Genetics, 3rd edn.* Garland, New York.

- Alberts B, *et al* (2005) *Molecular Biology of the Cell.* Garland, New York.

Earlier editions of both these books are freely available as searchable text on the NCBI Bookshelf – http://www.ncbi.nlm.nih.gov/entrez/query.fcgi?db=Books

Useful websites

ENSEMBL genome browser: http://www.ensembl.org/Homo_sapiens/

Human Gene Mutation Database: http://www.hgmd.org/

PFAM protein structure database: http://www.sanger.ac.uk/Software/Pfam/

SANTA CRUZ genome browser: http://genome.ucsc.edu

3.6. Self-assessment questions

(1) Consider the DNA sequence:

CCAGCTTCGCAAGTC

Which base is immediately downstream of a CpG dinucleotide (a) in the strand shown (b) in the complementary strand?

(2) A partial gene sequence from the database reads:

CAGCTGGAGGAACTGGAGCGTGCTTTTGAG

Write out the sequence of the template strand and the mRNA.

(3) The sequence of a 150-nucleotide section of chromosome 7 is shown. It is written in groups of 10 to make counting easier. The sequence in upper case is exon 1 of a gene. Flanking nucleotides shown in lower case are not part of the exon. The initiation codon is double-underlined.

```
  1   gcagccaatg gagggtggtg ttgcgcgggg ctgggattag ggccggggcg
                                    a
 51   aaatgGGATC CTCCAAGGCG ACCATGGCCT TGCTGGGTAA GCGCTGTGAC
                  b               c
101   GTCCCCACCA ACGGCgttag acctcagtac tgaatcagga cctcactcct
                  d                        e
```

a) What number nucleotide in the sequence is the first one to be transcribed into mRNA?

b) Name the parts of the sequence underlined and labeled a–e, choosing from the following list:

    3′ untranslated region
    3rd codon
    5′ untranslated region
    9th codon
    acceptor splice site (the 3′ end of an intron)

> donor splice site (the 5′ end of an intron)
> part of exon 2
> part of intron 1
> part of intron 2
> part of promoter

(4) Here are two nucleic acid sequences. Sequence (A) is a genomic sequence and (B) is the corresponding mRNA.

(A)

```
ATGACCACGCTGGCCGGCGCTGTGCCCAGGATGATGCGGCCGGGCCCGGGGCAGAACTACCCGCGTAGC
GGGTTCCCGCTGGAAGGTAAGGGAGGGCCTCAGCGCGCCGCGCTTCTCTTTTTCACCTTCCCACAGTGT
CCACTCCCCTCGGCCAGGGCCGCGTCAACCAGCTCGGCGGTGTTTTTATCAACGGCAGGTACCAGGAGA
CTGGCTCCATACGTCCTGGTGCCATCGGCGGCAGCAAGCCCAAGGTGAGCGGGCGGGCCTTGCCCTCCT
CGCCTGCCCGCCTGTTCTCTTAAAGCAGGTGACAACGCCTGACGTGGAGAAGAAAATTGAGGAATACAA
AAGAGAGAACCCGGGCGTGCCGTCAGGTACTAGGCCCATTAACCTCTCCCCGCTTCCTTCCTCCTCCCG
CCCCCAGTGAGTTCCATCAGCCGCATCCTGAGAAGTAAATTCGGGAAAGGTGAAGAGGAGGAGGCCGTC
CTGAGCGAGCGAGGTAAGCGGTGGCGCCTTGGGCGGCGGTTGAAGTAGCTTTTATGCCCTCAGGAAAGG
CCCTGGTCTCCGGAGTTTCCTCGCATTAAAGGAGAGAGAGAGAGAGTACTCTTTTGACTGGT
```

(B)

```
AUGACCACGCUGGCCGGCGCUGUGCCCAGGAUGAUGCGGCCGGGCCCGGGGCAGAACUACCCGCGUAGC
GGGUUCCCGCUGGAAGUGUCCACUCCCCUCGGCCAGGGCCGCGUCAACCAGCUCGGCGGUGUUUUUAUC
AACGGCAGGUACCAGGAGACUGGCUCCAUACGUCCUGGUGCCAUCGGCGGCAGCAAGCCCAAGCAGGUG
ACAACGCCUGACGUGGAGAAGAAAAUUGAGGAAUACAAAAGAGAGAACCCGGGCGUGCCGUCAGUGAGU
UCCAUCAGCCGCAUCCUGAGAAGUAAAUUCGGGAAAGGUGAAGAGGAGGAGGCCGUCCUGAGCGAGCGA
GGAAAGGCCCUGGUCUCCGGAGUUUCCUCGCAUUAAAGGAGAGAGAGAGAGAGUACUCUUUUGACUGGU
```

> How many exons does this gene have? Make a little table, showing the nucleotide number (in the genomic sequence) of the start and end of each exon, and the length of each exon and intron. Note that in real genes the introns are likely to be much longer than here.

(5) Look up the following genes using a genome browser such as the Ensembl or Santa Cruz browser: *BRCA1, GJB2, DYS*.

(a) How many transcripts are recorded for each?

(b) Choosing one transcript for each gene, note its ID number and report how many exons it has.

(c) What is the relationship between the different transcripts?

(d) What is the size of the gene, from the 5′ end of exon 1 to the 3′ end of the last exon? Note that nucleotides are counted from the tip of the short arm of the chromosome. Because the two strands of the double helix are antiparallel, genes on one strand are transcribed from the short arm tip towards the long arm tip, while those on the other strand are transcribed in the opposite direction. Therefore for genes on one strand the numbering of the nucleotides goes up as you move 5′→3′ through the sense strand, for those on the other strand the numbering goes down.

Chapter 4

How can a patient's DNA be studied?

Learning points for this chapter

After working through this chapter you should be able to:

- Describe the main applications of nucleic acid hybridization
- Describe a microarray and how it might be used
- Draw a diagram showing the principles of the polymerase chain reaction
- Describe appropriate applications of PCR, Southern blotting, Northern blotting, FISH and array-CGH
- Describe what information can and cannot be predicted by analyzing DNA with these techniques, and what additional information can be obtained through studying RNA or proteins

4.1. **Case studies**

CASE 11	Kavanagh family	81	97	152

- Healthy first baby boy
- Second child, Celia, pale with low hemoglobin levels
- Sickle cell disease

Ken and Carol are a healthy couple whose first child Keith was born when they were living in their native Kenya. He thrived and soon after Carol became pregnant again. This coincided with the family moving to England for Ken to undertake postgraduate studies and, soon after they arrived, baby Celia was born. Things didn't go so well for her; at three months of age she developed swelling of her fingers which seemed painful and she was referred to a pediatrician who noticed that she seemed pale and found she had an enlarged spleen. Her hemoglobin levels were low, only 7 g/dl, and the reticulocyte count was 12%, indicating she had a hemolytic anemia. The diagnosis of sickle cell disease was made on examination of a blood film which revealed sickled erythrocytes. Carol had trained as a nurse in Kenya and knew a lot about sickle cell disease and was devastated about the implications for Celia. She knew she would be likely to have crises leading to serious bone and abdominal pain necessitating hospital admissions and that she may need transfusions as well as lifelong penicillin. The next few months were very difficult for the family trying to settle in a new country and adjust to the news about Celia. Although they hadn't planned any more children yet, Carol found that she was pregnant again. Ken and Carol were very upset; they had always wanted three children but were really concerned about the risk of sickle cell disease in the new baby. They thought that their only option would be an abortion. However, when they went to see the gynecologist he explained that it would be possible to have tests early in pregnancy to see if a child were affected or not. They knew the risk of an affected child was 1 in 4 and of a child who was unaffected or a carrier 3 in 4, so they began to feel more optimistic.

(a) (b) (c)

Figure 4.1 – Sickle cell disease.
(a) Blood film showing a sickled cell, marked poikilocytosis (abnormally shaped red cells) and a nucleated rell cell. (b and c) Bony infarcations in the phalanges and metacarpals can result in unequal finger length. Photos courtesy of Dr Andrew Will, Royal Manchester Children's Hospital.

| CASE 12 | Lawton family | 82 | 98 | 376 |

- Family history of hemophilia
- Baby boy, Lennox, with cephalohematoma

Lennox was the first child born to Lillian and Leslie Lawton. Lillian had always been aware that her uncles had hemophilia, but it wasn't until she was pregnant that her mother told her more about her family history and the possible implications to Lillian's baby. She had one sister who was fine, but their mother had three brothers, two of whom had been diagnosed as having hemophilia in childhood. Lillian's affected uncles both had mobility problems due to repeated bleeds into their ankle and knee joints which occurred after activity or minor injuries, but both still managed to get around and attended their local Hemophilia Center as soon as problems occurred and for follow-up. One of them who used to have a motor bike ended up in intensive care after his bike slipped on an icy road and needed many months of care and rehabilitation. Lillian knew that hemophilia only happened in boys. During the pregnancy she asked to be referred to the genetic clinic and they explained to her that the risk of her present pregnancy resulting in the birth of an affected boy was 1 in 16 (her risk of being a carrier was 1 in 4, and the risk to a pregnancy if she was a carrier was 1 in 4, i.e. $\frac{1}{4} \times \frac{1}{4} = 1/16$). Lillian decided to look into things further when the baby was born.

(a) (b) (c)

Figure 4.2 – Effects of hemophilia.
(a) Bleeding around elbow. (b) A retinal bleed. (c) Repeated bleeds into joints produce severe arthritis. Photos (a) and (c) courtesy of the Medical Illustration Department, Manchester Royal Infirmary, and (b) Dr Andrew Will, Royal Manchester Children's Hospital.

Labor was slow and Lillian needed a forceps delivery. Lennox seemed fine but he had a large swelling on one side of his skull which the midwife said was a cephalohematoma which would gradually disappear. When he heard about the family history the pediatrician thought the cephalohematoma might indicate that the baby was affected and suggested tests were undertaken soon. He reasoned that if Lillian knew Lennox had hemophilia, then any symptoms of bleeding into joints could be identified early and problems minimized.

CASE 13	Murphy family	83	100	376

- Baby girl, Michelle, with dysmorphic features
- ? Unbalanced chromosome abnormality

Michelle was the third child born to Max and Millie. Their two sons were healthy and developing normally. The couple were delighted when their daughter, Michelle was born even though it had been a worrying pregnancy. Ultrasound scans had shown some swelling at the back of her neck at 18 weeks' gestation and later scans showed a swelling in the pelvis of one kidney. However, their minds had been put at rest after an amniocentesis showed the baby to have a normal chromosome pattern. Sadly, Max and Millie's delight was short-lived; the pediatrician heard a heart murmur and the first of many tests was requested. Over the next few months Michelle's development gave cause for concern; she needed tube feeding and was late smiling and sitting. The pediatrician referred her to the genetic clinic for a diagnostic assessment. The clinical geneticist had a special interest in dysmorphology (the study of patterns of birth defects, as described in *Box 4.1*). She felt that, in addition to the heart and kidney problems and microcephaly which had become apparent, Michelle also had a significant number of dysmorphic features. These included epicanthic folds, widely spaced eyes, a short philtrum and low-set ears. She also had incurved 5th fingers and short distal phalanges.

(a)   (b)

Figure 4.3 – A child with multiple congenital abnormalities suggestive of a chromosome abnormality.
She has severe mental retardation, growth retardation, microcephaly and dysmorphism of the face and hands (epicanthic folds, hypertelorism, arched eyebrows, low-set ears, short philtrum, open mouth appearance, full lips, irregular position of the lower teeth, clinodactyly of the 5th finger and distal brachydactyly). Courtesy of Dr Bert de Vries, Nijmegen.

Michelle has the combination of learning difficulties and dysmorphic features that suggests an unbalanced chromosome abnormality. As with Gillian Green (Case 7; ?22q11 deletion), her karyotype was grossly normal, but unlike Gillian, her phenotype did not provide any clue as to which part of which chromosome might carry a submicroscopic change. She therefore required a test that could scan her whole genome for copy number changes (duplications or deletions).

Malformations, deformations, dysplasias, syndromes

Malformation: a morphologic abnormality that arises because of an abnormal developmental process. A primary error in morphogenesis, e.g. cleft lip.

Malformation sequence: a pattern of multiple defects resulting from a single primary malformation, e.g. talipes and hydrocephalus can result from a lumbar neural tube defect.

Malformation syndrome: a pattern of features, often with a unifying underlying cause, that arises from several different errors in morphogenesis ('syndrome' from the Greek 'running together').

Deformation: distortion by a physical force of an otherwise normal structure.

Disruption: destruction of a tissue that was previously normal.

Dysplasia: abnormal cellular organization within a tissue resulting in structural changes e.g. within cartilage and bone in skeletal dysplasias.

Box 4.1

4.2. **Background**

A diploid human cell contains 6×10^9 bp of DNA, all chemically identical, all consisting of A, G, C and T nucleotides. Progressing the analysis of most of our cases will require us to examine specific genes or chromosomal regions in DNA samples provided by the patients. How can we achieve this, against a background of so much chemically identical but irrelevant DNA?

All the many laboratory methods boil down to one of two essential approaches:

a) hybridize the sequence to a labeled matching sequence (a **probe**).
b) amplify the sequence of interest; it is repeatedly copied to generate a large excess of just that sequence.

The principles and the applications that will be used in this chapter's investigations are described below. Some further applications that are important in clinical genetics are described in the final section of the chapter.

Nucleic acid hybridization

The two strands of a double helical DNA molecule are held together by relatively weak chemical bonds (hydrogen bonds) between paired bases. The bonds can be broken by boiling the solution containing the DNA, or by exposing it to a high pH. This is called **denaturing** the DNA. The process is reversible. Complementary single-stranded nucleic acids will **hybridize** or **anneal** (stick together to form a double helix) if they are mixed in solution at a moderate (typically below 50–60°C) temperature and pH (*Figure 4.4*). The ability of matching strands to hybridize is the basis of much of DNA technology.

Figure 4.4 – Denaturation of double-stranded DNA; hybridization of two complementary single strands.

Hybridization does not necessarily require a perfect match between the strands. Two strands will hybridize if there are enough correctly matching base pairs that can form hydrogen bonds, even if some bases are mismatched. Strands with mismatches will denature at a lower temperature than perfectly matched strands, and equally will require a lower temperature to hybridize successfully. Short strands will denature more easily than long strands because there are fewer hydrogen bonds holding them together. They need a lower temperature for hybridization, and hybridization is more sensitive to mismatches. By manipulating these variables, hybridization can be used in various different ways for DNA testing.

Using hybridization as the basis for DNA testing

Hybridization tests used in clinical genetics fall into two general types:

- Sometimes a test is used to check for a point mutation or very small sequence change in the test DNA. In the Kavanagh family (Case 11; sickle cell), if we are to check their fetus for the sickle cell mutation by a DNA test, we need to look for a substitution of one specific nucleotide out of the 3 000 000 000 in its genome. One way to do this is to use a short synthetic **oligonucleotide** (a piece of DNA typically 15–30 nucleotides long) as the hybridization probe. For such a short probe, the hybridization conditions can be such as to require a perfect match. Even a mismatch of a single nucleotide will be enough to prevent hybridization. Highly specific hybridization is also a prerequisite for the polymerase chain reaction (PCR, see below), which therefore also depends on using oligonucleotides. Although PCR is not primarily a test for hybridization, it does depend on specific hybridization for its ability to amplify just one specific sequence.
- At other times we want a hybridization test that will work on anybody's DNA, regardless of any minor differences between the DNA of different people. When we use a hybridization test to check for chromosomal microdeletions in Gillian Green (Case 7; ?22q11 deletion) or Michelle Murphy (Case 10; ?microdeletion), we don't want hybridization to fail

just because the corresponding sequence in the patient has a few variant nucleotides. Lack of hybridization should mean that the whole sequence is deleted. For these tests we use a much longer hybridization probe, typically a cloned piece of natural DNA. A probe 1 kb long will hybridize to its cognate sequence even if this varies a bit between individuals.

Whichever procedure we use for a hybridization test, we need to be able to tell whether or not the probe has hybridized to the test DNA. Most commonly this is achieved by labeling one of the two hybridizing partners, then separating out the other partner and seeing whether or not the label has accompanied it. In former times DNA was usually labeled by incorporation of radioactive ^{32}P; nowadays it is more usual to tag it with a fluorescent dye. Usually the separation is achieved by fixing one partner to a solid support – a piece of nitrocellulose film or a microscope slide, for example. This is immersed in a solution containing the labeled partner, left to hybridize, then taken out and washed. The label will then mark any areas of the solid support where hybridization has taken place. The investigations in this chapter use the following procedures.

- **Dot blotting** – for the **Kavanagh family** (Case 11, sickle cell) fetal DNA is spotted onto a nitrocellulose film that is immersed in a solution containing labeled oligonucleotide probes specific for the normal and sickle cell sequences. This is illustrated in *Figure 4.11*.
- **Southern blotting** – for the **Lawton family** (Case 12, hemophilia) the question is whether or not the affected boy has a large inversion that disrupts the *F8* gene on his X chromosome. The procedure is summarized in *Box 4.2* and *Figure 4.5*. Southern blotting can be used to check for the presence or absence of a sequence of interest, or to check the size of restriction fragment on which it is located. In the 1980s this was the main technique used in clinical genetic laboratories. It has largely been superseded by PCR, which is much quicker and easier to do and uses far less DNA. Southern blotting is still needed to examine DNA segments larger than a few kb. It is needed in this case because the position of the inversion breakpoints cannot be closely specified in advance. PCR becomes increasingly difficult as the size of the target increases.
- **Fluorescence *in situ* hybridization (FISH)** is used to check the presence or absence, copy number and chromosomal location of a particular DNA sequence in chromosomes of a patient. For **Gillian Green** (Case 7; ?22q11 deletion) we want to check for a megabase-sized deletion at a specific chromosomal location. If a deletion is present it will affect only one of the two homologous chromosomes. To retain the information about the chromosomal location the hybridization target is a spread of her chromosomes on a microscope slide, rather than extracted DNA. By very careful treatment the DNA in the spread-out chromosomes can be denatured without destroying the recognizable form of the chromosomes. Although each sequence has its partner nearby, because they are stuck down on the glass slide, the partners cannot move to find each other, so the chromosomal DNA remains single-stranded. The slide is exposed to a solution containing the labeled probe. A cloned piece of the relevant DNA, tens of kilobases long, is used as the probe so that, as mentioned above,

(a)

ca. 1 million identical molecules of genomic DNA

digest with a restriction enzyme

(b)

ca. 1 million identical sets of restriction fragments

gel electrophoresis

(c)

⊕ ⊖

fragments sorted by size along the gel

1 denature the DNA
2 transfer the pattern of fragments to a plastic film

(d)

reveal the fragment of interest by hybridizing to a labeled probe

(e)

Figure 4.5 – Southern blot analysis of DNA
The test DNA (a) is digested with a restriction endonuclease (b). The fragments are separated by size by gel electrophoresis (c), denatured by immersing the gel in alkali, and then transferred to a nitrocellulose film (d). The nitrocellulose sheet is then immersed in a solution containing the labeled probe, revealing any fragments that hybridize (e). See *Box 4.2* for more details.

Box 4.2

Principle of Southern blotting

The test DNA is first cut into specific fragments using a special enzyme (a restriction endonuclease – see *Box 4.3* and *Figure 4.5b*). These enzymes cut the DNA in a reproducible way, so that every molecule gives the same set of fragments. The mixture of fragments is subjected to gel electrophoresis (*Box 4.4*) so that fragments of different sizes are located at different positions in the gel (*Figure 4.5c*). The fragments, still in their size-dependent pattern, are denatured in alkali to make them single-stranded. We want to see which fragments will hybridize to our probe, but the hybridization reaction will not work efficiently on DNA immobilized in a gel. The molecules cannot move about to find partners. The next step is therefore to transfer the fragments on to nitrocellulose paper, while retaining their spread-out pattern. This is the actual Southern blotting procedure. It is usually done by laying the sheet of nitrocellulose paper on top of the gel, putting a stack of dry paper towels on top of that, and very carefully pressing so that the liquid in the gel is sucked through the nitrocellulose paper into the towels. The denatured DNA sticks to the nitrocellulose (*Figure 4.5d*). As before, this is immersed in a solution containing a labeled probe that will stick to just the fragment of interest and reveal its position (*Figure 4.5e*). Depending on the label used, the location of the probe is detected by autoradiography or by fluorescence. The technique provides information on whether a sequence matching the probe is present and, if so, on what size restriction fragment it is located.

minor sequence variations do not affect the hybridization. The probe is labeled with a fluorescent dye. After hybridization the slide is washed and examined under the microscope. Where the probe has hybridized, a pair of fluorescent spots is seen over the relevant chromosome (a pair of spots because at this stage in the cell cycle each chromosome consists of two sister chromatids, see *Chapter 2*). *Figure 4.6* shows the principle, *Figure 4.14* an actual example.

- **Interphase FISH** – Helen Howard (Case 8, Down syndrome) has been offered a prenatal test to see if her fetus has Down syndrome. Fetal cells have been obtained by amniocentesis (see *Chapter 14*). Interphase FISH allows specific chromosomes to be counted without waiting for the cells to divide in culture. As with the standard FISH protocol (above), the cells are immobilized on a microscope slide, the DNA carefully denatured and a fluorescently labeled probe applied. The probe consists of a sequence specific for the chromosome in question. The number of fluorescent spots in the cell nucleus is counted. Spots are counted in several dozen cells to get a reliable result.

- **Comparative genomic hybridization (CGH)** is a general method of looking for copy-number variants. That is, it checks for any sequence that is present in a greater or smaller number of copies per genome in the test DNA compared to a normal control DNA. It can detect variants that are too small to be seen under the microscope and, unlike FISH, it does not require prior knowledge of the chromosomal location of any variant. It is used in Case 13 (Michelle Murphy, dysmorphic and mentally retarded) to see if she has a submicroscopic deletion or duplication anywhere in her genome.

(a)

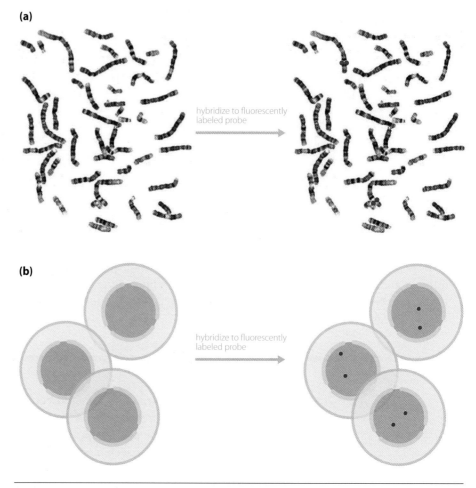

(b)

Figure 4.6 – Fluorescence *in situ* hybridization (FISH).
FISH can be used on either a chromosome spread (a) or on non-dividing cells (b).
In either case the material, on a microscope slide, is very carefully denatured and
then hybridized to a fluorescently labeled probe. See *Figures 4.14* and *4.15* for
examples.

The probes are in the form of a **microarray**. Microarrays use the dot
blot principle on a massively parallel scale. In this case it is the probe
rather than the test DNA that is anchored to a solid support, and the
test DNA rather than the probe that is labeled with a fluorescent dye.
Thousands of different probes are anchored in a grid pattern to a glass
slide, which is then immersed in a solution containing the labeled test
DNA. The slide is divided into thousands of cells, like the pixels of a
digital image. Each cell contains thousands of molecules of one particular
probe. CGH uses competitive hybridization. DNA from the patient and
DNA from a normal control are labeled with two different fluorescent
dyes, for example, the patient green and the control red. The two labeled
DNAs are mixed in equal proportions and allowed to hybridize to the
microarray (*Figure 4.7*). Green DNA fragments from the patient compete
with red fragments from the control for hybridization to the molecules of
the probe in each cell of the array. After hybridization and washing, the

Figure 4.7 – Principle of CGH using a microarray of genomic clones (array-CGH).
Adapted with permission from an original by Dr Joris Veltman, Nijmegen.

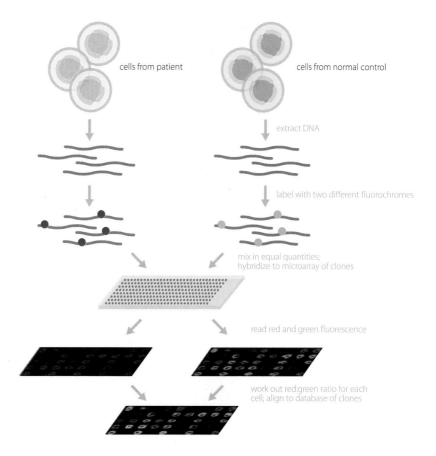

slide is examined under a microscope to determine the relative amounts of red and green fluorescence bound to each cell. Where the two are present in equal amounts the cell fluoresces yellow. Sequences where one or both copies are deleted in the patient give cells with more red fluorescence, because for that sequence there is relatively more control DNA. Duplications give green cells (*Figure 4.8*).

Array-CGH has many powerful features. The availability, through the Human Genome Project, of huge numbers of precisely mapped and characterized clones allows total control over the specificity and resolution of a CGH array. Arrays can be constructed that are specific for one particular chromosome, or that cover the entire genome. The resolution depends on the number and size of clones used and their distribution across the genome. Because each clone is precisely mapped on the human genome sequence, any deletion or duplication detected can be immediately linked to a list of the genes involved. An earlier version of CGH used a spread of normal chromosomes on a microscope slide in place of the microarray. This has now been superseded by array-CGH. CGH is a very powerful tool but it has two main limitations in clinical testing. It cannot detect balanced chromosomal rearrangements such as translocations or inversions, only copy number changes, and it is too expensive to be used in a completely routine way.

Figure 4.8 – Example of array-CGH output.
The test DNA (labeled green) and control DNA (labeled red) were mixed and
hybridized to a microarray containing over 30 000 Bacterial Artificial Chromosome
(BAC) probes, each from a known chromosomal location. The ratio of green to
red signal for each cell of the array is plotted on the vertical axis. Ratios above the
upper normal limit indicate a duplication in the test DNA; ratios below the lower
normal limit indicate a deletion. The results are arranged along the horizontal axis
according to the chromosomal location of the probe. Here only results from probes
from chromosome 15 are shown. The circle shows a set of contiguous clones
from 15q11–q13 that are present in only a single copy in the test DNA, indicating
heterozygosity for a deletion. Courtesy of Dr Joris Veltman, Nijmegen.

Restriction endonucleases

These bacterial enzymes cut double-stranded DNA whenever they encounter some specific
short sequence, usually 4, 6 or 8 bp long. Bacteria use them as part of a defense mechanism
against foreign DNA. Many different restriction enzymes have been isolated from a wide range
of bacterial species. Each has its own recognition sequence – for example, the enzyme *Eco*RI
cuts GAATTC.

For molecular biologists, restriction enzymes are very valuable tools. They provide a means
to cut a DNA molecule reproducibly into large fragments. It is easy to forget that virtually
everything one does with DNA involves a large collection of identical molecules. For example, a
Southern blot would typically use 5 μg of DNA extracted from blood. One human cell contains
6.4 pg of DNA, so 6.4 μg of DNA would be the DNA content of 1 million cells. Thus the starting
material is a very large collection of identical molecules. Unless the restriction enzyme cuts
each molecule in exactly the same places, the fragments would be a complete jumble and
would not run as sharp bands on a gel. The average size of fragment depends on the choice
of restriction enzyme. On average, a 4-bp restriction site will occur by chance once every $4^4 =$
256 bp, while a 6-bp site will occur on average every 4096 bp. Restriction sites are randomly
distributed in human DNA so there will be a wide spread of fragment sizes around these
averages.

Box 4.3

Box 4.4

Gel electrophoresis

Along with PCR, gel electrophoresis is a central tool of molecular genetics. DNA molecules carry a negative charge because of the phosphate groups (see *Box 3.2*). In an electric field a DNA molecule will move towards the positive pole. If the DNA is contained in an agarose or polyacrylamide gel, the DNA molecules have to fight their way through a jungle of long polymer molecules. How fast a double-stranded DNA molecule moves depends almost entirely on its size, and hardly at all on its sequence. Small molecules move quickly, large ones move slowly. Molecules of a given size will form a sharp band. The position of a fragment, revealed by hybridization or staining, is a measure of its size. As mentioned later, single-stranded DNA, or double helices containing mismatched bases show anomalous migration rates, which is the basis of some methods for detecting mutations.

Figure – loading an electrophoretic gel.
The DNA samples, mixed with blue dye to make them visible, are pipeted into wells formed in the agarose gel. The gel is submerged in a buffer solution to cool it and make electrical contact.

Amplifying the sequence of interest

When the sequence of interest forms only a very small fraction of a DNA sample, it may be made visible and followed by means of specific hybridization, as described above. Alternatively, it can be studied after selective amplification. Traditionally this was done by cloning the sequence in a living cell, usually in *E. coli* bacteria. This enabled the researcher to obtain many copies of the sequence in pure form, uncontaminated by all the other DNA originally present. This method is described in *Box 4.5*. For most clinical purposes cloning in living cells has been superseded by PCR. This is a form of *in vitro* cloning. Like conventional cloning, it works by making many copies of just the sequence of interest, but in a much quicker and easier way. Unlike conventional cloning, the PCR process does not separate the amplified sequence from the original mixture. If necessary this can be done in a separate step, but for many purposes this is not necessary. The amplified sequence is present in such large excess that the whole product can be treated as a slightly impure preparation of just the sequence of interest. PCR has several advantages over *in vivo* cloning – it is easier and quicker, but crucially, it is selective. With PCR you choose which bit of the DNA you want to amplify. With *in vivo* cloning you clone everything, then have to search through thousands or millions of clones to find the one you want.

Box 4.5

Amplifying a sequence by cloning

Until the mid 1980s, cloning was the only way to isolate a DNA fragment for study. It exploited the idea that if a DNA fragment was put into a cell in the right way, and then the cell was allowed to grow to form a colony of daughter cells, each of the daughter cells would contain a copy of the inserted fragment. The cells used are usually *E.coli* bacteria, but can be yeast, mammalian cells, or other types.

Cloning requires a **vector**. Getting a DNA fragment into a cell is surprisingly easy, but a loose DNA fragment inserted into a cell will normally be rapidly degraded and will certainly not be replicated when the cell divides. Vectors are pieces of DNA containing features that cause the host cell to tolerate their presence and replicate them. They are derived from naturally occurring viruses or plasmids. The fragment to be amplified is ligated into the vector so that together they form a single recombinant DNA molecule. A vast amount of ingenuity has gone into engineering vectors optimized for specific tasks. Engineered vectors incorporate various ingenious arrangements for identifying host cells that contain the recombinant vector, and for isolating the cloned DNA after the host cells have been grown up. For present purposes the only important point to note is that each type of vector has a maximum size of inserted fragment that it can accommodate (*Table*). This maximum size is always very much smaller than a chromosome, and smaller than many individual human genes:

Some vectors used for cloning DNA fragments.

Vector	Host cell	Maximum cloning capacity	Comments
Plasmid	*E. coli*	5–10 kb	Simple vectors for cloning small fragments
Cosmid	*E. coli*	45 kb	Mainly historical importance
Bacterial artificial chromosome (BAC)	*E. coli*	150 kb	Workhorse of the Human Genome Project
Yeast artificial chromosome (YAC)	Yeast	1000 kb	Technically tricky; special purposes only

The ability to cut and patch DNA, so central to genetic engineering, depends on the restriction endonucleases, described above, and on another enzyme, DNA ligase. Many restriction enzymes make a staggered cut when they cut a double helix, leaving short single strands ('sticky ends') protruding. Fragments with complementary sticky ends can hybridize end-to-end (see figure). DNA ligase then joins the abutting strands permanently with a standard (covalent) chemical bond.

Cloning is an essentially random process. A large collection of molecules of the test DNA is broken into random fragments. These are incorporated *en masse* into millions of vector molecules which in turn are used to infect millions of host cells. Vectors are engineered so that host cells containing a recombinant vector can be selected, usually through a particular pattern of antibiotic resistance. Next, single cells are picked and used to grow colonies. Each colony is an inexhaustible source of one specific human DNA fragment. The resulting collection of clones is called a **library** and ideally would contain cloned examples of every sequence in the test DNA. 'Library' is a very misleading name – in a real library the books are ordered on shelves and there is a catalog that enables you to go straight to any book you want.

Box 4.5 – continued

Creating a recombinant DNA molecule.
Two different molecules are digested with the same restriction enzyme to create complementary sticky ends. They hybridize, and are permanently joined by DNA ligase.

Recombinant DNA libraries might better be called haystacks, that may or may not contain the needle you want.

During the period 1970–1990, the rate of progress of human molecular genetics was largely determined by the rate at which interesting clones could be found by screening libraries. For a view of this heroic phase of human genetics, flip through any human genetics or molecular biology textbook from the 1980s. Nowadays the Human Genome Project has made available a complete collection of fully characterized and mapped BAC clones covering the entire genome. We also have a much easier way of amplifying selected DNA fragments from the genome of a patient, by PCR. As a result, making and screening recombinant DNA libraries is no longer part of mainstream clinical investigation, though it is still an important research activity.

The polymerase chain reaction

PCR revolutionized molecular genetics. Before PCR, only skilled researchers could amplify and characterize DNA. From around 1990, improved PCR methods allowed selective amplification of sequences from patient samples to become a routine tool in diagnostic laboratories.

PCR depends on three features of DNA replication.

(1) A new chain requires a **primer**. DNA polymerase (the enzyme that replicates DNA by synthesizing a strand complementary to a single-stranded template) cannot simply start assembling isolated nucleotides; it can only work by extending an existing chain. The primers used in PCR are chemically synthesized single-strand oligonucleotides, normally around 20 nt long.

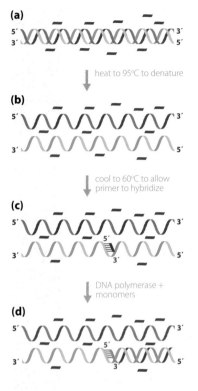

Figure 4.9 – Using a synthetic primer to force DNA polymerase to synthesize just a strand complementary to a specified part of a large DNA molecule.
(a) The primer (red) is present in a large molecular excess. (c) It hybridizes only to one specific sequence. (d) Only sequence downstream of the primer is copied.

(2) Chain extension can only proceed in the 5′→3′ direction (see *Box 3.2*)

(3) The two strands of a DNA double helix are anti-parallel, as shown in *Figure 3.5a*.

The requirement for a primer makes it possible to force DNA polymerase to copy just a selected sequence in a human DNA sample. A chemical oligonucleotide synthesizer is used to make a large number of molecules of a specific single-stranded oligonucleotide, whose sequence is such that it will hybridize to only one particular sequence in the human DNA. A large excess of this primer is added to the DNA. The whole sample is denatured by brief heating to 95°C, then cooled to a temperature at which hybridization can take place (typically 55–60°C). Some of the original double helices in the human DNA will re-form, but because there are so many more molecules of the primer, the sequence that matches the primer will most likely end up hybridized to the primer, rather than to its original partner. If the starting material consists of DNA from many cells, as is usually the case, some copies of the relevant sequence may re-hybridize to their original partner, but most will end up hybridized to a molecule of the primer. If DNA polymerase is then allowed to act on the mixture, most of the action will consist of adding nucleotides on to the 3′ end of the primer, building up a strand complementary to that bit of the genomic DNA. *Figure 4.9* summarizes this process.

The PCR uses this principle, but converts the linear reaction of *Figure 4.9* into an exponential chain reaction by using two primers and multiple cycles of denaturation, hybridization and synthesis. *Figure 4.10* shows how it works. The primers hybridize specifically to opposite strands of the DNA either side of the sequence to be amplified, and are oriented so that 5′→3′ chain extension from each primer runs towards the other primer. Thus each strand being synthesized by extending the forward primer comes to include the sequence to which the reverse primer can hybridize, and each strand made by extending the reverse primer comes to include the sequence to which the forward primer can bind. *Box 4.6* explains the process in more detail.

PCR has certain limitations:

- you need to know enough about the sequence to be amplified to be able to design specific primers
- PCR works best for amplifying sequences of 100–400 bp. Sequences longer than 1–2 kb are difficult, and sequences above 20 kb almost impossible to amplify

At the end of the PCR reaction, although all the original irrelevant DNA is still present, the amplified sequence is present in such excess that the product can be treated as a slightly impure preparation of just the target sequence.

Similarly to Southern blotting, PCR can be used to detect the presence or absence of a sequence or to measure its size. Examples of both those applications are shown below. Additionally, PCR products are suitable for sequencing and testing for point mutations, as we shall see in *Chapter 5*.

Box 4.6

Figure 4.10 – Principle of PCR.
The PCR reaction contains the target DNA, the DNA polymerase enzyme, large amounts of both primers and a supply of mononucleotides. (1) The starting DNA is denatured by heating to 95°C. (2) At 55–60°C the primers anneal to their target sequences. Note the 5′ and 3′ directions. (3) At 72°C the polymerase extends the primers in the 5′→3′ direction. (4) Another round of denaturing and annealing primers. (5) Another round of polymerization. After two rounds of PCR we have four strands where originally we had one.

Understanding PCR

In each round of denaturation, hybridization and synthesis, not only the original template but also all the copies made in previous rounds are replicated. Thus the amount of target DNA is doubled in each round – 20 rounds of PCR should suffice to amplify the target sequence one million-fold. Cycles of PCR are controlled by varying the temperature. A few seconds at 95°C denatures everything. Then a few seconds at around 55–60°C allows the primers to anneal to every possible template. Finally a few seconds at 72°C, the optimum temperature for the special polymerase used, sees each primer extended by adding nucleotides to the 3′ end. A typical amplification of 20–25 cycles with each stage lasting 30–60 seconds can be set up and completed in under 2 hours. A programmable heating and cooling block is used that will hold 20 or more individual reaction tubes, so that a number of samples can be PCR-amplified in parallel.

The selectivity of PCR depends on having primers that will anneal only to the desired target and not to any other sequence in the whole genome. The necessary specificity is achieved by using short primers (usually 18–22 nt) and fine-tuning the temperature. If the annealing temperature is too low, the primers may be able to hybridize to mismatched targets, while if it is too high they will not hybridize at all. Usually a temperature in the 55–60°C range allows specific hybridization. Possible primers are checked against the complete genome sequence database to make sure that no other sequence matches the primer. The

A typical thermocycler, used to carry out PCR amplification.
When in use an insulating lid covers the tubes.

length and nucleotide composition of the primer can affect the efficiency of the PCR process, and there are computer programs to assist with primer design.

When working out what goes on in PCR it is useful to think of two classes of PCR product:

- Product A is synthesized using the original DNA as the template. Molecules of Product A have a defined 5′ end (the 5′ end of the primer) but are of indeterminate length.

Box 4.6 – *continued*

- Product B is synthesized using Product A as template. Both ends of Product B are defined. The 5′ end is the 5′ end of the primer used to make it, and the 3′ end is defined by the end of its template (the 5′ end of Product A). All molecules of Product B are exactly the same size.

In later cycles of the PCR reaction, Product B is also used as the template for the next round of synthesis (*Table*). The end of a strand made by extending primer 1 is complementary to primer 2, and so in the next cycle primer 2 can hybridize to it and prime synthesis of a complementary strand. The end of this strand, in turn, is complementary to primer 1. The newly synthesized strand is exactly the same length as its template. After the first few cycles, virtually all the product is made in this way, using Product B as the template.

The best way to understand how PCR works is to take a large sheet of paper and draw out what happens in the first three or four cycles of the reaction. Check your effort against *Figure 4.10*. Take care to mark 3′ and 5′ ends. Make sure that hybridized strands are always anti-parallel and that strand extension is always 5′→3′.

Progress of the PCR reaction.

	Starting DNA	Product A template is starting DNA; 1 defined end		Product B template can be Product A or Product B; 2 defined ends		
	Single strands	Made in this cycle	Cumulative total	Made in this cycle using Product A as template	Made in this cycle using Product B as template	Cumulative total
After 1 cycle	2	2	2			
After 2 cycles	2	2	4	2	–	2
After 3 cycles	2	2	6	4	2	8
After 4 cycles	2	2	8	6	8	22
After 5 cycles	2	2	10	8	22	52

We imagine starting with one molecule of double-stranded DNA. After the first few rounds, almost all the product consists of just the sequence between the outside ends of the two primers. The numbers are numbers of single strands that are present when all the DNA is denatured.

4.3. Investigations of patients

We will first consider cases that were investigated by hybridization. The DNA regions involved range from a single nucleotide in the first case through successively larger parts of the genome until in the fourth case the entire genome was surveyed. The final three cases use PCR to check for the presence or absence of a sequence and to measure its size. In *Chapter 5* we will see examples of using PCR to check the actual nucleotide sequence.

Cases studied using a hybridization procedure

| CASE 11 | Kavanagh family | 81 | **97** | 152 |

- Healthy first baby boy
- Second child, Celia, pale with low hemoglobin levels
- Sickle cell disease

Sickle cell disease is caused by a single nucleotide substitution in exon 1 of the β-globin gene on chromosome 11. This changes a codon for glutamic acid into one for valine. Hemoglobin consists of two α-globin and two β-globin chains (plus four heme groups). The amino acid substitution in the β-globin affects the properties of the hemoglobin, causing it to aggregate and distort red blood cells. Heterozygotes have sickling trait, demonstrable in the laboratory, but they are normally healthy. Homozygotes have sickle cell disease, an autosomal recessive condition. Sickle cell disease and sickling trait are readily identifiable by standard hematological analysis; DNA tests are not needed to make the diagnosis. However, prenatal diagnosis requires testing of the DNA. Fetal blood sampling is difficult, not available in many centers and carries risks to the pregnancy; in any case, fetuses produce γ-globin instead of β-globin.

There are several alternative methods that could be used to check for the sickle cell mutation. The test used here is a dot-blot with two allele-specific oligonucleotides (ASOs) to distinguish the normal and sickle sequences. Some of the alternative methods that could have been used are discussed in *Chapter 5*.

The normal β-globin gene sequence reads (in part):

CTGACTCCTG**A**GGAGAAGTCTG

while the mutant version that is the cause of sickle cell disease reads:

CTGACTCCTG**T**GGAGAAGTCTG

Fetal DNA was obtained by chorion villus biopsy at 11 weeks of gestation (see *Chapter 14*). To increase the sensitivity of the test, a fragment containing the β-globin gene was amplified by PCR. The PCR product was denatured and spotted on to two slips of nitrocellulose film, together with control samples of known genotype (*Figure 4.11*). One slip was immersed in a solution containing each labeled probe. The result showed that the fetus was heterozygous for the mutation and therefore would not have sickle cell disease. Greatly relieved, Carol continued with the pregnancy and eventually delivered a healthy baby.

NORMAL SEQUENCE

normal-specific oligo A·C·T·G·A·G·G·A·C·T·C·C·T·C·T·T·C·A·G
C·T·G·A·C·T·C·C·T·G·A·G·G·A·G·A·A·G·T·C·T
sickle-specific oligo A·C·T·G·A·G·G·A·C·**A**·C·C·T·C·T·T·C·A·G

SICKLE SEQUENCE

A·C·T·G·A·G·G·A·C·^T·C·C·T·C·T·T·C·A·G
C·T·G·A·C·T·C·C·T·G·T·G·G·A·G·A·A·G·T·C·T
A·C·T·G·A·G·G·A·C·**A**·C·C·T·C·T·T·C·A·G

DOT BLOTS

Figure 4.11 – A dot blot test for sickle cell disease.
Denatured DNA from the fetus is immobilized on a sheet of plastic film and checked for hybridization to labeled oligonucleotides specific for the normal or sickle sequence.

This case carries a lesson for health service planners. The genetic intervention achieved the best of all possible results: a worried couple were reassured, an abortion was avoided and a healthy child was born. It would be all too easy to record the outcome of the genetic intervention as 'no action'. Clinical geneticists are very concerned not to have their achievements measured by the number of abnormal fetuses detected and aborted.

CASE 12	Lawton family	82	**98**	376

- Family history of hemophilia
- Baby boy, Lennox, with cephalohematoma

Hemophilia A is caused by mutations in the *F8* gene at Xq28 that encodes Factor VIII of the blood clotting cascade. A typical pedigree showing X-linked recessive inheritance was shown in *Chapter 1*, SAQ 3. Different families have different mutations in this gene, but about 40% of all severe cases are caused by an inversion. Though small in chromosomal terms, it involves 500 kb of DNA. One breakpoint is within the *F8* gene. Its effect is to disrupt the gene and so prevent production of Factor VIII (*Figure 4.12*). Because the breakpoint is deep within the 32 kb intron 22, and all the gene sequence is present, each exon can be amplified by PCR and has the correct sequence. Thus normal PCR tests do not pick up the inversion. A Southern blot can be used to check the size of a large DNA fragment spanning the usual breakpoint region. If the inversion is present the fragment is an abnormal size (*Figure 4.13*).

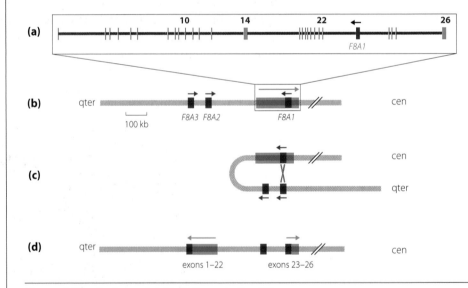

Figure 4.12 – An inversion that disrupts the *F8* gene.
(a) The *F8* gene has 26 exons spanning 187 kb of genomic DNA on the X chromosome at location Xq28. (b) The red boxes show a sequence present in intron 22 of the *F8* gene, of which two additional copies are located 360 kb and 435 kb away from the start of the gene. The arrows show the orientation. Note that these are inverted repeats (compare with the repeats in *Disease box 3*, which are direct repeats). (c) During male meiosis this part of the X chromosome has no matching partner. The DNA may loop round to allow two copies of the repeated sequence to pair in the same orientation. Occasionally there is recombination between the paired sequences. (d) The result is a chromosomal inversion of about 500 kb of DNA that disrupts the *F8* gene.

Figure 4.13 – Detecting the *F8* inversion using a Southern blot assay.
Genomic DNA is digested with the restriction enzyme *Bcl*1, run out on an agarose gel and Southern blotted onto a nitrocellulose filter. The filter is hybridized to a probe containing the F8A1 sequence from intron 22. In lanes C (normal control) and 4 (patient with a point mutation in *F8*) the autoradiograph shows bands of 21.5, 16 and 14 kb, representing fragments containing the F8A1, F8A3 and F8A2 sequences, respectively. In track 2 the 21.5 and 14 kb bands are altered, showing that the environments of F8A1 and F8A3 have been changed by recombination between them, as in *Figure 4.12*. In track 3 the 21.5 and 16 kb bands have been changed because of recombination between F8A1 and F8A2. Reproduced from Lakich *et al.*, (1993) (*Nature Genetics* **5**: 238) with permission from Macmillan Publishers Ltd.

| CASE 7 | Green family | 25 | 38 | 68 | **99** | 376 |

- Girl (Gillian) aged 3 years
- Slow to develop
- ? Chromosome abnormality
- Order tests to check for microdeletion at 22q11

Although conventional cytogenetic analysis showed a normal karyotype (*Figure 2.9*), this did not rule out a chromosomal deletion or duplication smaller than the 3–5 Mb resolution of standard preparations. Gillian's appearance was suggestive of a deletion of band 22q11. This is caused by recombination between misaligned low-copy repeat sequences on 22q11, as explained in *Disease box 3*. The usual deletion covers about 3 Mb and includes over 20 genes. One of these is the *TUPLE1* gene. A probe containing the *TUPLE1* sequence was used for FISH on a preparation of Gillian's chromosomes. The result showed a deletion on one copy of chromosome 22, confirming the diagnosis (*Figure 4.14*).

Figure 4.14 – 22q11 metaphase FISH.
The green spots are a control probe, used to identify the two copies of chromosome 22 and confirm that hybridization has taken place. The red spots are the *TUPLE1* probe. Only one of the two copies of chromosome 22 contains the sequence that hybridizes to this probe.

| CASE 8 | Howard family | 26 | 38 | 68 | **100** | 275 | 376 |

- Helen – new-born daughter of Henry and Anne (33 years old)
- Down syndrome
- Risk of recurrence if they have more children?

Helen's mother was offered a prenatal test in her next pregnancy. Although the risk of a recurrence of Down syndrome is low, someone who has already had one affected child is naturally extremely anxious in subsequent pregnancies. Waiting for the test result is also stressful. The fetal sample is cultured, but it takes two weeks for the cells to divide in sufficient numbers for conventional chromosome analysis. Two methods are available that give a rapid result on uncultured cells: QF–PCR is described in the final section of this chapter; in this case interphase FISH was used (*Figure 4.15*). As described above, DNA was denatured in non-dividing cells on a microscope slide and hybridized to a fluorescently labeled probe from chromosome 21. The average number of fluorescent dots, averaged over 50 cells, was 1.8. This suggests that the fetal cells had two copies of chromosome 21, although the hybridization failed in a few cases.

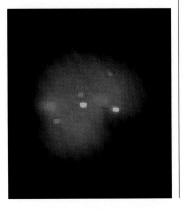

Figure 4.15 – Interphase FISH test for trisomy 21.
The chromosome 21 probe is labeled with a red fluorochrome and a control probe (for chromosome 18) is labeled in green. The two green dots show that the hybridization has worked for this cell, and the three red dots show that there are three copies of chromosome 21. The clinical report is based on examining a large number of cells. For prenatal diagnosis a mix of differently colored probes from chromosomes 13, 18, 21, X and Y is often used.

| CASE 13 | Murphy family | 83 | **100** | 376 |

- Baby girl, Michelle, with dysmorphic features
- ? Unbalanced chromosome abnormality

As with Gillian Green, the Murphy's daughter Michelle had features that suggested a chromosomal abnormality, but no abnormality was detectable on conventional cytogenetic analysis. Michelle's combination of mental retardation and dysmorphic features did not suggest any specific syndrome, so it was not possible to decide on one FISH probe that would give a useful test. Instead, array-CGH was used. In about 10% of similar cases this technique identifies submicroscopic chromosomal deletions or duplications. The precise abnormality seen varies widely between different cases. DNA was extracted from a blood sample and sent for analysis. The result (*Figure 4.16*) showed a duplication of material at 12q24.1. Michelle's DNA showed an increased dosage for 39 contiguous clones from 12q24.1 on the CGH microarray. The size of the duplication could be estimated by checking the precise chromosomal locations of these 39 clones in the human genome sequence. The data suggested that Michelle's duplication involved 2.3 Mb of material.

Before communicating this result to Michelle's parents, it was important to try to decide whether or not the duplication was the cause of her problems. As more and more samples are analyzed by array-CGH, it has become apparent that some small chromosomal segments show common copy number variations among normal people. Michelle's duplication was not one of these known non-pathogenic polymorphisms, but it could be a novel one. The first question was whether either parent carried the duplication, or whether it arose *de novo* in

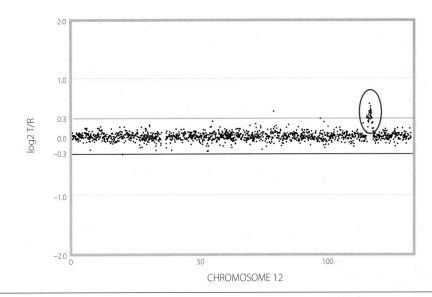

Figure 4.16 – Array-CGH result on the patient shown in *Figure 4.3*.
The whole genome was surveyed, but only results for the probes from chromosome 12 are shown. There is a duplication involving 39 contiguous clones from 12q24.1. Courtesy of Dr Joris Veltman, Nijmegen.

Michelle. Since her parents are normal, if either of them has the duplication it is not likely to be the cause of Michelle's problems.

It turned out that this was a *de novo* event. That does not prove that it is pathogenic, but makes it more likely. A check was made against the sequence database to see if the duplication involved any gene where an increased dosage was known to be associated with clinical problems. No clear candidate was identified, but the duplication involved a large number of genes, making it quite plausible that it could produce these effects. The strong balance of probabilities was that this was the cause of Michelle's problems. This was an important conclusion because it suggested that the recurrence risk was very low. The duplication was a *de novo* event and there was nothing to suggest any factor in either parent that might predispose to a recurrence. Counseling was that the recurrence risk was not zero but was very low. Because of all the unknown factors, it was not possible to give a precise figure – however, it was small compared to the general risk of a problem that attaches to any pregnancy. It would be possible to test for this specific abnormality in future pregnancies if the parents so wished.

Cases studied using PCR

| CASE 9 | Ingram family | 26 | 41 | 68 | **101** | 182 | 376 |

- Isabel – first daughter of Irene and Ian
- Small stature despite tall parents
- ? Turner syndrome

The diagnosis in Isabel has been clearly established from her karyotype (*Figure 2.13*). However, as explained in *Chapter 2*, it is important to check whether she has any 46,XY cells, as such cells in the gonads have the potential to become malignant. Such cells might be present if the cause of the syndrome in Isabel's case were loss of the Y chromosome during an early mitotic division of a 46,XY embryo. To check for the presence of XY cells a PCR reaction using

Y-specific primers is performed to see if there is any product. This is a very much more sensitive method than looking for XY cells in a conventional cytogenetic preparation. Ideally the test would be done on tissue from her streak gonads, because that is the tissue we are concerned about developing a malignancy, but usually this is done on blood samples.

In Isabel's case, no Y chromosome sequence could be amplified, reassuring us that it is unlikely she has XY cells in her gonads.

| CASE 4 | Davies family | 4 | 10 | 66 | **102** | 151 | 181 | 279 | 376 |

- Boy (Martin) aged 24 months, parents Judith and Robert
- Clumsy and slow to walk
- Family history of muscular dystrophy
- Pedigree shows X-linked recessive inheritance
- Order diagnostic DNA test

As we saw in *Chapter 1*, Martin had features (muscle weakness and calf pseudohypertrophy) suggestive of DMD. The pedigree reinforced the suspicion because there were two uncles who had a progressive neuromuscular disease. The geneticist had obtained their clinical notes. Their clinical course and muscle histology results were all consistent with DMD. The neurologist took a muscle biopsy from Martin and a blood sample to measure the level of creatine kinase (CK). CK is an enzyme present within muscle cells. If there is damage to the external cell membrane CK leaks out. The level is often raised in normal people after vigorous exercise, and tends to be permanently raised in female carriers of DMD (it can be used to give a probabilistic indication of a woman's carrier status). In affected boys it is strongly and unambiguously elevated.

These tests confirmed the bad news: Martin had Duchenne muscular dystrophy. At present there is no cure for this disease, only symptomatic treatment, and his prognosis was grave. Martin is unlikely to live much beyond age 20 unless in the meantime some new effective treatment is developed (the prospects for gene therapy are considered in *Chapter 14*). Initially Martin's parents Judith and Robert were entirely taken up with the emotional shock, and with planning how best to cope with a child with a severe progressive disability. But of course the diagnosis also had implications for any future pregnancies and for the wider family. When they were ready to consider such matters, the geneticist arranged a discussion. It seemed highly likely that Judith was a carrier, in which case any subsequent son would be at 1 in 2 risk. Other female relatives might very well also be carriers. To resolve all these questions it was necessary to identify the dystrophin gene mutation in Martin.

As we saw in *Chapter 3*, the dystrophin gene is huge, but about two-thirds of all mutations are deletions of one or more complete exons (see *Figure 3.9*). These deletions are relatively easy to detect in an affected male. If no deletion is found, this would not rule out the diagnosis because one-third of DMD cases have point mutations or duplications that would not be detected by this test. Further, more complex, tests would be necessary.

This is an X-linked condition, so a boy has only a single copy of the dystrophin gene. To check for partial deletions, individual exons of the gene are amplified by PCR. The 79 exons are all under 300 bp long (except for exon 79, the last exon, which is 2703 bp long – the last exon in a gene is often large, but consists mainly of the 3′ untranslated region). Thus individual exons are a suitable size for amplification by PCR. Primers are designed to match sequences in the introns flanking an exon, so that the product contains the complete exon and some intronic sequence. Experience shows that testing 18 carefully chosen exons picks up 98% of all deletions. By varying the amount of intron included, primers are designed so that each exon gives a differently sized product. A series of PCR reactions can then be performed in one operation (multiplexed), using all the primer pairs together in one reaction tube. The mix of products from all the PCR amplifications is run on an electrophoretic gel and shows a ladder of bands (*Figure 4.17*).

Figure 4.17 – PCR deletion screen in Duchenne muscular dystrophy.
Nine selected exons of the dystrophin gene have been amplified from the DNA of a panel of 20 affected boys. When the product is run on an electrophoretic gel each exon gives a band of a characteristic size. Because a boy has only a single X chromosome, any deletion shows up as missing bands. Different exon deletions can be seen in lanes 1, 5, 11, 12, 19 and 20. Lane 3 may be a large deletion or a technical failure. The boys with no deletion on this gel may have others of the 79 dystrophin exons deleted, or may have point mutations or duplications to cause loss of function of the gene.

The result (*Figure 4.17 Lane 5*) showed that Martin has a deletion of exons 45, 47 and 48. Exons 43 and 50 are present. Exons 44, 46 and 49 were checked in individual PCR tests, which showed that exons 44 and 46 were deleted but exon 49 was present. Thus Martin's deletion encompasses exons 44–48. The implications of this deletion for function of the dystrophin gene are considered in *Chapter 6*.

Now that we know exactly what mutation is segregating in this family, women can be offered an accurate carrier test, and if necessary accurate prenatal diagnosis. Judith and her mother are obligate carriers (see the pedigree in *Figure 1.10*) and the family includes at least eight women or girls who may be carriers. Judith's two daughters and her sister's daughter are all too young for any intervention at present. They will be re-contacted in their late teens. Through Judith, her three sisters and her two cousins (her mother's sister's daughters) were invited to contact the geneticist now. Carrier testing in women is more difficult than testing a boy because a carrier would be heterozygous and every exon of the dystrophin gene would amplify from her normal X chromosome.

A quantitative test is required, as described in the final section of this chapter and in *Chapter 5*. Before this test was available, many carrier women opted for fetal sexing and aborted all male fetuses, even though there was only a 1 in 2 chance of them being affected. With prenatal diagnosis they can be confident, if the tests are normal, of delivering boys free of the disease.

| CASE 1 | Ashton family | 1 | 7 | 65 | **104** | 150 | 376 |

- John – 28-year-old son of Alfred Ashton
- ? Huntington disease
- Other family members with similar symptoms
- Autosomal dominant inheritance shown in pedigree
- Diagnostic test ordered

The next step in investigating this family is to perform a diagnostic test on John's father Alfred. Alfred is already showing signs of disease. Although it seems highly probable that the family disease (see the pedigree in *Figure 1.7*) is Huntington disease, this needs to be proved before John can be given accurate counseling or offered a predictive test. His doctor takes a 10 ml blood sample from Alfred and sends it to the laboratory, where DNA is extracted.

As mentioned in the previous chapter, the laboratory will want to check the size of a run of glutamine codons (CAG) in exon 1 of the *HD* gene on chromosome 4. The normal range is 5–35 codons (15–105 bp) and anything over 37 codons is pathogenic. Expansions are normally in the 40–60 codon range, but are virtually never over 100 codons or 300 bp. This sort of test is easy to perform by PCR. Primers are designed that flank the region of interest. They need to be spaced far enough apart on the sequence to give a product that can be accurately sized on an electrophoretic gel: 100–300 bp would be ideal. The result (*Figure 4.18*) shows two bands because, of course, the DNA sample includes DNA from both Alfred's copies of the *HD* gene. Comparing the positions of Alfred's bands and control samples with known expansions in adjacent lanes of the gel, we see that Alfred's two copies of the gene have 15 and 65 CAG repeats, respectively (*Figure 4.18, Lane 1*). A repeat size over 37 is pathogenic. This result therefore confirms the diagnosis.

Now that Alfred's diagnosis was definite, it followed that John was at 50% risk of developing Huntington disease himself. If he wished, a PCR test on his DNA would tell him for sure whether or not he had inherited the *HD* gene mutation. Over several sessions with the genetic counselor, John and his wife pondered long and hard over whether or not to take the test. Initially John thought it would be a bad idea because having a genetic test could affect his ability to get insurance and maybe his job.

Figure 4.18 – Testing for the Huntington disease mutation.
This is a typical PCR application, amplifying a sequence a few hundred bp long using specific primers, and running the product on an electrophoretic gel. Smaller molecules move faster through the gel so the position of a band is a measure of the size of the PCR product. Bands are made visible by silver staining. Although all the other DNA in the genome is still present, the specific PCR product is present in so many more copies that under these conditions all the background genomic DNA is invisible. Each sample shows two bands, corresponding to the different sized PCR products produced by the two copies of chromosome 4. Lanes marked M carry size markers to calibrate the band sizes. The dotted line shows the upper limit of normal variation (36 repeats).

On discussion, he became convinced that these anxieties were misplaced. If he applied for insurance in the UK he would have to reveal his family history of Huntington disease, and many companies would see this as a reason for heavily loading the premium. In fact a genetic test might help John: if it was negative, the family history would no longer count, while in the UK, if it was positive he wouldn't have to declare the result for life policies up to a certain ceiling under a moratorium agreed by the insurance industry; in any case most of the bad news was already present in the family history. In the US, many states have enacted legislation to prevent genetic discrimination in insurance. As for employment, in the UK it would be illegal for an employer to discriminate against him on the grounds of his genetic risk. Unless he developed symptoms that prevented him doing his job properly, his genotype would be of no interest to any employer. John's wife was then worried about his existing insurance policy. He had a life insurance policy to pay off the mortgage on his house should he die. But when John took out that insurance he was unaware of the nature of the family problem. He had, however, answered all the questions on the form honestly, to the best of his then knowledge, and so that policy was valid and was not affected by later developments.

Having disposed of those concerns, the discussion returned to the basic question of whether or not John and his wife wanted to know. This is a very personal and difficult decision, but about 70% of people in John's position make the choice not to know. Of course a negative test would be a great relief, and a positive test would at least allow John and his wife to start planning for the future. But most of us like to see our lives as open-ended. Few of us would wish to know, at the age of 28, when and how we will die. After long reflection, John and his wife chose not to know. The counselor would have supported them whichever way they chose. Now she arranged to see them over the coming months to continue her support, and assured them that she was always available at any time for further discussion. She also pointed out that if, over the coming years, a treatment was developed that could slow the very early development of the disease, it might be in John's interest to have the test, and she promised to contact them should any such development occur.

The final discussion concerned what to do about John's other at-risk relatives. His sister Helen, her two young sons, and his aunt Alice in Australia were all at risk as a result of the positive test on Alfred. It was agreed that John should contact Helen and Alice, explain the situation and give them contact details of their local genetics service. Whether or not they chose to take up the contact was then up to them. Had John chosen to take the test, the geneticist would not have revealed that fact or the result to any other family member. Since John was close to Helen, he might choose to discuss with her his own thoughts and decisions, but there was absolutely no obligation on him to do this.

4.4. **Summary and extension**

Table 4.1 summarizes the techniques covered in this chapter so far and the type of problem for which each is appropriate.

Among the techniques described above, an adaptation of Southern blotting can be used directly to identify mRNA molecules. This variant of the technique is called **Northern blotting.** (The name is a joke: Southern blotting was developed by Dr Ed Southern in Oxford, UK.) mRNA is extracted from the relevant tissue, run out on a gel and blotted on to nitrocellulose. The probe is a labeled DNA corresponding to exons of the gene in question. The result shows whether an mRNA is present, and if so, how big it is. Absence of the expected transcript might show that the gene is somehow being silenced, while an unexpected size could indicate a disturbance of normal splicing.

Making cDNA

RNA cannot be cloned, amplified by PCR or sequenced like DNA. Most RNA studies therefore first make a DNA copy of the RNA, and study the copy. This is a reversal of the normal DNA → RNA flow of information, as described in the Central Dogma (*Figure 3.3*). Some viruses encode an enzyme, reverse transcriptase, that makes DNA copies of a template RNA. The final product is a double-stranded **cDNA** (complementary DNA). In **RT-PCR** (reverse transcriptase-polymerase chain reaction), reverse transcription is performed on total extracted mRNA, and gene-specific primers are then used in a PCR reaction on the total cDNA to amplify the chosen gene. RT–PCR can be performed as a single operation and is a powerful tool, provided a tissue can be sampled where the gene of interest is expressed. **cDNA libraries** are made by reverse transcribing total mRNA and cloning the resulting population of cDNAs *en masse*. Tissue-specific cDNA libraries are a very important resource for identifying genes and their pattern of expression.

The complete mRNA repertoire of a cell type or tissue can be studied by hybridizing the bulk mRNA (or more usually, bulk cDNA) to a microarray. Suitable **expression arrays** carry anchored oligonucleotides corresponding to exons of a whole number of genes – maybe the entire genome. The mRNA or cDNA is labeled with a fluorescent dye and allowed to hybridize to the array. Usually a protocol of competitive hybridization is used, as described for CGH (*Figure 4.7*). The test sample is labeled with one color dye and mixed with a control sample labeled with a different color. The ratio of the two dyes bound to each cell of the array shows the ratio of expression of that gene in the test tissue compared to the control. An example is shown in *Chapter 12*.

Testing protein

If a disease is caused by absence of a particular protein, which in turn may be the result of any one of a large number of mutations in the relevant gene, might it not be simpler to test directly for the protein rather than hunting through the whole gene for any possible mutation? In principle the answer should be yes. However, while DNA from any sample can be used to test any gene, the relevant protein may be present only in an inaccessible tissue. Also DNA tests are generic while protein tests are specific. That is, a laboratory can apply the same well-tried techniques to test the DNA of any gene, whereas each protein needs a specific assay that must be developed, set up and optimized. Protein testing is best done using commercial kits, where the company will optimize the reagents and protocol. However, companies will only develop these for relatively common conditions. We will see examples of protein testing used for population screening in *Chapter 11*, and used for diagnostic testing in *Chapter 12*.

Chromosome painting

This technique is a variant of FISH in which the fluorescently labeled probe is a whole cocktail of sequences from one particular chromosome. In a metaphase spread that chromosome appears brightly colored. Its use is in identifying the origin of abnormal chromosomes seen on standard karyotyping. For example, if we used a chromosome 1 paint on cells from Elizabeth Elliot (Case 5, *Figure 2.15*), the paint would highlight both copies of her normal chromosome 1 plus that part of her translocated chromosome that was derived from chromosome 1. In this particular case we don't need chromosome painting to understand the karyotype, but patients sometimes show small extra 'marker' chromosomes, or extra material inserted into a chromosome, whose origin can be impossible to identify without chromosome painting. Extending the concept, M–FISH or SKY use a mix of paints, one for each chromosome, each labeled with a different mix of fluorescent dyes, so that each chromosome is painted a different color. We will meet this technique when considering the very complex chromosomal changes typical of leukemia and cancer cells (*Chapter 12*).

Diseases caused by expanding nucleotide repeats

The mutation in Huntington disease is unusual but it is not unique. Starting with Fragile-X syndrome in 1991, a growing list of human diseases have been identified that are caused by expansions of a nucleotide repeat. Mostly the repeats are trinucleotides, as in Huntington disease, but examples are known that involve 4, 5 and 12 nucleotide repeats. In every case the repeat is present in normal people, where it is stable and non-pathogenic. The number of repeat units varies among normal people as a result of occasional rare mutations, but is always below some threshold number. If one of these rare mutations creates a repeat that is above the threshold, it becomes unstable and has a high probability of expanding yet further on transmission from parent to child. The higher the repeat number, the more unstable it is. Separately from this, repeats above a certain size cause disease. Repeats that are big enough to be unstable but not big enough to cause disease are called **premutations**. People carrying premutations are healthy but are at high risk of having affected children. The main examples are shown below.

A feature of many of these diseases is **anticipation**. This describes the way a disease may get more severe going down the generations. It happens because the expanded repeats are very unstable and tend to expand still further on transmission. The size of expansion is often correlated with the severity of symptoms and/or with onset at younger ages. Thus an expanding repeat is suspected to lie at the root of any genetic disease that shows anticipation. However, reports of anticipation must be viewed with considerable skepticism. If a dominant disease is naturally very variable, as many are, then clinicians will often see severely affected children born to a mildly affected parent. Mildly affected children born to a severely affected parent will be less frequently seen. This is because severely affected people may not have children, and if they do, they may not feel there is anything wrong with a mildly affected child. Thus a common bias of ascertainment often mimics anticipation.

Disease box 4

Diseases associated with pathogenic expanded nucleotide repeats.

SCA, spino-cerebellar ataxia; DRPLA, dentatorubral pallidoluysian atrophy; SBMA, spinobulbar muscular atrophy.

Disease	OMIM no.	Mode of inheritance	Location of gene	Location of repeat	Repeat sequence	Normal range (repeats)	Pathological range (repeats)
Huntington disease	143100	AD	4p16	Exon 1	$(CAG)_n$	5–35	37–120
DRPLA	125370	AD	12p13	Exon 5	$(CAG)_n$	7–34	58–88
SCA1	164400	AD	6p23	Exon 8	$(CAG)_n$	19–38	40–81
SCA2	183090	AD	12q24	Exon 1	$(CAG)_n$	15–29	35–59
SCA3 (Machado–Joseph disease)	109150	AD	14q24-q31	Exon 10	$(CAG)_n$	14–40	68–82
SCA6	183086	AD	19p13	Exon 49	$(CAG)_n$	6–17	21–30
SCA7	164500	AD	3p21-p12	Exon 3	$(CAG)_n$	7–17	38–130
SCA17	607136	AD	6q27	Exon 3	$(CAG)_n$	25–44	50–55
SBMA	313200	XLR	Xq11	Exon 1	$(CAG)_n$	11–33	38–62
Fragile-X site A (FRAXA)	309550	XL	Xq27.3	5'UTR	$(CGG)_n$	6–54	200–>1000
Fragile-X site E (FRAXE)	309548	XL	Xq28	Promoter	$(CCG)_n$	6–25	>200
Friedreich ataxia (FRDA)	229300	AR	9q13-q21.1	Intron 1	$(GAA)_n$	7–22	200–1700
Myotonic dystrophy 1 (DM1)	160900	AD	19q13	3'UTR	$(CTG)_n$	5–35	50–4000
Myotonic dystrophy 2 (DM2)	602668	AD	3q21	Intron 1	$(CCTG)_n$	12	75–11 000
SCA8	603680	AD	13q21	Untranscribed RNA	$(CTG)_n$	16–37	110–>500
SCA10	603516	AD	22q13	Intron 9	$(ATTCT)_n$	10–22	Up to 22 kb
SCA12	604326	AD	5q31	Promoter	$(CAG)_n$	9–18	66–78
Progressive myoclonic epilepsy (PME)	254800	AR	21q22.3	Promoter	$(CCCCGCCCCGCG)_n$	2–3	40–80

The first nine diseases in the table all involve expanding $(CAG)_n$ runs within the coding sequence of a gene. CAG is the codon for glutamine (see *Table 6.1*) so the effect is to encode a protein with an expanded polyglutamine tract. These proteins are in some way toxic to neurons. The cumulative death of neurons leads to a late onset neurodegenerative disease. SBMA is described in more detail in *Disease box 6*. For most of the other diseases in the table the expanded repeat prevents expression of a gene, and the disease is the result of lack of the gene product. The two forms of myotonic dystrophy, however, are the result of the toxicity of mRNA containing the expanded repeat. Toxic RNA may also be part of the molecular pathology of FRAXA, SCA8 and perhaps other diseases. Thus although all these diseases are caused by expanded repeats, the mechanisms by which they cause disease are quite diverse and for the most part, poorly understood.

(a)   (b)   (c)

Anticipation in myotonic dystrophy.
(a) A 'blue-dot' cataract may be the only sign of the disease in the first affected generation. (b) A three generation family showing the grandmother who has bilateral cataracts but no muscle symptoms or facial weakness; her daughter has moderate facial weakness with ptosis and cataracts; the child has the congenital form. Reproduced from *Myotonic Dystrophy* by Peter Harper (Saunders, 3rd edition, 2001) with permission. (c) A baby with the congenital form showing hypotonia. The congenital form is seen only when the child inherits the disease from its mother. It is caused by very large expansions of the CTG repeat, which are never found in sperm.

Clinically, the polyglutamine diseases are all late onset neurodegenerative conditions. The precise symptoms probably depend on the pattern of expression of the mutant gene and of genes whose products interact with the mutant protein. Friedreich ataxia is also a result of progressive death of neurons, with die-back affecting cerebellar function. The two fragile X diseases (so called because when cells are cultured in a special medium a proportion of X chromosomes show an abnormal decondensed region, a 'fragile site') present with mild to moderate mental retardation, often behavior problems, a characteristic face and macro-orchidism. Unlike in most X-linked diseases, carrier females often show mild to moderate mental retardation. Finally, the two forms of myotonic dystrophy are multisystem diseases with muscle myotonia, cataracts, testicular atrophy and frontal balding. Myotonic dystrophy shows especially striking anticipation:

A Southern blot.
Shows unstable expanded CTG repeats in several members of the same family. The lowermost two bands are a non-pathogenic 10/11 kb polymorphism. Pathogenic CTG expansions produce the bands higher up the gel. Photo. courtesy of Dr Simon Ramsden, St Mary's Hospital, Manchester.

4.5. **References**

General descriptions of the techniques covered here can be found in many textbooks, for example Strachan T and Read AP (2004) *Human Molecular Genetics, 3rd edn.* Garland, New York – available on the NCBI Bookshelf http://www..ncbi.nlm.nih.gov/antrez/query-fcgi?.db=Books.

Useful websites

The University of Utah Genetic Science Learning Center has an excellent animated explanation of gel electrophoresis at http://gslc.genetics.utah.edu/units/biotech/gel/

The Access Excellence Resource Center has elementary descriptions of Southern blotting (http://www.accessexcellence.org/RC/VL/GG/southBlotg.html) and other techniques – lacking detail at this level, but good for graphics.

For a large amount of detailed information and pictures of FISH see Tavi's Multicolor FISH Page at http://info.med.yale.edu/genetics/ward/tavi/FISH.html

4.6. **Self-assessment questions**

(1) Design 10-nucleotide-long primers to amplify each of the 50 bp sequences underlined so as to produce a 50 bp product.

(a) - guidance provided.

CCACTCCCCTCGGCCAGGGCCGCGTCAACCAGCTCGGCGGTGTTTTTATCAACGGCAGGTACCAGG
AGACTGGCTCCATACGTCCTGGTGCCATCGGCGGCAGCAAGCCCAAGGTGAGCGGGCGGGCCTTGC

(b)

AAGAGAGAACCCGGGCGTGCCGTCAGGTACTAGGCCCATTAACCTCTCCCCGCTTCCTTCCTCCTC
CCGCCCCCAGTGAGTTCCATCAGCCGCATCCTGAGAAGTAAATTCGGGAAAGGTGAAGAGGAGGAG

[Note that real primers would be 16–25 nucleotides long and would be designed to give a product of a few hundred bp; this is an exercise in getting the position and orientation of your primers correct. Do it by hand even if you have access to a primer design program.]

(2) Extend *Table 4.1* to show the progress of the PCR reaction up to cycle 10. (It would be neat to make a spreadsheet to do this). How many cycles would it take to produce 100 000 copies of Product B?

(3) There are four different nucleotides in DNA, 16 different dinucleotides, 64 different trinucleotides and 4^n different sequences n nucleotides long. If a restriction endonuclease cuts DNA whenever it encounters a particular five-nucleotide sequence, and assuming these occur at random throughout the human genome, into how many fragments might it cleave the DNA of a human cell?

(4) Assuming the human genome consisted entirely of unique sequence DNA, how long would an oligonucleotide probe need to be in order to hybridize to just one sequence in the genome? [Guidance provided.]

(5) For each of the following sequence changes or effects, choose possible testing methods from the list below that could be used to check for the presence of the change or effect (more than one method may be appropriate for some cases):

- a G>A change in exon 2 of the *PAX3* gene that results in replacement of valine 60 by methionine in the gene product
- a heterozygous 3 bp deletion in exon 6 of the *BRCA1* gene
- an A>T nucleotide substitution that changes the codon for arginine 214 (AGA) into a stop codon (TGA) in exon 7 of the *MITF* gene
- a GT>GA change in the donor splice site at the end of exon 4 of the *PAH* gene, which encodes the liver enzyme phenylalanine hydroxylase
- a C>A change in an intron near a splice site in the ubiquitously expressed actin gene: the question is whether or not it affects splicing of the primary transcript
- deletion of several contiguous genes on one copy of chromosome 17 in a child with suspected Smith–Magenis syndrome
- a duplication of one or more exons in the dystrophin gene in a boy with Duchenne muscular dystrophy
- deletion of one or more exons of the *HYP* gene in a boy with hypophosphatemia (an X-linked dominant condition)
- insertion of three nucleotides in the promoter of a gene – the question is whether this affects expression of the gene
- any material extra or missing on a copy of chromosome 7 in a patient – the cytogeneticist reported that the banding pattern on one copy of chromosome 7 was abnormal but could not work out exactly what events had produced the change

Options:

(a) PCR amplification, check for the presence / absence of product
(b) PCR amplification, check the size of the product
(c) PCR amplification followed by sequencing
(d) PCR amplification followed by dot-blot hybridization to an allele-specific oligonucleotide
(e) RT–PCR
(f) real-time quantitative PCR
(g) Southern blotting
(h) FISH
(i) chromosome painting
(j) array-CGH

Chapter 5

How can we check a patient's DNA for gene mutations?

Learning points for this chapter

After working through this chapter you should be able to:

- Describe the principle of DNA sequencing and read a straightforward DNA sequencer trace
- Describe the circumstances in which a DNA test involves scanning a gene for mutations or checking for a specific change
- Describe briefly the principles of two methods (apart from sequencing) by which a gene can be scanned for mutations
- Describe briefly the principles of two methods by which a person's DNA can be checked for a specified mutation
- Describe briefly the principles of two methods by which a person's DNA can be checked for deletion or duplication of exons of a gene

5.1. Case studies

| CASE 14 | Nicolaides family | **115** | 129 | 153 | 376 |

- ? β-thalassemia carriers

Spiros Nicolaides is an IT graduate who was born in the UK but whose family originally came from Cyprus. He is healthy, and on a recent trip to see his grandparents in Cyprus met and fell in love with Elena, who recently returned there from the USA where she was studying. Both of the families are delighted and a big engagement party is planned. However, Elena's older sister tells her that before she married she was advised to have some blood tests to see if she was a carrier for β-thalassemia. Luckily, although Elena's sister was shown to be a carrier, her future husband was not and they now have a healthy son. Naturally Elena and Spiros are concerned and request an appointment in the genetic clinic to discuss their risks.

(a)   (b)   (c)   (d)

Figure 5.1 – Effects of thalassemia.
(a) Blood film with very marked hypochromia and many nucleated red cells. (b) osteoporotic appearance of hands due to bone marrow extension (c) 'hair on end' skull. (d) liver biopsy with Perl's stain, showing iron overload. Courtesy of Dr Andrew Will, Royal Manchester Children's Hospital.

5.2. **Background**

In the previous chapter we saw how PCR or various hybridization methods can be used to examine any chosen small piece of the DNA in a sample. Sometimes no further investigation is needed. That was the case for several of the families:

- for Case 4 (Davies family), PCR identified and characterized a partial deletion of the dystrophin gene, confirming the diagnosis of Duchenne muscular dystrophy.
- in Case 1 (Ashton family), the size of the PCR product identified the pathogenic Huntington disease allele.
- for Case 12 (Lawton family), Southern blotting showed that the Factor VIII gene was disrupted by an inversion, causing hemophilia A.

But many disease mutations are substitutions of one nucleotide for another somewhere within the DNA of a gene, which would not generate any visible difference in a PCR product or Southern blot. Insertion or deletion of a nucleotide or two would also not make a noticeable difference to the size of a PCR product. We need therefore to consider how to check a gene for such point mutations.

The available methods fall into three classes:

- DNA sequencing
- methods that check for a specific sequence change
- methods that rapidly scan a gene for any change, without identifying the nature of the change

DNA sequencing – the ultimate test

Rather like PCR, DNA sequencing uses a DNA polymerase to make many copies of the fragment of interest. The stages are as follows.

(1) The starting material is a collection of identical DNA molecules – usually a PCR product, or sometimes a cloned copy of the fragment of interest.
(2) Unlike in PCR, for sequencing we want to make copies of just one of the DNA strands. Therefore a single primer is used (as in *Figure 4.9*). Rather than denaturing the template DNA to make it single-stranded, a special cloning procedure is often used. This involves using a specialized vector, M13, that reels off copies of just one of the two DNA strands.
(3) Having got our single-stranded template, we add the primer, the four nucleotide monomers A, G, C and T, and a DNA polymerase enzyme to synthesize the complementary strand. However, the pool of monomers is spiked with chain-terminating molecules. This is the key to the sequencing technique. The idea was developed by Fred Sanger, and earned him the Nobel prize (his second! – he had already won one for determining amino acid sequences of proteins).

The chain terminating molecules are modified versions of the standard A, G, C and T nucleotides (*Figure 5.2*). They are incorporated into a growing polynucleotide chain just like their regular counterparts, but they then prevent the chain growing any further. The chemical trick that does this is to remove

(P) = phosphate

Figure 5.2 – Formulae of (a) a ribonucleotide (b) a deoxyribonucleotide (c) a dideoxynucleotide. The dideoxynucleotide can be added to a growing DNA chain through its 5′ phosphate, but because it lacks a 3′ hydroxyl group, no further growth of the chain is then possible. In sequencing reactions the dideoxynucleotides are normally labeled, either radioactively or by tagging with a fluorescent dye.

the hydroxyl group on position 3 of the deoxyribose sugar: chain terminators are *dideoxy* nucleotides. Since this hydroxyl group provides the link to the next nucleotide in the chain, its absence means that no new nucleotide can be added to that particular chain.

To make the whole thing work, we need to add just the right amount of chain terminators. When it is incorporating an A into the growing chain the polymerase will randomly pick a normal or a dideoxy version of the A nucleotide. If there is 1% as much dideoxy-A as normal A, then at each A position around 1% of the growing chains will incorporate the chain terminator and grow no further. As a result, a series of nested fragments accumulate, each terminated by a dideoxy-A. Putting this into a concrete example: suppose we use a 20-nucleotide primer and the DNA we are copying has Ts 7, 10, 15, 21, etc. nucleotides from the start position (the 3′ end of the primer). Opposite each T in the template strand, the polymerase will incorporate an A in the growing strand. A proportion of growing strands will terminate at each of these positions. Thus there will be fragments of length 27, 30, 35, 41, etc. nucleotides. When the product is size-separated by electrophoresis, if we can read off the lengths of the fragments, we can read off the positions of the As in the newly synthesized strand. If dideoxy-A was the only dideoxy nucleotide used, there would not be fragments 28, 29, 31, 32, etc. nucleotides long, because at those positions the polymerase would not be incorporating an A into the growing chain, and so there would be no risk of a dideoxy-A preventing the chain from growing further.

The original version of the Sanger sequencing technique worked exactly as we have just described, using radiolabeling of the chain terminators and manual analysis (*Box 5.1*). Nowadays most sequencing is done using fluorescent labeling of the dideoxynucleotides, as shown in *Figure 5.3*. This brings several benefits, apart from avoiding the hazards of radioactive work. The four dideoxynucleotides are tagged with four different colored fluorescent dyes; the standard nucleotides

Figure 5.3 – Principle of DNA sequencing.

(a) Each time a nucleotide is incorporated into the growing chain, there is a small chance that it will be a dideoxynucleotide, which will terminate growth of the chain. The result is a series of nested fragments. (b) Electrophoresis separates the fragments by length. Each dideoxynucleotide carries a different colored fluorescent dye.

(c) Sequencing machines such as this Applied Biosystems Prism 377 automate the separation, detection, sizing and quantitation of the fragments.

(a)

sequence to be copied

5′ A G C T T G A A G A C T T A A T G A C C A A C T T G A T T A T C A T A A G T A C G G C T A G C 3′

direction of growth   3′ A T G C C G A T C G 5′   primer

C A T G C C G A T C G
T C A T G C C G A T C G
T T C A T G C C G A T C G
A T T C A T G C C G A T C G
T A T T C A T G C C G A T C G
G T A T T C A T G C C G A T C G
A G T A T T C A T G C C G A T C G
T A G T A T T C A T G C C G A T C G
A T A G T A T T C A T G C C G A T C G
A A T A G T A T T C A T G C C G A T C G
T A A T A G T A T T C A T G C C G A T C G
C T A A T A G T A T T C A T G C C G A T C G
A C T A A T A G T A T T C A T G C C G A T C G
A A C T A A T A G T A T T C A T G C C G A T C G
G A A C T A A T A G T A T T C A T G C C G A T C G

Products of the reaction: a nested set of fragments, each terminated by a color-labeled dideoxynucleotide

(b)

C T T A T G A T A A T C A A G T T G G T C A T T

SMALL ⟶ LARGE

(c)

The original manual Sanger sequencing technique

The original version of the technique used radiolabeling of the dideoxynucleotides. The four nucleotides all carry the same ^{35}S label, therefore it is necessary to run four separate reactions in parallel, each using just one of the chain terminators. The four products are run in adjacent lanes of a sequencing gel, which is then sandwiched with a sheet of X-ray film to reveal the sizes of the labeled fragments in each track by autoradiography (see figure). [35]S is used rather than ^{32}P because its lower-energy radiation gives sharper bands on the autoradiograph.

Manual sequencing using radiolabeled dideoxynucleotides. The sequence is read off from the autoradiograph, from the bottom upwards (because the smallest fragments migrate furthest down the gel). The first 15 nucleotides read TCCAAGATCCTGTGC.

T C G A

Box 5.1

(a)

C T C C G A TA A T TA A G C TG A T TA A C A T T TG T T C C T C T C C A A AG A A T T TG G T C A C A C C A G G C T
90   100   110   120   130   140

(b)

G G TG T C TC A T GT G A C A G A C C A C C A G C G A C C C T C A C C C A G T T A T G
129   137   145   153   161

Figure 5.4 – Examples of DNA sequencer traces.
(a) Sequence of part of exon 15 of the *OCRL* gene. (b) Sequencing requires high quality DNA. If the DNA used is not carefully purified, the result may be a trace that cannot be reliably interpreted. (Track (a) courtesy of Dr Andrew Wallace, University of Manchester; track (b) anonymous.)

are unlabeled. Now small amounts of all four terminators can be included in a single reaction mix. Each fragment that ends with an A will be (say) green, each fragment ending in C will be blue, and so on. DNA sequencing machines separate the fragments by length using gel or capillary electrophoresis and read the color. The result is displayed as a series of colored peaks (*Figure 5.4*). Sophisticated software interprets the sequence and can provide other information, such as quantitating each peak and defining the length of each fragment. These features make automated sequencers useful for other tasks as well as sequencing. Increasingly, PCR-based tests are formatted to use fluorescently labeled primers, so that the PCR product can be sized and quantitated on a sequencing machine, rather than run on a manual electrophoretic gel. A number of the tests illustrated below by photographs of gels are nowadays commonly run on a sequencer (we used the gel photos here to give a more direct feel for the process).

Methods for detecting specific sequence changes

It often happens that the laboratory is looking for the presence or absence of one specific sequence variant in a sample. This happens under various circumstances.

- The disease in question may always be caused by exactly the same sequence change. The prenatal test for sickle cell disease in the Kavanagh family (Case 11) relied on the fact that sickle cell disease is always caused by precisely the same sequence change. The reasons why some diseases are always caused by one specific mutation are discussed in *Chapter 10*.
- A disease may be caused by various different mutations, but one or a few mutations may be so frequent in a particular population that it is worth first checking for these before going on to a more general search. An example is cystic fibrosis. Over 1000 different mutations have been reported, but 80% of all mutations in Northern Europeans are one particular deletion of three nucleotides (see *Table 11.1*); 80% of all β-thalassemia mutations in Greek Cypriots are c.93–21G>A (see *Table 5.2*);
- The test may be to check a patient for a family mutation that has already been identified and characterized in other family members.

The same techniques are also used for genotyping people for non-pathogenic single nucleotide polymorphisms (SNPs), for example, in linkage and association analysis (*Chapter 9*) and in anthropological investigations.

Many methods are available to detect a specific sequence change. These include:

- Sequencing the DNA, usually in the form of a PCR product. A standard Sanger sequencing run as described above delivers several hundred nucleotides of sequence, which is not what is required here. A special variant method, Pyrosequencing®, sequences just a few nucleotides from a given starting point. Pyrosequencing requires a special machine and reagents but, once set up, it is good for checking one specific nucleotide in samples from a large collection of individuals. *Figure 5.16* shows an example.
- Hybridizing the PCR-amplified sample to an allele-specific oligonucleotide probe, as was done for sickle cell disease (*Chapter 4, Figure 4.11*).
- Digestion with a restriction enzyme. If the mutation happens to either create or destroy a sequence that is the recognition site for a restriction enzyme, this allows an easy test. The relevant region is PCR amplified, the product is digested with the appropriate restriction enzyme and then run out on a gel. The size of the fragments shows whether the restriction site was present. Heterozygotes show both the cut and uncut fragments. Examples are illustrated below for LHON (Case 6 – Fletcher family, *Figure 5.15*) and β-thalassemia (Case 14 – Nicolaides family, *Figure 5.14*).

- Performing an allele-specific PCR reaction. PCR primers may work even if there are slight mismatches to their target, provided the primer is long enough to hybridize, but the 3′ end nucleotide of the primer is critical. Unless it correctly base-pairs to the template the reaction will not work. We can therefore check whether a given nucleotide is A or G by setting up a PCR reaction where this nucleotide must pair with the 3′ end nucleotide of one of the primers. A primer ending in T will amplify only the A allele, while one ending in C will amplify only the G allele. As with ASOs, two parallel reactions are run with the two different primers, or alternatively the primers are differently labeled (e.g. with different dyes) so as to give identifiable products in a single mixed reaction. *Figure 5.5* shows the principle; *Figures 5.10* and *5.13* show applications.
- Oligonucleotide ligation analysis (OLA). The enzyme DNA ligase was mentioned in *Box 4.5*. This enzyme will covalently seal a single-strand gap in a DNA double helix. To test for an A/G change by OLA, two oligonucleotides are hybridized to the test DNA. One has its 3′ end at the variable position, the other has its 5′ end at the next nucleotide. DNA ligase will join the two if they perfectly match the test strand, but not if either of the two end nucleotides to be linked is not correctly base-paired with the test DNA. The oligonucleotides are subsequently isolated and checked for size to see whether a ligation product is present. OLA has been developed commercially as a convenient kit for checking for a panel of specific sequence changes in a single operation. *Figure 5.6* shows the principle.

The choice of method depends to a large extent on how many samples require the test. Allele-specific oligonucleotides and oligonucleotides for OLA have to be custom-synthesized. This makes those methods unattractive for a one-off test. Primers for allele-specific PCR also have to be custom-synthesized, but this is less of an extra expense because whatever technique is used, primers for PCR amplification will be needed. Restriction enzyme digestion is simple in principle, but if the particular sequence change requires the use of an unusual enzyme

Figure 5.5 – Principle of allele-specific PCR reaction.
A PCR reaction will not yield product if the 3′-most nucleotide of a primer is not correctly base-paired. Mismatches elsewhere in the primer sequence may be tolerated, but the 3′ end must match. One primer (not shown, off to the left) is standard; the second primer is specific for one allele of a T/A single nucleotide polymorphism (green). Two reactions are set up, one using the common plus T-specific primers, the other using the common plus A-specific primers. See *Figures 5.10* and *5.13* for examples.

Figure 5.6 – Using the oligonucleotide ligation assay to genotype a C/T variant.
DNA ligase can only seal the gap between the two abutting oligonucleotides if the two ends are correctly base-paired with a template strand. One oligonucleotide is labeled with a fluorescent dye, and after the ligation reaction the size of the labeled product is measured on a DNA sequencer. OLA tests can be multiplexed by designing oligonucleotides to give different sized ligation products, and/or by labeling them with different fluorescent dyes.

this can be expensive. Also, not all changes create or remove a restriction site. Pyrosequencing is a good general method for testing many samples, but it requires expensive special equipment.

Methods for scanning a gene for any sequence change

The most common task for a diagnostic DNA laboratory is to check the entire sequence of a gene for any possible mutation. Increasingly, the laboratory will simply sequence every exon and splice junction of the gene. Sequencing provides the gold standard for such mutation scanning – but it is not the method of choice in every case. Although costs are falling, it is still a relatively expensive technique. Skill and good quality DNA are needed to get results clear enough to detect heterozygotes reliably. The structure of genes also makes scanning by sequencing relatively inefficient. Individual human exons average only 145 bp, well below the 400–800 bp that can be read in one sequencing run. But most introns are too large to allow more than one exon to be amplified from genomic DNA as a single PCR product. Thus testing a gene usually involves a separate PCR reaction and sequencing run for each exon. For a gene like fibrillin (see Case 10, Johnson family) with 66 exons, this is a lot of work. Studying mRNA by RT–PCR would solve that problem (see *Chapter 4*), but RNA is hard to handle, and obtaining it may be excessively invasive (what if the relevant gene is expressed only in the brain?).

For these reasons, a variety of other methods are used as adjuncts to sequencing. These perform a quick scan of a DNA fragment such as a PCR-amplified exon, and report whether its sequence differs in any way from the normal version. Using these can save time and money. The commonest methods are based on either of two principles:

- *Properties of heteroduplexes.* If a person is heterozygous for a sequence variant in an exon, PCR amplification of the exon will give a mix of the mutant and normal sequences. If the mix is heated to denature the DNA and then slowly cooled, some of the resulting double helices will be **heteroduplexes**, containing one strand from each of the two alleles.

Heteroduplexes have bulges or kinks compared to perfectly matched DNA (*Figure 5.7a*). This makes them run slower through an electrophoretic gel than the corresponding homoduplexes. Their presence can be revealed as extra bands on the gel. Heteroduplexes also denature more easily than

(a)

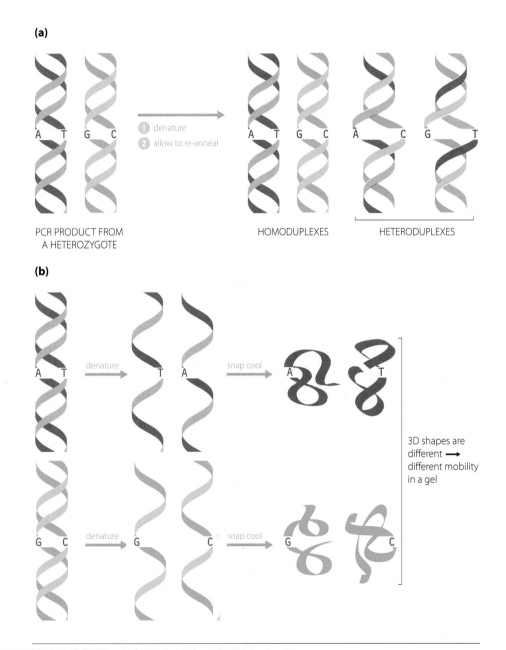

(b)

Figure 5.7 – Two techniques for mutation scanning.
(a) Heteroduplexes are formed when the PCR product from a heterozygous person is heated then allowed to renature. Heteroduplexes can be detected by their slower rate of migration on an electrophoretic gel, or by their lower denaturation temperature on a denaturing high-performance liquid chromatography column. (b) Single-stranded DNA adopts a conformation that depends on its sequence. Samples from people with different sequence variants may fold in different, though unpredictable, ways and have different mobilities in a gel. A real example is shown in *Figure 5.11*.

fully matched duplexes. This can be noted in various ways, for example, by their altered mobility on a <u>d</u>enaturing <u>h</u>igh-<u>p</u>erformance <u>l</u>iquid <u>c</u>hromatography (dHPLC) column. dHPLC is widely used when the same sequence needs to be tested in a large number of samples.

- *Properties of single-stranded DNA*. Single-stranded DNA ties itself into knots as bases in different parts of the strand pair with each other. The precise shape of the knot depends on the sequence, and affects the rate at which the knot migrates through an electrophoretic gel. <u>S</u>ingle <u>s</u>trand <u>c</u>onformation <u>p</u>olymorphism (SSCP) analysis looks for any differences between the migration of the test sequence and a normal sequence (*Figures 5.7b* and *5.11*). Compared to dHPLC, SSCP requires no expensive equipment and is simple to set up, but probably misses more mutations (claimed sensitivity is 80–90%). It is particularly useful for testing small numbers of samples.

Laboratories often use these or similar methods for a preliminary scan of each exon of a gene. Any exon showing a departure from the normal version is then sequenced. Compared to simply sequencing every exon, this two-stage approach saves the cost and labor of sequencing the normal exons. However, none of these methods picks up 100% of the changes in a sequence, and as the cost of sequencing keeps falling, the use of these alternatives is diminishing.

Methods for detecting deletion or duplication of whole exons

As described in *Chapter 3* (*Figure 3.9*), large deletions or duplications in genomic DNA usually cause deletion or duplication of whole exons. Exons form only a very small part of the whole human genome sequence, so a random breakpoint is unlikely to fall within an exon. Even if the breakpoint is within a gene, it is much more likely to be within an intron than an exon. In a heterozygous person, a deletion or duplication of one or more whole exons would not be detected using any of the methods described above. For example, Judith Davies (Case 4) is heterozygous for a deletion of several exons of the dystrophin gene. But if we individually PCR-amplified each exon of her dystrophin gene, the appropriate sequence would amplify from her normal X chromosome, and the PCR product would appear entirely normal by any of the tests described above. Special techniques are needed to detect whole exon deletions or duplications.

- *Quantitative PCR* was described in *Chapter 4*. When major life decisions hang on the result of a single test, as with the at-risk females in the Davies family (Case 4), a very accurate and reliable test is essential. Various commercial systems using real-time quantitative PCR are used most often.
- *Multiplex ligation-dependent probe amplification (MLPA)* uses the specificity of the OLA (*Figure 5.6*) to increase the accuracy of simple quantitative PCR. *Figure 5.8* shows the principle and *Figure 5.9* an example. MLPA has rapidly gained acceptance in genetic diagnostic laboratories due to its simplicity compared to other methods, relatively low cost, capacity for reasonably high throughput and perceived

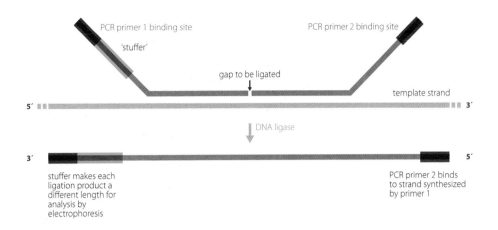

PCR primer 1 binding site

'stuffer'

PCR primer 2 binding site

gap to be ligated

template strand

5′ ━━ ━ ━━━ ━ ━ ━ 3′

↓ DNA ligase

3′ ━━━━━━━━━━━━━━━━━━━━━━━━━━━━━━━━━━━━━ 5′

stuffer makes each
ligation product a
different length for
analysis by
electrophoresis

PCR primer 2 binds
to strand synthesized
by primer 1

Figure 5.8 – Principle of the multiplex ligation-dependent probe amplification (MLPA) method for detecting deletions or duplications.
Each probe consists of a pair of oligonucleotides that can be ligated only if their matching sequence is present in the test sample, as in the oligonucleotide ligation assay (*Figure 5.6*). After ligation the mixed probes are PCR-amplified using a single pair of primers that hybridize to sequences present on the ends of every probe pair. Only ligated molecules can be amplified because only they possess both primer sites. One of the primers is fluorescently labeled, and the reaction mix is analyzed on a fluorescence DNA sequencing machine. Each probe has an amplification product of different length, giving a unique peak on the sequencer trace.

robustness. MLPA is a multiplex procedure, testing up to 45 short (typically 60 bp) sequences simultaneously for copy number variation. This makes it well suited to checking a large multi-exon gene for any whole exon deletion, but equally it could be used to test selected exons from several different genes. Establishing a new MLPA assay is time-consuming because each individual probe needs to be carefully designed, so it is mostly used for frequently investigated genes, where probe sets are commercially available. MLPA probes are expensive because they are much longer than normal PCR primers, but overall the technique is cheaper than most alternatives.

Figure 5.9 – An example of MLPA.
Each peak is the amplified ligation product for one exon of a gene. The upper trace shows a copy-number reduction in three peaks, corresponding to three probe pairs. Reproduced with permission from MRC-Holland.

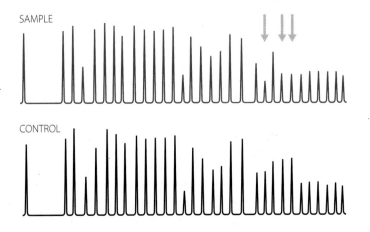

SAMPLE

CONTROL

5.3. **Investigations of patients**

The stories so far...

Table 5.1 summarizes the achievements and requirements for testing in the cases described so far. This section describes the further tests performed on Cases 2, 6 and 14, which illustrate the various techniques described above.

Table 5.1 – **Summary of testing performed to date in the cases featured, and further tests required.**

Case	Problem	Tests so far	Tests needed
1	Huntington disease	Size of expansion checked by PCR	None needed
2	Cystic fibrosis		**Check *CFTR* gene for mutations**
3	Deafness		Identify gene and mutation (see *Chapter 9*)
4	Duchenne muscular dystrophy	Deletion of exons 44–48 defined by PCR	None needed
5	Chromosomal translocation	Identified by karyotyping	None needed
6	Leber's hereditary optic neuropathy		**Check for mitochondrial mutation**
7	? Deletion of 22q11	Deletion confirmed by FISH	None needed
8	Down syndrome	Confirmed by karyotyping. Prenatal test by FISH	None needed
9	Turner syndrome	Confirmed by karyotyping. Check for Y sequences by PCR	None needed
10	Marfan syndrome		Molecular testing not undertaken – clinical diagnosis suffices
11	Sickle cell disease	Prenatal test using allele-specific oligonucleotides	None needed
12	Hemophilia	Check for inversion by Southern blot	None needed
13	? Chromosomal abnormality	Check for chromosomal imbalances by array-CGH; check if it is *de novo*	No further routine investigation
14	β-thalassemia		**Identify mutation**

CASE 2	Brown family	2	8	65	**126**	151	279	376

- Girl aged 6 months, parents David and Pauline
- ? cystic fibrosis
- Order molecular test?
- Define mutations in *CFTR* gene

David and Pauline indicated that they might consider having more children in the future but would definitely wish for prenatal tests because they felt that coping with the extra needs of one child with cystic fibrosis was as much as they could do. Before that could be done, it would be necessary to define both mutations in Joanne. Additionally, after discussion at family reunions, other members of the large extended family became concerned about their own carrier risk and several relatives expressed a desire for carrier testing. Again, this has to be done by checking for the mutations present in Joanne. Although over 1000 different mutations in the *CFTR* gene have been described in cystic fibrosis patients, most of these have been seen only in one or a very few cases. A small number of mutations are relatively common. Mutation testing in cystic fibrosis therefore starts by checking for these common mutations. Several commercial kits are available for this purpose. Joanne's DNA was screened using a multiplex allele-specific PCR assay (see *Figure 5.5* for the principle). The result (*Figure 5.10*) shows that she has the p.F508del mutation (see *Box 5.2* for a brief explanation of this nomenclature – though this one is often called by the non-standard name delta-F508). This mutation is the commonest cystic fibrosis mutation in Northern Europeans, comprising 70–80% of all cystic fibrosis mutations in many populations.

Figure 5.10 – A multiplex allele-specific PCR test for 29 common *CFTR* mutations.
The same seven samples are amplified with different cocktails of primers in the two gels. No mutation is detected in lanes 3 or 4. Extra bands in the other lanes define particular mutations by their presence and size. Courtesy of Victoria Stinton and Roger Mountford, Liverpool Women's Hospital.

Joanne is heterozygous for the p.F508del mutation because the test shows that she also has the corresponding normal allele. No second mutation was detected. Given her diagnosis she should have a second mutation, but it might be anywhere in the gene. Rather than immediately sequencing all 27 exons of the *CFTR* gene, the laboratory PCR-amplified each exon and used the SSCP method (see *Figure 5.7b*) to identify exons containing sequence variants. The result (*Figure 5.11*) showed that something was different in exons 3 and 14b in Joanne's DNA compared to a normal control. Either or both of these may well be non-pathogenic sequence variants. (For historical reasons the 27 exons of the gene are numbered 1–5, 6a, 6b, 7–13, 14a, 14b, 15, 16, 17a, 17b, 18–24 in the main mutation database).

Figure 5.12 shows one of the sequencer traces, with a control for comparison. The following changes were identified:

- exon 3   c.368G>A
- exon 14b   c.2752–15C>G

In *Chapter 6* we will see how the laboratory attempted to decide whether either of these changes was likely to be pathogenic.

(a)

(b)

Figure 5.11 – SSCP analysis of exons of the CFTR gene.
Each exon was amplified in separate PCR reactions from each of a series of samples from cystic fibrosis patients. Results from exons 3 (a) and 14b (b) are shown. In Joanne's sample the products (lane 4 on each gel) show a different band pattern from the other samples, indicating that they have some difference in their sequence. The samples in lanes 2 and 3 (from other cystic fibrosis patients) also show abnormalities in exon 3. It is then necessary to sequence (*Figure 5.12*) in order to identify the change and decide whether it is pathogenic. Using this procedure reduced the sequencing requirement for Joanne from 27 to 2 exons.

A T G G A A C A A N A C A C A G T T G A T

Figure 5.12 – DNA sequencer trace of part of the exon 14b PCR product from Joanne Brown's CFTR gene.
At the arrowed position G and C nucleotides are both present, showing that Joanne is heterozygous for a nucleotide substitution (remember that the products of PCR and sequencing are normally a mix of the products from the two alleles). Control samples show only the G. It is usual to sequence both strands of the DNA separately to confirm any change. In this case the sequence shown is of the reverse strand, so in the sense strand the change in Joanne is C>G.

Box 5.2

A brief guide to nomenclature of mutations

A mutation can be described in terms of the change in the genomic DNA, the cDNA or the encoded protein. The description is prefixed with g., c., or p. according to which of these it describes.

For DNA, > means 'changes to'. Thus G>A means the normal G is replaced by an A nucleotide. Deletions and insertions are symbolized by del and ins respectively. The affected nucleotide is numbered from an agreed starting point and database file. For cDNA, nucleotides are counted from the A of the AUG start codon. A nucleotide in an intron is given the number of the last nucleotide of the preceding exon, a plus sign and the position in the intron, such as c.77+1, c.77+32, etc. If it is near the end of a large intron it may be given the number of the first nucleotide of the following exon, a minus sign and the position (*Tables 5.2* and *11.1* show examples). For genomic DNA, the start nucleotide position must be specified.

For protein level changes the one-letter or three-letter amino acid abbreviations are used (see *Box 3.6*). X means a stop codon. Amino acids are counted from the initiator methionine of the protein (even though this is usually removed in post-translational processing).

Examples:

c.76A>C means that at nucleotide 76 an A is changed to a C
c.76–78del means a deletion of 3 nucleotides, from nucleotides 76 to 78 inclusive
p.Ala26Val or p.A26V means that amino acid alanine-26 is changed to a valine
p.Cys318X or p.C318X means the codon for cysteine 318 is changed to a stop codon

This level of detail is sufficient for understanding everything in this book. Nomenclature has been defined for describing every possible sequence variation. You can find full details at the Human Genome Variation Society website,
http://www.genomic.unimelb.edu.au/mdi/mutnomen/

| CASE 14 | Nicolaides family | 115 | **129** | 153 | 376 |

- ? β-thalassemia carriers
- Check mutations

Hemoglobinopathies are the most intensively studied of all genetic diseases, and rightly so, because they affect millions of people in many countries. Children homozygous for β-thalassemia have a difficult life. They require endless blood transfusions, but then have major problems with iron overload. Among Greek Cypriots, it has been estimated that one person in seven is a carrier of β-thalassemia. Thus we would expect one in 49 marriages to be between carriers. This has triggered a national population screening program. The reasons why hemoglobinopathies are so remarkably common in some populations are discussed in *Chapter 10*. Carrier testing is carried out using routine hematological methods. This indicated that both Spiros and Elena were carriers, though entirely healthy in themselves. They were offered molecular tests to identify their precise mutations, and because they thought they might wish for prenatal diagnosis in any pregnancy, they took up the offer. It was better to do it now, when there was no urgency, than to wait until Elena was pregnant and require urgent testing.

Spiros and Elena each provided a mouthwash sample from which DNA was extracted. Five specific mutations in the β-globin gene make up 98.4% of all β-thalassemia mutations among Greek Cypriots (*Table 5.2*). Their DNA was therefore first tested for each of these mutations. Had the results been negative, their β-globin genes would have been sequenced to look for the mutations. Because the β-globin gene is small (3 exons and 2 introns; only about 1500 bp in total), it can be a routine procedure to sequence the exons, introns and promoter to check for mutations.

Table 5.2 – **Common β-thalassemia mutations among Greek Cypriots**

Mutation	Percentage of all β-thalassemia mutations in Greek Cypriots	Sequence change: (normal, mutant)
c.93–21G>A	79.8	ctatt**g**gt ctattttccc ctatt**a**gt ctattttccc
c.92+6T>C	5.5	AGgttgg**t**at AGgttgg**c**at
c.92+1G>A	5.1	AG**g**ttggtat AG**a**ttggtat
c.316–106C>G	5.1	cag**c**taccat cag**g**taccat
p.Gln39X	2.9	TGGACC<u>**C**AG</u>AGGTTC TGGACC<u>**T**AG</u>AGGTTC

Exon sequences are in upper case, intron sequences in lower case. All but the last of these mutations are in an intron of the β-globin gene. See *Box 5.1* for the nomenclature of mutations and *Chapter 6* for discussion of how these mutants cause disease. Data from HbVar database (http://globin.cse.psu.edu/globin/hbvar).

Neither of them carried the most common Cypriot mutation, c.93–21G>A, so the DNA was then checked for the other four common mutations. Spiros turned out to be carrying the p.Gln39X mutation while Elena carried the c.316–106C>G mutation. All these mutations could be checked by sequencing, allele-specific PCR or hybridization to allele-specific oligonucleotides; the c.316–106C>G mutation also creates a restriction site for the enzymes *Rsa*I (GTAC) and *Kpn*I (GGTACC). A convenient general method would be a **reverse dot blot**, in which a panel of allele-specific oligonucleotides is spotted onto a nitrocellulose filter, which is then hybridized to dye-labeled product of PCR–amplifying the patient's β-globin genes. *Figures 5.13* and *5.14* illustrate the use of different methods for detecting these mutations.

C-specific primer   3′ GTTTCCAAGAAACTCAGGAAACC 5′
5′ GGACC<u>C</u>AGAGGTTCTTTGAGTCCTTTGGGGATCTGTCCAC 3′

5′ GGACC<u>T</u>AGAGGTTCTTTGAGTCCTTTGGGGATCTGTCCAC 3′
T-specific primer   3′ ATTTCCAAGAAACTCAGGAAACC 5′

Figure 5.13 – Identification of the p.Gln39X mutation by allele-specific PCR.
The C>T change converts a codon for glutamine (CAG) into a stop codon (TAG). The C-specific and T-specific primers are used with a common primer that hybridizes to a sequence to the left of the region shown. A deliberate mismatch at position 3 of each primer increases the specificity of the reaction.

	KpnI site	undigested PCR product	*KpnI*-digested PCR product
normal sequence	absent	406 nt	406 nt
c. 316–106 C>G	present	406 nt	300 + 106 nt

Figure 5.14 – Identification of the c.316–106C>G mutation.
The mutation creates a *KpnI* restriction site (GGTACC) in intron 2 of the β-globin gene. A suitable size fragment including the mutation site is PCR amplified and the product incubated with the restriction enzyme.

CASE 6	Fletcher family	5	12	67	**131**	152	376

- Frank, aged 22, with increasingly blurred eyesight
- Family history of visual difficulties
- Pedigree suggests X-linked recessive inheritance but not conclusive
- ? LHON
- Order blood test to check for mutation in mtDNA
- Check mutations by Pyrosequencing

LHON (OMIM 535000) is the result of inadequate function of the mitochondria, caused by mutations in the mitochondrial DNA (mtDNA). Confirming the diagnosis in Frank depends on demonstrating the presence of a mutation. The molecular genetics of LHON is quite complicated. Eighteen different point mutations in the mtDNA have been associated with this one disease. Presumably there are many ways in which mitochondrial function can be impaired, leading to the disease. Five of the 18 have a sufficiently serious effect to cause LHON by themselves; the others are found in combination with each other and presumably the disease is caused by an accumulation of smaller effects.

Three point mutations cause the great majority of cases, at least in people of European origin (we use the usual mtDNA nomenclature here):

- G11778A – substitution of A for G at nucleotide 11778 of the 16.5 kb mitochondrial genome. This results in replacement of arginine 340 by histidine in the ND4 protein that is part of the oxidative phosphorylation machinery.
- G3460A – the G→A nucleotide change replaces alanine 52 in the ND1 protein with tyrosine.
- T14484C – this nucleotide substitution causes methionine 64 in the ND6 protein to be replaced by valine.

The usual diagnostic procedure is first to test for these three specific mutations. If none is present, then a wider search is needed, which may include sequencing parts of the mtDNA.

Any of the methods described previously could be used for checking for the common mutations. *Figure 5.15* shows a restriction enzyme-based method for the G11778A mutation. An alternative method uses Pyrosequencing (*Figure 5.16*). This has the advantage that the result is quantitative. As explained in *Chapter 1*, people can be homoplasmic or heteroplasmic for mitochondrial mutations, so a full mutation test includes checking the relative amounts of normal and mutant mitochondria. The result showed that Frank was homoplasmic for the G3460A mutation, thus confirming the diagnosis of LHON.

		SEQUENCE		FRAGMENT SIZES	
				*Sfa*NI	*Mae*III
	11770	11780	11790		
normal	CGAACGCACT	CACAGTCGCA	TCATAATCCT	417 + 91	233 + 218 +57
	11770	11780	11790		
G11778A	CGAACGCACT	CACAGTCACA	TCATAATCCT	508	233 + 131 + 87 + 57

Figure 5.15 – Detecting the G11778A mutation by its effect on restriction enzyme recognition sites.
The mutation abolishes a site for the enzyme *Sfa*NI (GCATC) but creates one for the enzyme *Mae*III (GTNAC, where N is any nucleotide). The assay shown here involves PCR amplifying a 508 bp portion of the mtDNA that includes nucleotide 11778. Separate samples of the PCR product are digested with the two enzymes and the fragments sized on an electrophoretic gel. Restriction sites are underlined, the changed nucleotide is highlighted in color and the sizes of fragments are shown.

5.4. **Summary and extension**

The three questions

The feasibility and methodology of mutation testing depends crucially on the precision of the question being asked. Consider these three possible questions:

(1) Does Joanne Brown (Case 2) have any mutation in any gene that would account for her condition?
(2) Does Joanne Brown have any mutation in the *CFTR* gene?
(3) Does Joanne Brown have the p.F508del mutation in the *CFTR* gene?

Question (3) is quick and cheap to answer, using any of the methods described in the section on detecting specific sequence changes. That section also describes the circumstances under which it is possible to ask such a specific question.

Question (1) is not answerable at present. In the next 10 years technical advances may make it possible to sequence every gene in a person, or even a person's whole genome, so easily and cheaply that it will become a routine procedure. Even so, it is not likely that having somebody's complete genome sequence would allow the geneticist to answer such an unfocused question. There are just too many individual differences between genomes. Most human characteristics depend on combinations of several, maybe many, variants. Getting enough knowledge to predict the effect of any combination of any of several million variants might eventually be possible, but is certainly not likely to happen soon.

Question (2) is always answerable in principle but the cost depends on the total number of exons to be screened. For **Nasreen Choudhary (Case 3)** there were over 50 known candidate deafness genes, totalling many hundreds of exons. Mutation screening was not feasible until the field could be narrowed down to one or a few genes. How this was done in that particular case is described in

Figure 5.16 – Detection of the G3460A mtDNA mutation by Pyrosequencing.
The Pyrosequencing machine tries adding each nucleotide in turn to the end of a primer. Successful addition triggers a bioluminescent reaction, recorded by the machine as a peak. Upper trace: mutant sequence GTGTCA; lower trace: normal control GCGTCA (the sequences are of the reverse strand).

Chapter 9. For Joanne Brown (Case 2) there is only a single candidate gene: cystic fibrosis is always caused by mutations in the *CFTR* gene. Testing that whole gene would still involve testing 27 exons. How far a laboratory will go in trying to answer question (2) depends on how much expense could be justified by the clinical importance of the answer. Increasing automation, and the use of some of the technologies described below, are rapidly increasing the size of mutation screen that a diagnostic laboratory can undertake for a given cost.

Mutation detection using chips

Microarrays ('DNA chips') offer a way of performing a large number of hybridization tests in parallel. As described in *Chapter 4*, microarrays consist of hundreds up to hundreds of thousands of different DNA probes anchored to

Long QT syndrome

It has long been recognized that sudden death can occur in apparently healthy young people without there being any clue on post-mortem examination as to why the tragedy happened. Occasionally more than one person in a family is affected. In recent years two main groups of conditions have been recognized that cause sudden adult death without obvious signs on post-mortem: Long QT syndromes and cardiomyopathies. In the latter group there may be preceding symptoms and, in some individuals, obvious hypertrophy at post-mortem. However, some individuals may have no symptoms and histological signs detected only by experts in the field.

Long QT syndromes are characterized by ECG abnormalities (*Figure 1*). These consist of QT prolongation (indicating prolonged or disordered ventricular repolarization) and T-wave abnormalities associated with a tendency to tachycardia (rapid beating of the heart) which may cause syncope (fainting). Twitching occurring during the syncope may lead to the misdiagnosis of epilepsy. Often these episodes self-terminate, but they can progress to ventricular fibrillation where the heart ceases to pump blood effectively and sudden death occurs. In 10–20% of all cases of drowning, Long QT or other genetic pro-arrhythmic conditions may be the cause (see Choi *et al.*, 2004). Long QT syndrome may also explain some cases of Sudden Infant Death Syndrome.

(a)

QRS T WAVE

QT INTERVAL

(b)

Figure 1 – (a) the QT interval and (b) part of an exercise electrocardiogram showing a long QT interval (535 ms). Courtesy of Dr Kay Metcalfe, St Mary's Hospital, Manchester.

Families have been described where the condition is compatible with dominant inheritance but others are reported where affected individuals have sensorineural deafness and autosomal recessive inheritance. The dominant types (*Figure 2*) are collectively called Romano–Ward syndrome (OMIM 192500) and the recessive types Jervell and Lange–Nielsen syndrome (JLN; OMIM 220400). JLN-affected individuals have profound sensorineural hearing loss and a long QT interval. Half of those untreated die before the age of 15 years.

The underlying problem is a malfunction of one or another of the ion channels that are important for regulating cardiac rhythm. Linkage studies revealed that both Romano–Ward and JLN syndromes are heterogeneous, with different loci implicated in different families. Mutations have been found that implicate the following ion channel genes.

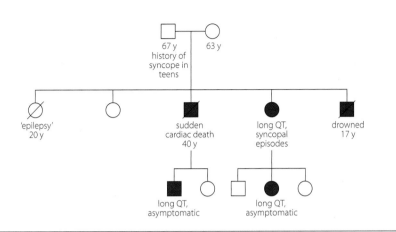

Figure 2 – A typical pedigree of a family in which dominant Long QT syndrome is segregating.

- *KCNQ1* and *KCNE1* – these encode components of the IKs potassium channel. Romano–Ward patients can be heterozygous and JLN patients homozygous for mutations in either gene. Syncope and sudden death are particularly triggered by physical exertion, especially swimming.
- *KCNH2* and *KCNE2* – these encode components of the IKr potassium channel. Heterozygous mutations in either gene have been described in some Romano–Ward patients. Emotional excitement or loud noise (especially noises that wake somebody up) are the commonest triggers of sudden death.
- *SCN5A* – encodes a cardiac sodium channel. Heterozygous mutations have been described in some Romano–Ward patients. Death most commonly occurs during quiet rest or sleep.

In *Chapter 6* we discuss the reason why mutations in *KCNQ1* and *KCNE1* can cause either of these syndromes, with different modes of inheritance. Up to 30% of families do not have a detectable mutation in any of these genes. The genotype–phenotype relationship is further complicated by the fact that an apparently separate condition, Brugada syndrome (OMIM 601144) can be caused by mutations in *SCN5A*. In this condition, ventricular fibrillation and sudden death occur but the ECG abnormalities are different (resembling right bundle branch block with variable ST segment elevation), or they may be absent without provocation.

After a catastrophic event such as sudden death, particularly in a young person, close relatives are usually anxious. Screening and genetic counseling can provide reassurance and help these individuals cope with the risk of sudden death. A detailed family history should be taken, particularly noting a history of syncope or unexplained 'seizures'. First degree relatives should be assessed for evidence of Long QT syndrome. It is highly desirable to identify a causative mutation, so that at-risk relatives can be clearly identified and those not at risk reassured. Treatment for all the Long QT syndrome disorders is directed at avoiding known precipitating factors, reducing the tendency to tachycardia by the use of beta-blocker medication, and, for some, the use of implantable cardioverter defibrillators. Knowledge of the specific mutation may enable anticipatory guidance about avoiding specific precipitating factors. However, because any one of several genes may be involved, molecular diagnosis encounters similar problems to those for families with deafness (see **Case 3, Choudhary family**).

5.6. **Self-assessment questions**

(1) For each of the following sequence changes or effects, choose possible testing methods from the list below that could be used to check for the presence of the change or effect (more than one method may be appropriate in many cases).
- A point mutation in any of the 26 exons of the *F8* gene
- Duplication of exons 50–54 of the dystrophin gene in a boy with Duchenne muscular dystrophy
- Expansion of the $(CAG)_n$ repeat in the *SCA3* gene in a woman suspected of having Machado–Joseph disease
- Identifying a small additional 'marker' chromosome seen in a dysmorphic baby
- Insertion of 4 nucleotides in exon 7 of the dystrophin gene in the sister of a boy known to have this mutation
- Deletion of any of 20 exons of the dystrophin gene in a boy with Duchenne muscular dystrophy
- An A>G mutation in exon 4 of the *OCRL* gene
- Deletion of any of 20 exons of the dystrophin gene in the mother of a boy who died of Duchenne muscular dystrophy
- A 1.5 Mb deletion at 7q11.23 in a child suspected of having Williams–Beuren syndrome
- Lack of expression in lymphocytes of an apparently intact gene that is normally expressed in these cells
- Deletion of exons 5–6 of a gene on chromosome 15 in a mentally retarded boy
- A point mutation anywhere (exons or introns) in the β-globin gene

Possible methods:
- Karyotyping
- FISH
- Array-CGH
- Southern blotting
- Northern blotting
- Multiplex ligation-dependent probe amplification
- PCR – check for presence / absence of product
- PCR – size product
- PCR – sequence product
- PCR – check for restriction digestion of product
- Allele-specific PCR
- Reverse transcriptase–PCR
- SSCP (single-strand conformation polymorphism)
- Hybridization to allele-specific oligonucleotide
- Sanger sequencing
- Pyrosequencing

(2) For each of the following tests, note whether it uses a property of single-stranded or double-stranded DNA:

- Checking for heteroduplexes by gel mobility
- Dot-blotting with an allele-specific oligonucleotide
- Conformation-sensitive gel electrophoresis
- Checking for creation / abolition of a restriction site
- Allele-specific PCR
- Denaturing high-performance liquid chromatography
- Sequencing using a microarray
- FISH

(3) The restriction enzyme *Eco*RI cuts the sequence GAATTC. Part of the coding sequence of a certain gene reads as follows:

```
CAA  AAC  CTC  AAG  TCA  ACG  AGT  TCG  GTA  ACG  TAC
Gln  Asn  Leu  Lys  Ser  Thr  Ser  Ser  Val  Thr  Tyr
```

This part of the gene is PCR amplified from DNA of a patient with a disease that is often caused by mutations in this gene. It is noted that the PCR product, which in normal people is not cut by *Eco*RI, is now cut into two fragments. Assuming the mutation changes a single nucleotide in the segment shown, identify it.

Chapter 6

What do mutations do?

Learning points for this chapter

After working through this chapter you should be able to:

- Describe and identify silent, mis-sense, nonsense and frameshift changes in coding sequences and splice site mutations
- Use a table of the genetic code to define the effect on the gene product of a change within a coding sequence
- Explain and give examples of loss of function, gain of function, haplo-insufficiency, dominant negative effects, nonsense-mediated decay and dosage sensitivity
- Discuss how far genotype–phenotype correlations can be established
- List ways in which a change in non-coding DNA may affect expression of a gene

6.1. Case studies

| CASE 15 | O'Reilly family | **141** | 154 | 376 |

- Family history of myopia and hip problems
- Orla has severe myopia, is short, and has hip problems
- ? Stickler syndrome

Orla O'Reilly, who is married to Raymond, has worn glasses for severe myopia since she was a young child. She is also only 4′ 11″ (150 cm) tall. Her brother Oliver is also short and myopic and he was born with a cleft palate. He also wears hearing aids. They take after their father who is short and stocky and has recently needed bilateral hip replacements; when he was 35 years old he underwent surgery for a retinal detachment in one eye, and laser treatment to prevent a detachment in the other eye. Orla went for a medical check for an insurance policy and mentioned that she had been getting some hip pain. The doctor doing the medical had just been on a genetics course and, after taking a family history, thought there might be a connection between Orla's and Oliver's medical problems and those of their father, so he referred her to the genetics clinic. There Orla had a detailed examination including an eye test which, in addition to the myopia, showed she had paravascular lattice retinopathy. The doctor also noted she had a short nose with a flat nasal bridge and rather knobbly joints. He told Orla he suspected she might have a condition called Stickler syndrome. This condition is due to mutations in genes encoding components of either type II or type XI collagen. See Snead and Yates (1999) for a review.

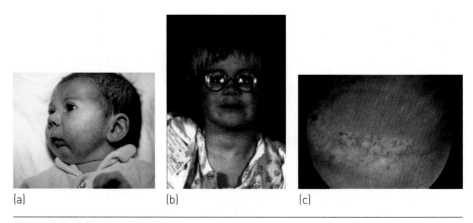

(a)　　　　　　　　　　　(b)　　　　　　　　　　　(c)

Figure 6.1 – (a) A baby with Stickler syndrome; note the small jaw (often associated with cleft palate) and rather flat face with prominent eyes. (b) Facial features of a 4-year-old child with Stickler syndrome. (c) Typical pigmented paravascular retinal lattice degeneration. (b) and (c) reproduced from Snead and Yates (1999) with permission from the BMJ Publishing Group.

6.2. **Background**

The word '**mutation**' can be used to describe either the event that produces a DNA sequence variant, or the resulting variant, whether produced then and there, or inherited maybe through many generations. In other words, it can describe the process or its product. Here we are using it to mean the product. Note, incidentally, that in genetic counseling the term 'mutation' is rarely used in discussion with patients, partly to avoid technical jargon but also because it has pejorative connotations (*mutants...*). A mutation may be described as a 'gene change', 'alteration', or 'fault'.

In the last two chapters we have seen some of the methods used to detect DNA sequence variants, and in some cases considered their effects, e.g. the large inversion in Case 12 (Lawton family) disrupts the *F8* gene. In this chapter we will look more systematically at the effects of sequence changes. There are two aspects to this:

- on the one hand we need to understand how a sequence change can affect the basic processes of transcription and translation
- on the other hand we want to think in terms of overall gene function
  – is there a loss of function or a gain of function, and how far does the genotype predict the phenotype?

In this section we will consider transcription and translation. If a protein-coding sequence is to function as proposed in the Central Dogma (*Figure 3.3*), a series of steps is necessary. Any of these steps might be affected by a mutation. *Box 6.1* summarizes the types of change discussed. *Section 6.3* provides a series of examples that lead on to a discussion of molecular pathology in the last section of the chapter, including loss and gain of function and the prospects for genotype-phenotype correlations. *Disease box 6* illustrates a particularly striking example of how loss, modification or gain of function in the same gene can produce a set of very different phenotypes.

Summary of types of mutation considered in this section

In terms of the DNA, mutations can be classified as:

- deletions of a whole gene
- duplications of a whole gene
- disruption of a gene by a chromosomal rearrangement
- deletions or duplications of one or more exons of a gene
- mutations in the promoter or other *cis*-acting regulatory sequence
- mutations that affect splicing by altering an existing splice site
- mutations that affect splicing by activating a cryptic splice site
- mutations that alter the triplet reading frame (frameshifts)
- mutations that introduce a premature stop codon (nonsense mutations)
- mutations that replace one amino acid in the protein with another (mis-sense mutations)
- mutations that alter one codon for an amino acid into another codon for the same amino acid (synonymous substitutions)

Alternatively, mutations can be classified as null or amorphic (no product is made, or there is no function), hypomorphic (too little product, or too little function) and hypermorphic (too much product or excessive function).

Deletion or duplication of a whole gene

These would be expected to decrease or increase the amount of gene product proportionally to the change in gene number, though this may be modified by feedback controls regulating the level of expression according to the need for the gene product. Not all deletions or duplications are pathogenic. It has recently become apparent that there is considerable variation among normal people in the copy number of some genes. Comparative genomic hybridization (*Figure 4.7*) has revealed unexpected large-scale copy number variants that are common and not evidently pathogenic. Other examples of common non-pathogenic duplications or deletions include the following.

- people vary in the number of tandemly repeated green color vision pigment genes on the X chromosome
- people vary in the number of beta-defensin genes at 8p23
- some major histocompatibility complex haplotypes at 6p21 (see *Chapter 8*) contain different numbers of HLA genes

For most genes, however, copy number changes are abnormal and often pathogenic. A gene is called **dosage-sensitive** if a 50% decrease or increase in copy number (having 1 or 3 copies of a gene that is normally present in 2 copies) causes a phenotypic change. Duplications are much less common than deletions and are less likely to be pathogenic (although chromosomal trisomies must produce their pathogenic effect through increased dosage of genes on the relevant chromosome – see *Section 6.4*).

Disruption of a gene

If a gene is disrupted by a chromosomal rearrangement the 5′ fragment of the gene retains the promoter and may still be transcribed, but there can be no production of the normal full-length transcript. The Factor VIII inversion that was found in Lennox Lawton (Case 12, see *Figure 4.12*) is an example. Stability of an mRNA is largely mediated by the 3′ untranslated region, and a partial mRNA is unlikely to be stable or to encode any product. Occasionally a chromosomal rearrangement may create a novel chimeric gene by bringing together exons of two different genes. Changes of this sort are important in cancer (see *Chapter 12*) and form a partial exception to the rule that disruptions prevent expression of a gene.

Mutations that affect the transcription of an intact coding sequence

Here we are concerned with **cis-acting** effects – specific effects of a DNA sequence change on an immediately adjacent gene. These are logically different from **trans-acting** effects where the causative mutations affect the expression of distant genes, often on different chromosomes. *Trans*-acting effects are normally the downstream consequence of a *cis*-acting event. We saw an example with ATRX (*Disease Box 2*). In that disease, mutations affecting a chromatin-remodeling complex caused changes in the expression of many genes. Similarly, mutations in genes encoding transcription factors can affect expression of many other genes. *Cis*-acting changes directly affect only the gene immediately adjacent to the changed sequence (or occasionally other genes nearby on the same chromosome), although changes in the expression of that gene may have all sorts of *trans*-acting downstream effects on other genes.

Promoter changes. An active initiation complex (see *Section 3.4*) must be assembled on the promoter, allowing RNA polymerase to make the primary transcript. Mutations that remove or alter binding sites for transcription factors can abolish, reduce or sometimes increase transcription of a gene. The gene product is normal, but present in the wrong quantity (or none may be produced), or it may be produced in the wrong tissue. Unfortunately, it is very difficult to predict the likely effect of a sequence change upstream of a gene. Programs are available that identify likely transcription factor binding sites – but these tend to report large numbers of possible binding sites, and they do not take account of the protein–protein interactions between the various factors, so they have limited predictive power.

The effect of promoter changes can be investigated in the laboratory using a so-called transient transfection assay. A gene whose activity is easily monitored (β-galactosidase is often used) is placed in a vector where its expression is governed by the promoter under investigation. The recombinant vector is introduced into a cell and the level of expression is measured. This can be compared to the level seen when the wild-type promoter is used. Transient transfection assays are valuable research tools, but their results must be viewed with great caution because the experimental system is quite artificial. Needless to say, such tests are not part of routine diagnostic investigations.

Changes in other regulatory sequences. As well as the promoter region, which lies immediately upstream of the transcription start site, *cis*-acting regulatory elements can be located much further away, and in either direction from the coding sequence. As mentioned in *Chapter 3* these are currently very poorly understood or cataloged. The ones we know about have been discovered by chance observations of deletions or chromosomal rearrangements that have breakpoints tens or hundreds of kilobases away from a gene and yet affect its expression. A large international collaborative project, the ENCODE project (Encyclopedia of DNA Elements, www.genome.gov/10005107) is trying to define all the regulatory elements in a 1% sample of the human genome, and ultimately across the entire genome. The main strategy is to look at non-coding sequences that are highly conserved across a range of organisms, the assumption being that sequence conservation implies sequence-specific function. Eventually ENCODE may provide the knowledge necessary to direct searches for long-range regulatory mutations – but at present we have only scattered examples.

In summary, regulatory mutations are hard to identify and characterize. They may have their main relevance in complex multifactorial disease (*Chapter 13*) where many susceptibility factors probably slightly change the expression level of an intact gene, rather than mendelian diseases, which tend to have mutations of large effect.

Mutations that affect splicing of the primary transcript

Abolition or modification of existing splice sites. Any change to the (almost) invariant GT...AG dinucleotides that mark the beginning and end of introns will prevent the affected site from being used. What the cell will do in response to this is hard to predict. The exon involved may be skipped, or sequence from the intron may be retained within the mature mRNA. Often some other nearby site is used as a replacement splice site, with consequent changes to the sequence of the mature mRNA. Other changes close to an exon–intron junction also often affect splicing, but less predictably. As mentioned in *Chapter 3* (*Figure 3.11*) GT...AG sequences only function as splice sites when they are embedded in a loosely defined consensus sequence. Additionally, correct functioning of a splice site depends on splicing enhancer or suppressor sequences nearby that bind components of the splicing machinery. Again these are not rigidly defined. Enhancers may be located in the intron near a splice site, but they may also lie in the exon. If a change within a coding sequence alters an exonic splicing enhancer, it may be pathogenic for reasons unconnected with any predicted amino acid sequence change. Two examples will illustrate these effects.

- Near the 3′ end of intron 8 of the *CFTR* gene is a run of T nucleotides. In different people there may be 5, 7 or 9 Ts. The 5T variant causes inefficient use of the nearby splice site; exon 9 is often skipped, leading to loss of function. The loss of function is only partial because a proportion of transcripts are correctly spliced. Thus the 5T variant is associated with mild and atypical forms of cystic fibrosis.
- Spinal muscular atrophy (SMA or Werdnig–Hoffmann disease, OMIM 253300) is caused by loss of function of the *SMN1* gene on 5q13. A

duplicate copy of the gene (*SMN2*) lies only 500 kb away on the same chromosome, and at first sight should be able to replace the function of the mutated gene. The two genes have only apparently insignificant sequence differences. One of these is a T>C change in exon 7, six nucleotides downstream of the 5′ splice site. The substitution apparently only replaces one phenylalanine codon with another (TTT>TTC). But in fact this change inactivates an exonic splicing enhancer, so that exon 7 is correctly spliced in only a very small minority of transcripts, and the *SMN2* gene is largely non-functional. Interestingly, some SMA patients have several copies of this gene. Although each one produces very little protein, together they make enough to render the disease in these patients milder and of later onset.

Creation of novel splice sites. Some sequence changes affect splicing by activation of a **cryptic splice site**. That is, there is a sequence that by chance has many of the features of a splice site, but is sufficiently different for the cell not to mistake it for a real splice site. A change may increase the resemblance to the point where the cell does start using it. The cryptic site can be either in an exon or an intron, as the following examples show.

• In hemoglobin E the β-globin gene has a G>A substitution 14 nucleotides upstream of the 3′ end of exon 1. This would be predicted to cause an amino acid substitution Glu26Lys. However, the pathogenic effect is on splicing. Changing this one nucleotide causes the changed sequence to be used as an alternative splice site. Transcripts that use this site are non-functional, and the effect is β-thalassemia.
• One cause of cystic fibrosis is a single base change c.3849+10kb C>T, 10 kb inside intron 19 of the *CFTR* gene. This activates a cryptic splice site, causing aberrant splicing and loss of function of the gene.

Changing the balance of splice isoforms. Rather than prevent production of any functional transcript, splicing mutations may simply alter the balance between isoforms. Many transcripts are subject to alternative splicing. The average number of different transcripts per locus found by the ENCODE project is 5.4 (although some of these are due to the use of alternative promoters and first exons, rather than to alternative splicing of a single transcript). If a change in a consensus splice sequence or a splicing enhancer changes the efficiency of a splice site, it may affect the balance of splice isoforms, and this may produce a phenotype. Again, such changes are more likely to act as susceptibility factors for common disease rather than mendelian disease mutations.

In summary, effects on splicing are widespread but, apart from changes to the invariant GT...AG dinucleotides, very hard to predict. Undoubtedly they are under-reported because they may only be recognized if mRNA is studied, rather than genomic DNA. Computer programs are available that try to predict the effect of a sequence change on splicing, but the results to date are indicative only.

Mutations that cause errors in translation

Effects on translation of a sequence change in a protein-coding sequence need to be considered in relation to the genetic code (*Table 6.1*).

Table 6.1 – **The genetic code**

1st base in codon	2nd base in codon				3rd base in codon
	U	**C**	**A**	**G**	
U	Phe	Ser	Tyr	Cys	**U**
	Phe	Ser	Tyr	Cys	**C**
	Leu	Ser	STOP	STOP	**A**
	Leu	Ser	STOP	Trp	**G**
C	Leu	Pro	His	Arg	**U**
	Leu	Pro	His	Arg	**C**
	Leu	Pro	Gln	Arg	**A**
	Leu	Pro	Gln	Arg	**G**
A	Ile	Thr	Asn	Ser	**U**
	Ile	Thr	Asn	Ser	**C**
	Ile	Thr	Lys	Arg	**A**
	Met	Thr	Lys	Arg	**G**
G	Val	Ala	Asp	Gly	**U**
	Val	Ala	Asp	Gly	**C**
	Val	Ala	Glu	Gly	**A**
	Val	Ala	Glu	Gly	**G**

Some amino acids such as serine and arginine have multiple codons, whereas tryptophan and methionine have only one each. AUG doubles as the initiator codon and as the codon for internal methionines. Note the three stop codons.

Frameshift mutations. Insertion or deletion of any number of nucleotides that is not a multiple of three produces a **frameshift mutation**. The effect is to change completely the reading of all the message downstream of the mutation (see *Box 3.3*). In principle, a completely novel polypeptide might be produced by translation of the frameshifted mRNA. Even if such a protein were produced, it would probably be unstable. Only a very small subset of all the myriad possible polypeptide chains can fold so as to produce a stable protein. Cells detect and degrade those that fail to fold correctly. More commonly, however, no novel polypeptide is produced. It is usually not long before the frameshifted message includes a stop codon. As explained below, mRNAs containing premature termination codons are normally degraded and do not produce protein. Thus one way or another, no protein is produced. *Figure 6.2* shows an example of a common frameshift mutation that produces a premature stop codon.

Whole exon deletions or duplications. When one or more complete exons of a gene are deleted or duplicated, the effect will partly depend on whether or not this produces a frameshift. Whole-exon deletions in the dystrophin gene provide a classic example. *Table 6.2* lists the sizes of the exons shown in *Figure 3.9*. Exons

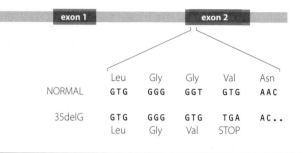

Figure 6.2 – The c.35delG mutation in the connexin 26 (*GJB2*) gene.
This gene is a frequent cause of autosomal recessive congenital deafness. One G
nucleotide out of a run of 6 Gs is deleted. Reading the frameshifted message the
ribosome quickly hits a stop codon. The *GJB2* gene has only two exons. Coding
sequence is shown in black; the colored parts of exons 1 and 2 encode the 5′ and 3′
untranslated regions of the mRNA. Diagram is not to scale.

41, 42, 47, 48 and 49 have exact multiples of three nucleotides. Deleting any one
of those exons will not cause a frameshift. The other exons have either one
nucleotide more than a multiple of three (+1) or one fewer (–1). Deleting any one
of these will cause a frameshift. The dystrophin protein is still partly functional
if an internal segment is missing or duplicated, but a frameshift will of course
completely wreck it. As a result, non-frameshifting deletions or duplications
cause a milder disease, Becker muscular dystrophy (BMD – OMIM 300376),
while frameshifting deletions or duplications (and other major mutations) cause
the severe Duchenne muscular dystrophy (DMD – OMIM 310200) as in Case 4
(Davies family). Because of the frameshift effect, deletions of several exons
can have a counter-intuitive effect: combining a lethal mutation with a second

Table 6.2 – Sizes of exons of the dystrophin gene

Exon	Size (bp)	Frame	Disease
41	183	0	BMD
42	195	0	BMD
43	173	–1	DMD
44	148	+1	DMD
45	176	–1	DMD
46	148	+1	DMD
47	150	0	BMD
48	186	0	BMD
49	102	0	BMD
50	109	+1	DMD

Deletions of exons produce the severe Duchenne muscular dystrophy (DMD) or the milder Becker
muscular dystrophy (BMD) depending whether or not the deletion produces a frameshift. See text
for further explanation.

lethal mutation can produce a non-lethal mutation. For example, deleting either exon 43 or 44 causes the severe DMD, yet somebody who has both these exons deleted has a frame-neutral deletion and will have the milder BMD.

Nonsense mutations. The three codons UAG, UAA and UGA in mRNA are stop codons (*Table 6.1*). A single nucleotide change that converts any other codon into a stop codon (TAG, TAA or TGA in the DNA) causes the ribosome to detach and protein synthesis to terminate at that point. Such mutations are called **nonsense mutations**. Contrary to common belief, mRNAs containing nonsense mutations do not normally produce truncated proteins. Cells have a very interesting mechanism (**nonsense-mediated decay**) for detecting and degrading mRNAs that contain premature termination codons (*Figure 6.3*). In some cases a certain amount of a truncated protein may be produced, but the usual effect of a nonsense mutation is the same as a complete deletion of the gene.

Nonsense-mediated decay probably evolved to protect cells against possibly toxic dominant negative effects of truncated proteins (see below). It presumably explains why the last exon of many genes is very large – you can't split the 3′ untranslated region between several exons. Some rather mystifying differences between the effects of nonsense mutations in different parts of the same gene are the result of nonsense-mediated decay operating in the red zone (*Figure 6.3*) but not in the green zone (see OMIM 602229 for an example). For further details see the review by Holbrook *et al.* (2004).

exon junction complex proteins

50 nt

5′   3′

STOP codons in this region trigger NMD

STOP codons in this region do not affect mRNA stability

Figure 6.3 – Nonsense-mediated decay.
When a spliced mRNA is exported from the nucleus to the cytoplasm certain components of the splicing machinery (the exon junction complex, EJC) remain attached to each splice site. As the first ribosome moves along the mRNA it displaces each EJC until it reaches the stop codon and detaches. If this happens in the red segment of the mRNA, one or more EJCs will remain in place. This triggers degradation of the mRNA. Thus mRNA molecules are only stable if the first stop codon lies within the green segment. Equally, nonsense mutations in the red segment are detected and no truncated protein is produced, but any mutation in the green zone is able to direct production of a truncated protein that may be pathogenic.

Mutations that cause amino acid substitutions

A single nucleotide change within a coding sequence will change one codon into another. Assuming the changed codon is not a stop codon, there are two possible results.

- *synonymous substitutions* are single-nucleotide changes that replace a codon with a different one that encodes the same amino acid – for example, a T>G change in the DNA that converts a UUU codon in the mRNA to UUC. Both code for phenylalanine.
- *Mis-sense mutations* replace one amino acid with another by changing a codon. Use *Table 6.1* to identify the effect of a codon change on the amino acid sequence.

It is important to remember, as mentioned above, that seemingly innocuous synonymous or mis-sense changes may have a major pathogenic effect by disrupting splicing.

Table 6.3 in *Section 6.4* gives a general guide to the likely effect of the various types of mutation.

6.3. Investigations of patients

Here we consider the molecular pathology of the mutations that have already been identified, as well as the investigation of Case 15 (O'Reilly family).

| CASE 1 | Ashton family | 1 | 7 | 65 | 104 | **150** | 376 |

- John – 28-year-old son of Alfred Ashton
- ? Huntington disease
- Other family members with similar symptoms
- Autosomal dominant inheritance shown in pedigree
- Diagnostic test ordered

The trinucleotide repeat expansion was described in *Chapter 4*. Formally this is an insertion in the coding sequence of the *HD* gene. The mutant gene is transcribed and translated. The expansion adds CAG triplets, thus it does not disrupt the reading frame. The protein product is the normal 3142 amino acid huntingtin protein with an expanded run of glutamines near the N-terminal end (CAG is a codon for glutamine). Affected people are normally heterozygotes, but rare homozygotes have been described and they are usually clinically indistinguishable from heterozygotes. This suggests that it is the presence of the mutant protein, rather than the absence of the normal protein, that is causing the problems. No Huntington disease patients have been described who have deletions, nonsense mutations or other changes in the gene. Additionally at least one person has been described who does not have Huntington disease despite having a chromosomal rearrangement that disrupts one copy of the Huntington disease gene. Together, these observations make clear that Huntington disease must be caused by a gain of function. The mutant protein is somehow toxic to neurons, especially in the striatum and caudate nucleus of the brain. Gradual cell death leads to the late-onset disease. Exactly why the mutant protein is toxic is controversial. It forms aggregates inside neurons but it is not clear that the aggregates are themselves harmful. More probably an intermediate in the aggregation process is toxic. The normal protein interacts with many other proteins – it probably functions as some sort of scaffold for assembling multiprotein complexes – making it very difficult to identify one key altered function.

| CASE 2 | Brown family | 2 | 8 | 65 | 126 | **151** | 279 | 376 |

- Girl (Joanne) aged 6 months, parents David and Pauline
- ? Cystic fibrosis
- Order molecular test?
- Define mutations in *CFTR* gene

Cystic fibrosis is a recessive disease caused by complete loss of function of the chloride channel encoded by the *CFTR* gene. Being affected, Joanne must have no functional copy of the gene (what matters is having no functional copy, rather than having two mutant copies, although of course normally these amount to the same thing). DNA testing (*Chapter 5*) revealed three sequence changes: c.368G>A in exon 3, p.508del in exon 10 and c.2752–15C>G in the exon 14b PCR product. Of these, p.F508del is very well understood, being by far the commonest mutation in Europeans with cystic fibrosis (see *Table 11.1*). The mutation is an in-frame deletion of three consecutive nucleotides in the coding sequence. A virtually full-length protein is produced with 1479/1480 correct amino acids – but the one missing amino acid affects the structure. The mutant protein is not correctly processed after synthesis, and fails to locate to the apical cell membrane where it is needed. The result is a complete loss of function (see *Table 6.4*). Joanne's other two mutations were not common and required further analysis. The exon 14b change was thought to be non-pathogenic for two reasons.

(1) The C>G change was in intron 14a, 15 nucleotides before the start of exon 14b. Intronic changes can sometimes be pathogenic by affecting splicing. This mutation did not have any features suggesting it might do so, but without RNA studies an effect on splicing could not be ruled out. However, in this case there was a second line of evidence:

(2) When DNA from Joanne's parents David and Pauline was checked, both the p.F508del and c.2752–15C>G mutations came from David. They must both be in the same gene copy. Even if the c.2752–15C>G mutation was pathogenic, it would not explain Joanne's disease, because the gene she inherited from Pauline must also be mutated.

Joanne's other mutation, c.368G>A did come from her mother. The nucleotide change is within exon 3 and converts the codon for tryptophan 79 (TGG) into a stop codon (TAG). This is an unambiguously pathogenic change. Because of nonsense-mediated mRNA decay (see above) it is unlikely that the mutant gene would produce any protein, and any that it did produce would certainly be non-functional since the stop codon occurs very early in the sequence. Additionally, a search of the *CFTR* mutation database at www.genet.sickkids.on.ca/cftr/ showed that it had previously been identified in other CF patients.

| CASE 4 | Davies family | 4 | 10 | 66 | 102 | **151** | 181 | 279 | 376 |

- Boy (Martin) aged 24 months
- Family history of muscular dystrophy
- Pedigree shows X-linked recessive inheritance
- Order diagnostic DNA test
- Frameshift mutation in the dystrophin gene

Martin has a deletion of exons 44–48 of the dystrophin gene (*Chapter 4*). The long dystrophin molecule functions within the muscle cell a bit like a rope with hooks at each end (*Figure 6.4*). The body of the rope consists of repeated units, the precise number of which is not critical to dystrophin function. If Martin simply made slightly smaller than normal dystrophin molecules, he would have a relatively good prognosis. But adding up the exon lengths in *Table 6.2*, we can see that his deletion produces a frameshift. Any protein produced would have a completely wrong amino acid sequence downstream of the frameshift – but in fact a ribosome reading the message in this novel reading frame would soon encounter a stop codon. As before, nonsense-mediated decay means that Martin's gene would produce no protein product, rather than a truncated protein. Studying a muscle biopsy with labeled dystrophin antibody would confirm the absence of dystrophin protein (see *Figure 1.4*). In Martin's case this adds no useful new information, but in boys where the PCR deletion screen identifies no mutation it is a valuable diagnostic test. Searching all through the huge dystrophin gene (79 exons, 11 kb of coding sequence, 2.4 Mb of genomic DNA) for a point mutation can be impossibly laborious, and a muscle biopsy provides a much easier confirmation of the diagnosis.

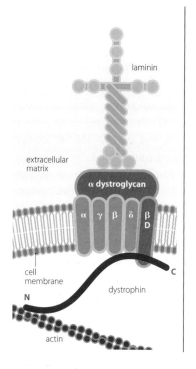

Figure 6.4 – The dystrophin molecule anchors the cytoskeleton of muscle cells to the extracellular matrix, via the dystrophin glycoprotein complex.
This includes the sarcoglycans (mutations in which cause limb-girdle muscular dystrophies) and dystroglycans. Muscle cells that lack dystrophin are mechanically fragile, and fail after a few years, hence the progressive muscle weakness.

| CASE 6 | Fletcher family | 5 | 12 | 67 | 131 | **152** | 376 |

- Frank, aged 22, with increasingly blurred eyesight
- Family history of visual difficulties
- Pedigree suggests X-linked recessive inheritance but not conclusive
- ? LHON
- Order blood test to check for mutation in mtDNA
- Check mutations by Pyrosequencing
- G3460 mutation in mtDNA

The causative mutation was identified as G3460A in his mitochondrial DNA (*Chapter 5*). Most mitochondrial proteins are encoded by nuclear genes, synthesized on cytoplasmic ribosomes and then imported into the mitochondria, but the 13 protein-coding genes in mitochondrial DNA are transcribed and translated within the mitochondrion in a way closely similar to the way nuclear genes are expressed. They encode components of the electron transport chain of oxidative phosphorylation (*Figure 3.10b*).

Mitochondrial mutations can be classified in the same way as nuclear mutations (*Box 6.1*). Large deletions and duplications are relatively more common, and splicing mutations are absent because mitochondrial genes do not have introns. Heteroplasmy introduces an extra layer of variability between genotype and phenotype. The three common LHON mutations are all mis-sense mutations affecting three different proteins in the electron transport system: p.Ala52Tyr in the ND1 protein, p.Arg340His in ND4 and p.Met64Val in ND6. Frank's mutation is the first of these.

| CASE 11 | Kavanagh family | 81 | 97 | **152** |

- Healthy first baby boy
- Second child, Celia, pale with low hemoglobin levels
- Sickle cell disease
- Single nucleotide mutation, Glu→Val

The single nucleotide change in the coding sequence of the β-globin gene changes the codon for amino acid 6 from a codon for glutamic acid into one for valine (*Figure 6.5*). The effect of this change has been studied in great detail. Glutamic acid is, chemically, a polar amino acid. The carboxy (–COOH) group in its side chain is acidic. It readily loses a proton forming a –COO⁻ anion.

		Val	His	Leu	Thr	Pro	Glu	Glu	Lys	Ser
NORMAL		GTG	CAT	CTG	ACT	CCT	GAG	GAG	AAG	TCT
SICKLE		GTG	CAT	CTG	ACT	CCT	GTG	GAG	AAG	TCT
		Val	His	Leu	Thr	Pro	Val	Glu	Lys	Ser

Figure 6.5 – In sickle cell disease an A>T nucleotide substitution causes glutamic acid to be replaced by valine at position 6 of the β-globin protein.

When a soluble protein chain folds, such charged groups tend to be located on the outside of the molecule, in contact with the aqueous environment. Valine is non-polar and naturally associates with other non-polar amino acids in the interior of the folded protein, away from water. Having a valine on the outer surface makes the mutant β-globin molecules tend to stick together. The resulting protein aggregates distort the red cells into a sickle shape, cause clumping and subsequent vascular ischemia. Thus the sickle cell change might be considered a gain of function mutation, because the mutant protein does something positively harmful. However, gain of function mutations would normally be expected to be pathogenic in heterozygotes, and people with sickling trait are healthy.

CASE 14	Nicolaides family	115	129	**153**	376

- ? β-thalassemia carriers
- p.Gln39X nonsense mutation for Spiros
- c.316–106C>G mutation for Elena

Spiros has the p.Gln39X mutation. This is a classic nonsense mutation. A single nucleotide substitution converts a codon for glutamine (CAG) into a stop codon (TAG) (*Figure 6.6*). The mutated gene produces no product, causing a β⁰ thalassemia in homozygotes.

INTRON 1		Leu	Leu	Val	Val	Tyr	Pro	Trp	Thr	Gln	Arg	Phe	Phe	Glu
ccacccttagG		CTG	CTG	GTG	GTC	TAC	CCT	TGG	ACC	CAG	AGG	TTC	TTT	GAG
ccacccttagG		CTG	CTG	GTG	GTC	TAC	CCT	TGG	ACC	TAG	AGG	TTC	TTT	GAG
INTRON 1		Leu	Leu	Val	Val	Pro	Pro	Trp	Thr	STOP				

Figure 6.6 – The p.Gln39X mutation in the β-globin gene near the start of exon 2 converts a glutamine codon into a stop codon. Lower case letters represent intron, upper case exon.

Elena's mutation (*Figure 6.7*) is more subtle. The change, c.316–106C>G, is a single nucleotide change deep within intron 2 of the β-globin gene, 106 nucleotides upstream of the start of exon 3. It is an example of the sort of mutation that could only be characterized by studying mRNA. This apparently innocuous change activates a cryptic splice site that is then preferentially used compared to the normal donor splice site. The result is a β⁺ thalassemia – that is, the mutant gene produces some correct β-chains, using the normal splice site, but not a sufficient quantity.

Table 5.2 listed three other β-globin mutations that are common causes of thalassemia in Greek Cypriots. Interestingly, all three affect splicing.

- The commonest mutation, c.93–21G>A, again activates a cryptic splice site in an intron, intron 1 this time. Studies of the mRNA showed that

NORMAL INTRON 2

ctaatagcagctacaatccagctaccattctgct

MUTANT-
part handled as exon,
with new donor splice site

CTAATAGCAGCTACAATCCAGgtaccattctgct

Figure 6.7 – The c.316–106C>G mutation activates a cryptic splice site deep within intron 2 of the β-globin gene. Lower case letters represent intron, upper case are the abnormal exon.

> 80% of the time the new splice site is used, so this allele produces only 20% of the normal quantity of β-globin. For many genes a 20% level of function would be sufficient, but β-globin is required in large amounts, so the result is a β⁺ thalassemia.

- The second mutation, c.92+6T>C, is an example of a mutation that reduces the efficiency of a normal splice site. The changed nucleotide is in intron 1, six nucleotides from the start of the intron (GGCAGgttggtatcaa.., where exon sequence is in upper case letters and the nucleotide that is mutated is underlined). The T nucleotide is not part of the invariant GT found at the 5′ end of every intron, but forms part of the context that is necessary for the splice site to be recognized efficiently. Again the result is a β⁺ thalassemia.
- The third common Greek Cypriot mutation is c.92+1G>A. This directly changes the obligatory GT at the exon 1 – intron 1 splice site to AT. No transcripts can be correctly spliced, so this mutation produces β⁰ thalassemia.

| CASE 15 | O'Reilly family | 141 | **154** | 376 |

- Family history of myopia and hip problems
- Orla has severe myopia, is short, and has hip problems
- ? Stickler syndrome
- Frameshift mutation in *COL2A1*

Orla's combination of high myopia and joint problems, inherited in autosomal dominant manner, is characteristic of people who have a mutation in Type II collagen (or occasionally Type XI collagen). Collagens are the major structural proteins of the human body. They play a variety of roles, mostly in connective tissue. There are at least 19 different human collagens, encoded by at least 30 genes. The number of genes is greater than the number of collagens because each collagen is a trimer of three polypeptide chains wound into a triple helix. *Box 6.2* shows how the mature collagens are synthesized. Collagen II forms fibrils that are major structural proteins of cartilage, and are also important in the vitreous of the eye and in the inner ear. Disorders of collagen II are one cause of chondrodysplasias – a group of some 150 clinically defined phenotypes with defects of cartilage, that often lead to defects of modeling of long bones.

Collagen II is a homotrimer of polypeptides encoded by the *COL2A1* gene on chromosome 12q13. The gene has 53 exons, of which exons 8–49 encode the triple helical region. Orla's mutation might be anywhere within these exons. Changes outside this region are not associated with her phenotype. Because collagen genes have large numbers of exons, mutation screening is extremely laborious and is available only in specialized laboratories. In Orla's case, after much work, sequencing of PCR-amplified exon 40 revealed a single nucleotide

Biosynthesis of collagens

The 30 or so human collagen genes are distributed around the genome. Collagens are large proteins – the collagen II that is mutated in **Orla O'Reilly** has 1418 amino acids. Despite having large numbers of exons (53 for *COL2A1*, 118 for *COL7A1*, the collagen VII gene) the genes are not particularly large (40 kb for *COL2A1*, 32 kb for *COL7A1*). An unusual feature is that all the exons encoding the central part of the protein that will form the triple helix are frame-neutral. For example, in *COL2A1* these exons are mostly 54 or 108 bp, with a few of 45 or 99 bp. Thus exon deletions in this region do not result in frameshifts; the protein is just rather shorter.

The initial product of translation is a preprocollagen. The future triple helical region has a repetitive structure Gly–X–Y where X and Y can be any amino acid, but are often proline or lysine. This undergoes extensive post-translational modification.

- In the rough endoplasmic reticulum a proportion of the lysines and prolines are hydroxylated by special hydroxylase enzymes that use oxygen, Fe^{2+} and ascorbic acid as cofactors. These modifications are essential for maturation of the collagen.
- Sugar residues are attached to some of the hydroxyl groups.
- Three chains are then wound together, starting at their C-terminal ends, to form a triple helix. Many collagen mutations disrupt this process, especially by replacing glycines with bulkier amino acids that will not fit into the interior of the triple helix.
- This procollagen is secreted, after which special enzymes cleave off the C-terminal and N-terminal propeptides. Some mutant collagens lack the necessary cleavage sites and hence cannot mature.
- Finally, the triple helical molecules are assembled into large multimers and crosslinked through lysine residues. Some collagens (I, II, III, V and XI) are fibrillar; others form meshworks that support membranes.

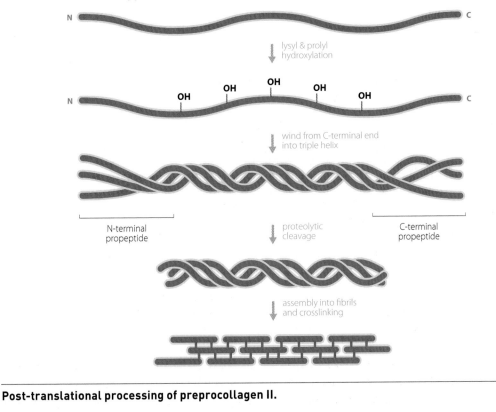

Post-translational processing of preprocollagen II.

deletion. This would cause a frameshift, leading to a premature termination codon and nonsense-mediated decay of the mRNA.

COL2A1 mutations cause autosomal dominant phenotypes of variable severity depending on how they interfere with collagen biogenesis. The *COL2A1* chondrodysplasias form a spectrum from achondrogenesis type II, an intrauterine or perinatal lethal condition, through hypochondrogenesis, spondylo-epiphyseal dysplasia (SED) and Kniest dysplasia, to Stickler syndrome, a relatively mild condition that is often diagnosed late. Interestingly, the mutations with the most drastic effect on protein synthesis are not the ones that produce the most severe phenotypes.

- The most severe phenotypes are caused by mis-sense mutations that replace glycines in the Gly–X–Y units of the triple helical region. Only glycine, the smallest amino acid, can fit into the interior of the tight-packed triple helix, so replacements prevent proper assembly of the fibril. The triple helix assembles from the C-terminal end and, in general, substitutions near that end have a more severe effect than those in more N-terminal positions.
- Whole exon deletions and exon skipping due to splicing mutations are also associated with relatively severe phenotypes. Heterozygous people try to combine chains of different lengths into the triple helix, which again disrupts the structure. Mutations located in exons 12–24, towards the N-terminus, tend to cause Kniest dysplasia which, whilst not lethal, is associated with severe short stature, retinal detachment, deafness and disabling joint abnormalities.
- Nonsense mutations and frameshifts cause Stickler syndrome. In a heterozygote there are no abnormal chains to interfere with the assembly of normal chains. The phenotype, which can be variable with short, normal or tall stature, is presumably caused by a quantitative deficiency of collagen II.

Figure 6.8 – A dominant negative effect.
The mutant allele produces an abnormal protein that disrupts the construction of a multiprotein complex. In heterozygotes dominant negative alleles produce more severe phenotypes than null alleles.

This series shows that it is better (in a heterozygote) to make no protein than one that can interfere with the function of its normal counterpart. Mutations are called **dominant negative** if the mutant product prevents the normal product from functioning (*Figure 6.8*). If molecules are selected at random from a 50:50 mix of normal and abnormal polypeptide chains for incorporation into triple helices, only one triple helix in eight would consist of three normal chains, compared to a 50% level of normal triple helices in a heterozygote for a null mutation.

6.4. **Summary and extension**

A central ambition of clinical molecular genetics is to be able to predict the phenotypic effect of any DNA sequence change. This goal, of establishing genotype–phenotype correlations, can be divided into two tasks:

- deciding how a mutation affects the function of a gene – does it cause loss of function (partial or total), gain of function, or does it have no effect?
- deciding how loss or gain of function of a gene will affect the phenotype.

Loss of function and gain of function changes

A first question to ask concerning the effect of a mutation is, does it cause a loss of function or a gain of function? To put it differently, does the mutated gene product simply fail to do its normal job (partially or totally), or does it do something positively harmful? *Table 6.3* summarizes the likely effects of different types of mutation.

Many of the changes in *Table 6.3* are likely to abolish the gene function. Some mis-sense mutations and in-frame deletions or duplications will reduce but not abolish the function of the gene product, like the exon deletions in the dystrophin gene that produce Becker muscular dystrophy (*Table 6.2*). It is

Table 6.3 – **Common types of mutation and their likely effects**

Type of mutation	Likely effect on a gene
Large deletion or inversion	Most likely to completely abolish function
Duplication of whole gene	Will increase the amount of product by 50% (from 2 to 3 gene copies); this will generally have no phenotypic effect, unless the precise level of the gene product is critical (dosage-sensitive gene); see for example Aitman *et al.* (2006)
Change in promoter or regulatory sequence	May reduce or increase the level of transcription, or alter the response to control signals; any protein produced has the normal structure and function
Change in intron	Most likely to have no effect – but can sometimes affect splicing
Change in 5′ or 3′ untranslated region of mRNA	Most likely to have no effect – but can sometimes affect the stability or translation efficiency of the mRNA
Splicing mutation	Mutation of the canonical GT...AG splice sites is likely to abolish function of that allele. Other mutations may have more subtle effects, causing a proportion of transcripts to be incorrectly spliced or changing the pattern of alternative splicing. This can produce a partial loss of function. A change deep within an intron may activate a cryptic splice site
Frameshift mutation	Likely to abolish function of that allele. The polypeptide downstream of the frameshift bears no resemblance to the correct sequence. Usually a stop codon will be encountered quite soon as the ribosomes read the frameshifted codons. The effect will then be the same as a nonsense mutation
Nonsense mutation	Likely to abolish function of that allele. Most mRNAs containing premature termination codons are not translated to produce a truncated protein. Instead, they are degraded and not used at all (nonsense-mediated mRNA decay)
Mis-sense mutation	Effect very variable, depending on the nature and function of the amino acids concerned. Could be loss or gain of function, or no effect. Replacing an amino acid by a chemically very similar one is likely to have less effect than a more radical change. Some amino acids in a protein are essential to its structure or function, others are not. Apparent mis-sense mutations may actually be pathogenic because of an effect on splicing
Synonymous substitution	Most likely to have no effect – but can sometimes affect splicing

difficult to predict what effect a mis-sense mutation would have on a protein. Many amino acid substitutions affect the stability of the 3-dimensional structure of the protein, rather than altering an active site or other directly functional part of the protein. Proteins are often cleaved, glycosylated, phosphorylated or otherwise modified after synthesis of the basic polypeptide chain. Any mis-sense mutation that replaces amino acids required for any of these modification steps will probably cause a loss of function. But as *Table 6.4* shows, mis-sense mutations can have a range of other effects.

Table 6.4 – Mutations in the *CFTR* chloride channel gene reduce or abolish function of the gene product in different ways. A loss of function in both copies of the gene leads to cystic fibrosis.

Class of mutation	Effect	Type of mutation	Example
I	No synthesis Reduced synthesis	Nonsense, frameshift or splicing Mutations that affect the efficiency of correct splicing	p.Gly542X c.3849+10kb C>T
II	Block in protein processing	Mis-sense or in-frame deletions	p.F508del
III	Chloride channel not correctly regulated	Mis-sense	p.Gly551Asp
IV	Altered conductance of chloride channel	Mis-sense	p.Arg117His

Gains of function are less common. Generally we are not talking about a gain of a completely novel function, but of the product functioning when it should not. It may become insensitive to signals that should shut it off, or be expressed at too high a level. A cell surface receptor may become constitutively active, transmitting a signal to the cell interior even when no ligand is present. Huntington disease is an example of a mutant protein having a toxic gain of function (see above). Gain of function mechanisms require the mutant allele to produce an abnormal protein. Gain of function mutations are therefore mis-sense or regulatory mutations, not nonsense or frameshift mutations.

Changes that create chimeric genes are a special class of gain of function mutation. As mentioned earlier, chromosomal rearrangements sometimes create a novel gene by juxtaposing exons of genes that are normally far apart in the genome. Such chimeric genes may gain novel functions. This type of exon shuffling has probably been important in evolution – many proteins can be seen to be made of varying combinations of a limited repertoire of functional domains, each encoded by separate exons (see figure in *Box 3.7*). Because chromosomal translocations cause major problems in meiosis (*Chapter 2*), such rearrangements are rarely the cause of inherited disease. However, cancers develop entirely by mitosis from mutant somatic cells, and so there is no obstacle to the propagation of chromosomal rearrangements. See *Chapter 12* for a much fuller discussion.

Dominant or recessive?

Dominance and recessiveness are properties of characters or phenotypes, not of genes. We should not really talk of 'dominant genes' and so on, though it is sometimes hard to avoid doing so. A character is dominant if it is seen in a heterozygote, and recessive if not.

- Gain of function mutations are expected to produce dominant characters. The gain of function is present in a heterozygote, regardless of the presence of the normal allele.
- Loss of function mutations can produce either dominant or recessive characters, depending how sensitive the organism is to a partial loss of that particular function (*Figure 6.9*). For most genes the threshold for pathology is below 50% and loss of function mutations cause recessive phenotypes. Sometimes there is **haplo-insufficiency**, meaning that 50% of the normal function is not sufficient. In that case, a mutation causing complete loss of function will produce a dominant phenotype, because the normal allele in a heterozygote cannot provide sufficient function on its own.
- Dominant negative mutations are a special class of loss of function mutations, where the abnormal product interferes with the function of the normal product (see *Figure 6.8*). The Long QT syndromes (*Disease Box 5*) are an example. Simple loss of function mutations in the ion channel genes produce the recessive Romano–Ward syndrome: a 50% level of the protein is adequate for normal function. The dominant JLN syndrome is the result of dominant negative mutations in the same genes. A single mutant allele produces more than 50% loss of function. Because dominant negative effects are so damaging, full-length but abnormal proteins are particularly dangerous to the organism. This probably provides the force that drove evolution of the nonsense-mediated decay mechanism.

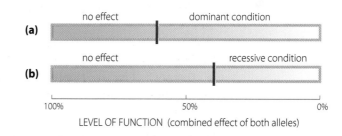

Figure 6.9 – Whether a loss of function mutation causes a dominant or a recessive condition depends on how sensitive the organism is to loss of that function. If the threshold for normal function is as shown in (a) a heterozygote with 50% function will be affected, and the condition will be dominant. This situation is called haplo-insufficiency. If the threshold is as in (b) the condition will be recessive.

Understanding the phenotype

There is often a wide gulf between the biochemical action of a gene product within a cell and the clinical result of mutations in the gene. Many of the cases discussed through this book illustrate this. Even when we know both the biochemistry and the phenotype it is often difficult to explain how the one leads to the other. Why, as one example among many, should lack of the FMR1 RNA-binding protein cause mental retardation, macro-orchidism and a long face in men with Fragile-X syndrome?

It is important to avoid thinking naively about 'the gene for...'. You would hopefully not describe your domestic freezer as a machine for ruining your stocks of frozen food. That is what happens when things go wrong. Similarly we don't have genes 'for' cystic fibrosis or muscular dystrophy. Many human genes were discovered through studies of the diseases that result when they go wrong, so there is a natural tendency to attach the disease name to the gene. It can be hard to avoid talking about 'the Huntington disease gene', etc. – but it is important not to be drawn into thinking that the disease defines the function of the gene.

Genotype–phenotype correlations

Accurately establishing predictive correlations between mutations and phenotypes is the Holy Grail of molecular pathology – highly desirable but seldom achieved. For the most part the chain of events between a DNA sequence change and a patient's problems is just too long to allow neat correlations. Genes do not act in a vacuum. All the other direct interactors with the gene and its product, the general biochemical milieu, the patient's history and lifestyle, and simple chance events – all conspire to prevent simple predictions of phenotypes. The mendelian diseases that have been the main topic of this book so far are simply the small subset of all diseases where the effect of a single genetic change happens not to be completely submerged by other genetic or environmental effects. Even mendelian diseases are seldom simple when investigated carefully. An excellent article by Scriver and Waters (1999) dissects the reasons why close correlations do not exist in one typical mendelian disease, phenylketonuria – see *Chapter 8* for further discussion.

In the light of this, diseases where a good genotype–phenotype correlation does exist appear as the interesting exceptions to the general rule.

- One such class is exemplified by the hemoglobinopathies. Sickle cell disease and thalassemia are defined in terms of the globin gene product, rather than by distant downstream effects of the mutations. Thus sickle cell disease is quite specifically the result of a p.Glu6Val mutation in β-globin, and other mutations lead predictably to β^0- or β^+-thalassemia.
- Gain of function mutations may produce highly specific effects that are not easily over-ridden by other genetic or environmental factors. The $(CAG)_n$ expansion in the Huntington disease gene always produces Huntington disease, and there is even a statistical (though not individually very predictive) correlation between repeat size and age of onset. Perhaps the most striking example of tight genotype–phenotype correlations in clinical genetics is seen with gain of function mutations in the fibroblast growth factor receptor genes (*Box 6.3*).

The concept of **syndrome families** has proved a productive way of exploring the relationship between genotypes and phenotypes. Before it was known

Box 6.3

Genotype–phenotype correlation in mutations of the *FGFR* genes

The nine fibroblast growth factors control the growth and differentiation of various mesenchymal and neuro-ectodermal cells. They act through four cell surface receptors. Each receptor consists of an extracellular portion with three immunoglobulin-like domains, a transmembrane segment, and an internal portion with two tyrosine kinase domains and a C-terminal transactivation region (see figure). On activation by the ligand, receptors dimerize. This triggers conformational changes that activate the intracellular tyrosine kinase. This in turn leads to activation of Stat1 signaling molecules and ultimately to cell cycle arrest.

Structure of a fibroblast growth factor receptor and position of major mutations. TM, transmembrane domain; TK, tyrosine kinase domain; Ap, Apert syndrome; Cr, Crouzon syndrome; TD, thanatophoric dysplasia; M, Muenke craniosynostosis; Ach, achondroplasia; Hypoch, hypochrondroplasia.

The four *FGFR* genes each encode at least 12 alternative splice isoforms. Receptors can heterodimerize as well as homodimerize, and they have different affinities for the nine FGFs. As a result they can mediate a large variety of subtly tuned responses to different combinations of FGFs in different cell types. Mutations cause a gain of function. The mutant receptor becomes constitutively active and transmits its signal, to a greater or lesser extent, even in the absence of ligand. The FGFR mutations show quite remarkably specific genotype–phenotype correlations (see table). Nearly all the mutations are in the *FGFR2* and *FGFR3* genes. They produce specific syndromes with craniosynostosis or skeletal dysplasias. Mutations occur particularly in the short linker between the second and third immunoglobulin domains, where they may affect the flexibility of the molecule and hence its dimerization potential, or in the transmembrane domain. Each immunoglobulin domain is held together by an S–S bridge. Other common mis-sense mutations either remove one of the cysteines or create another, and it is likely that these too make the molecules more likely to dimerize even in the absence of ligand.

Phenotypes and major mutations in the *FGFR2* and *FGFR3* genes

Gene	Disease (OMIM number)	Mutations
FGFR2	Apert syndrome (101200)	p.Ser252Trp (65%), p.Pro253Arg (34%)
	Crouzon syndrome (123500)	p.Cys342Tyr or Arg (50%)
	Beare–Stevenson Cutis gyrata (123790)	p.Ser372Cys (25%), p.Tyr375Cys (75%)
FGFR3	Achondroplasia (100800)	p.Gly380Arg (97%)
	Hypochondroplasia (146000)	p.Asn540Lys (50%), p.Asn540Thr, p.Ile538Val
	Thanatophoric dysplasia I (187600)	p.Arg248Cys (60%), p.Tyr373Cys (25%)
	Thanatophoric dysplasia II (187600)	p.Lys650Glu (100%)
	Muenke syndrome (see 134934.0014)	p.Pro250Arg (100%)

is found, there is a problem of interpretation. Is this the cause of the patient's disease, or is it a harmless variant? To resolve the problem, various lines of evidence are considered:

- Has the change previously been reported as a cause of the disease? And if so, is there a reason to believe the report?
- Is the change found in unaffected people? If it is not present in a few hundred randomly selected unaffected people from the same ethnic background as the case, then at least it is not a common polymorphic variant, but it still might be a previously undescribed rare neutral variant.
- If the patient is from a large family with several affected members, is the change found in all the affected people? If not, then it is unlikely to be pathogenic. However, even if it is found in all the affected people in the family, it may be that the real mutation has not been found, and this is just an irrelevant rare variant that is in the same gene. The c.2752–15C>G change in Joanne Brown (Case 2) would be an example if the true mutation in the same gene had not already been discovered.
- Does the amino acid that is replaced have a vital role in the function or structure of the protein? There is rarely enough detailed knowledge of the protein to allow a certain answer. If all related proteins in humans and other animals have the same amino acid at this position (evolutionary conserved residue), this would be evidence (but not proof) of a vital role.

After all these lines of inquiry have been exhausted, all too often the laboratory has to label the change as a 'variant of unknown significance'. This is of course deeply unsatisfactory for everybody concerned.

Dosage sensitivity and the pathology of chromosomal abnormalities

Although some large-scale copy number variants are harmless, and may even be common population polymorphisms, most chromosomal imbalances are pathogenic. Presumably the cause is having wrong numbers of certain dosage-sensitive genes. Since there are on average around 1000 genes per chromosome, even a small imbalance can involve many genes. Most genes are not dosage-sensitive. Relatively few loss of function mutations produce dominant phenotypes through haplo-insufficiency, and it is still less common for a 50% increase in the number of copies or level of product to cause problems. Nevertheless, all autosomal monosomies and trisomies are embryonic lethals or cause major congenital abnormalities. We can consider two possible explanations.

- In some cases imbalance of just two or three dosage-sensitive genes may explain much of the pathology. For example, the major problems of Down syndrome may be caused by just two genes on chromosome 21, *DSCR1* and *DYRK1A*. The products of these genes regulate certain transcription factors, and so indirectly affect expression of many genes. Chromosomal phenotypes must, however, always involve more than one gene. Clinicians can usually recognize 'chromosomal' patients even when they can't predict which chromosome is involved. Their phenotypes involve multiple independent developmental abnormalities and, except for a few specific cases, are not seen in patients with single-gene abnormalities.

- In other cases the problem may be an accumulation of many lesser effects. Genes encoding functionally related proteins are seldom located close together on the same chromosome. The individual components of multi-chain proteins like hemoglobin are usually encoded by genes on separate chromosomes. Similarly, the genes for a transcription factor and its target are more often than not on different chromosomes. Whether this is the result of some principle that we don't understand, or just an example of the apparently chaotic nature of our genome is not known, but it means that chromosomal imbalances almost always cause imbalances in multiple interacting systems. Having 50% extra of one partner of an interaction might result in only a subtle imbalance, but the cumulative effect of dozens of such imbalances could well derail development. The fact that patients with all sorts of different chromosomal imbalances tend to have rather the same spectrum of abnormalities (mental retardation, growth retardation, fits and dysmorphic face) supports this view of the pathology.

It is noteworthy that the three autosomal trisomies that are compatible with survival to term (trisomies 13, 18 and 21) involve chromosomes that are small and relatively poor in genes. These three chromosomes have 3.50, 4.23 and 5.77 genes per Mb of DNA respectively, compared to a genome-wide average of 7.32, according to data from the ENSEMBL genome browser (release 35, November 2005). Similarly, the low number of genes on the Y chromosome helps explain why most 47,XYY men are within the normal spectrum and remain undiagnosed. Nevertheless, the X chromosome carries large numbers of genes, and so the fact that normal people can have either one or two X chromosomes is unexpected and requires a special explanation. This is covered in the following chapter.

Somatic mutations

The case studies reviewed in this chapter have all involved inherited mutations. But mutations can affect any cell and so, by simple arithmetic, the majority happen in somatic cells and do not get passed on. Somatic mutations are only a problem in two circumstances.

- If a somatic mutation arises very early in embryogenesis, the one mutant cell may give rise to a substantial clone. The person is mosaic for the mutation. Whether this matters depends on what cells are affected and what the mutation does.
- If a mutation causes a somatic cell to start multiplying out of control, the result could be cancer. These mutations are considered in *Chapter 12*.

How do mutations arise?

Mutations arise through DNA damage or replication errors. DNA is a fairly stable molecule, but it is not immune to chemical change. Cytosine bases are liable to deaminate spontaneously – the consequences of this are described in the following chapter. Reactive oxygen species generated within cells as part of normal oxidative metabolism cause chemical modifications of the bases. Strand breaks are happening all the time as a result of errors in replication, chemical changes or natural radiation. The great bulk of all this damage is unrelated to industrial pollution, nuclear power plants or any other human activity. Cells have enzymes that are able to repair many types of DNA damage, so that much damage passes unnoticed, but they are not infallible. If damage is limited to one strand of the double helix, the complementary strand can be used as a template to make a correct repair. Double strand breaks, however, pose more problems, and often the repair process leaves errors in the sequence.

DNA replication is also a fallible process. The likelihood of the polymerase incorporating a mispaired base into a growing chain is simply a function of the relative binding energies of correctly paired and mispaired bases. That thermodynamic calculation suggests an error rate orders of magnitude higher than the observed rate. The higher accuracy is the result of proof-reading and mismatch detection mechanisms. The polymerase checks the newly synthesized DNA for mis-paired bases. If one is detected, the polymerase backs up, degrades a short stretch of the DNA and tries again. Interestingly, when mice were engineered to abolish the proof-reading capacity, but not the polymerase activity, of one minor DNA polymerase (specialized for replicating the mitochondrial DNA), they showed many features of accelerated aging (see Trifunovic *et al.*, 2004). One theory of aging ascribes it to accumulation of mutations. After the polymerase has moved on, special enzymes excise and repair mismatched bases in newly replicated DNA. In *Chapter 12* we will see what can happen when this mechanism fails. Even with all this, occasional errors persist. Runs of identical bases are particularly liable to lose or gain a base by slipped-strand mispairing. The 35delG mutation in the *GJB2* gene (*Figure 6.2*) is an example. Other mutations may occur endogenously, such as by deamination of methylated cytosines, and this is described further in *Chapter 7.*

Mutations can affect any piece of DNA at any time. We have focused on mutations affecting coding sequence because these are the ones studied in relation to genetic diseases, and where we can often predict the effect on the gene product. Because only 1.5% of our DNA is coding, these are actually a very minor subset of all mutations. Most mutations in non-coding sequence are unlikely to have any phenotypic effect. Very little of this sequence is conserved between humans and other species, implying that it could mutate over evolutionary time without the mutants suffering any selective disadvantage. No doubt certain changes are pathogenic but at present, with a few fortuitously discovered exceptions, we are unable to identify them.

Molecular pathology of variants in the androgen receptor gene

Mammals, including humans, develop by default as females. A specific cascade of events is necessary to produce males. In normal development the cascade starts with the *SRY* gene on the Y chromosome. This causes the early indifferent gonad to develop as a testis. The testis secretes the androgen (male sex hormone) testosterone. An enzyme, steroid 5-α reductase, converts testosterone to dihydrotestosterone (DHT). DHT activates the androgen receptor, a nuclear Class I steroid receptor. The activated androgen receptor stimulates transcription of a variety of genes whose effect is to produce the male sexual anatomy. The androgen receptor is encoded by the *AR* gene on the proximal long arm of the X chromosome at Xq11–q12. The gene has eight exons covering 178 kb of genomic DNA and encodes a protein of 920 amino acids. Different mutations in this gene have a surprisingly wide range of effects.

Loss of function mutations result in the X-linked androgen insensitivity syndrome (OMIM 300068), previously called testicular feminization syndrome. XY embryos develop testes as normal, and these secrete testosterone as normal. But if there is complete loss of function of the receptor, the tissues of the embryo are unable to react to androgens, and so anatomical development proceeds along the default female line. Affected patients are phenotypically female, with female external genitalia and breast development, but a blind vagina and absent uterus. The testes are inguinal or abdominal, and patients often come to medical attention because of a presumed inguinal hernia. It is advisable to remove the testes surgically because they have a propensity to develop malignancy. Apart from this, and their inevitable infertility, most affected people lead normal female lives.

Partial loss of function of the androgen receptor can result in a variety of sexually ambiguous states, often including hypospadias and micropenis with gynecomastia (Reifenstein syndrome; OMIM 312300). Such pseudohermaphroditism can have many other causes. Perhaps the most intriguing of these is the recessive condition (PPSH, OMIM 264600) caused by loss of function of the *SRD5A2* gene that encodes steroid 5-α reductase. Being unable to convert testosterone to dihydrotestosterone, affected infants have ambiguous genitalia but are normally raised as girls. However, at puberty an alternative 5-α reductase gene, *SRD5A1*, triggers a conversion to male phenotype. The patient's voice breaks, he grows a beard and usually takes on a male identity. It is reported that they live comfortably with their new male identity, which if true suggests that early masculinization of the brain by testosterone may be at least as important as social factors for determining a person's sexual identity.

Expansion of a (CAG)$_n$ repeat in exon 1 of the AR *gene* has very different effects. Spinal and bulbar muscular atrophy (SBMA, OMIM 313200) is one of the family of conditions caused by unstable repeat expansions (see *Disease Box 4*). Like Huntington disease, the CAG repeat is in the coding sequence and encodes an expanded run of glutamines in the receptor protein. As in the other diseases caused by expanded polyglutamine runs, there is a gain of function: the mutant protein is toxic to neurons. The result is an X-linked adult-onset slowly progressive muscular atrophy. However, there is a second effect. The expanded polyglutamine run is located in the N-terminal part of the protein, which is the transactivation domain through which the activated (androgen-bound) receptor stimulates transcription of its target genes. Expansion of the polyglutamine tract decreases the efficiency of transactivation. Males with SBMA therefore show mild signs of androgen deficiency, in particular gynecomastia.

Normal variation in the (CAG)$_n$ repeat mediates normal variation in response to androgens. Short repeats promote a strong response and longer repeats (within the normal range) a weaker response. This shows up in the incidence of prostate cancer, an androgen-dependent condition. Though the distributions overlap strongly, the average repeat size is lowest in African–Americans, intermediate in non-Hispanic white Americans and highest in the

Japanese and Chinese. The incidence of prostate cancer varies between these groups in inverse proportion to the average repeat length. Repeats at the upper end of normal (>27 repeats), on the other hand, are associated with a fourfold increase in the risk of male infertility.

Androgen receptor variation as a susceptibility factor for male baldness. For almost a century geneticists have studied the inheritance of balding in middle-aged men (androgenic alopecia, OMIM 109200). One clear conclusion is that though balding can run in families it is not a simple mendelian character. However, it has recently been shown that a major susceptibility factor lies somewhere within the androgen receptor locus. Variation at this locus may explain about half the overall genetic susceptibility. Precisely what variant confers susceptibility is not certain, but a strong candidate is variation in a run of glycines in exon 1. Unlike the polyglutamine run described above, this is variable but stable. A likely reason for the stability is that at the DNA level it is not a pure repeat, but includes various different glycine codons $(GGN)_n$, where N can be any nucleotide. This variation reduces the risk of slippage during DNA replication.

COMPLETE LOSS OF FUNCTION: androgen insensitivity syndrome, M>F sex reversal (OMIM 300068)

PARTIAL LOSS OF FUNCTION: male pseudohermaphroditism

178.80 Kb

exon 1

CAG repeat

GGN repeat

NORMAL VARIATION: role in susceptibility to male pattern baldness (?)

NORMAL VARIATION: low copy number increases susceptibility to prostate cancer
(11–33 repeats) high copy number associated with some cases of male infertility

ABNORMAL EXPANSION: spinal and bulbar muscular atrophy (OMIM 313200)
(38–62 repeats)

Different variations in the *AR* gene lead to a wide variety of different effects.
Loss of function or gain of function mutations cause distinct mendelian conditions, while normal variation affects susceptibility to several different common non-mendelian conditions.

6.5. **References**

Aitman TJ, Dong R, Vyse TJ, *et al.* (2006) Copy number polymorphism in *Fcgr3* predisposes to glomerulonephritis in rats and humans. *Nature* **439**: 851–855.

Brunner HG and van Driel MA (2004) From syndrome families to functional genomics. *Nat. Rev. Genet.* **5**: 545–51.

Donnai D and Read AP (2003) How clinicians add to knowledge of development. *Lancet,* **362**: 477–484.

Holbrook JA, Neu-Yilik G, Hentze MW and Kulozik AE (2004) Nonsense-mediated decay approaches the clinic. *Nature Genetics,* **36**: 801–808.

Scriver C and Waters PJ (1999) Monogenic traits are not simple: lessons from phenylketonuria. *Trends Genet.* 15: 267–272.

Snead MP and Yates JRW (1999) Clinical and molecular genetics of Stickler syndrome. *J. Med. Genet.* 36: 353–359.

Trifunovic A *et al.* (2004) Premature ageing in mice expressing defective mitochondrial DNA polymerase. *Nature,* **429**:357–359.

Useful websites

For more discussion of molecular pathology see Chapter 16 of Strachan and Read (2004), *Human Molecular Genetics* (3rd edn, Garland). The 2nd edition is freely available as searchable text on the NCBI Bookshelf: www.ncbi.nlm.nih.gov/entrez/query.fcgi?db=Books

For the nomenclature of mutations see www.hgvs.org/mutnomen/

6.6. **Self-assessment questions**

(1) Cystic fibrosis is caused by the absence from apical cell membranes of functional chloride ion channels that are encoded by the *CFTR* gene. Which of the following mutations might be a cause of cystic fibrosis?

(a) Deletion of the *CFTR* gene.

(b) A mutation in the gene encoding arginine-specific tRNA that causes the protein synthesis machinery to incorporate arginine in growing polypeptide chains in response to serine codons. Substitution of arginine for serine in the CFTR protein makes it non-functional.

(c) A mutation in the promoter of the *CFTR* gene that abolishes its ability to recruit the RNA polymerase machinery.

(d) A mutation in the coding sequence of the *CFTR* gene that replaces an essential serine with a non-functional arginine.

(e) A mutation in one of the small non-coding RNA molecules in the spliceosome that causes the splicing machinery to treat GA...AG as the signal for the start and end of introns, instead of GT...AG.

(f) A mutation in the RNA polymerase II gene that renders the polymerase non-functional.

(g) A mutation in the coding sequence of the *CFTR* gene that causes the ion channel to transport excessive quantities of chloride ions.

(2) *Box 6.4* shows the sequence of two exons (upper case), with flanking intron sequence (lower case), as amplified by PCR for mutation detection in the *PAX3* gene. For exon 1, only part of the 5′UT is included in the PCR product. Nucleotides are numbered as in the cDNA (with the first nucleotide of the initiator codon numbered +1), and the protein sequence is shown using single-letter codes (see *Box 3.6*).

Box 6.4

Partial sequence of *PAX3* gene for Self-assessment questions

Exon 1 (451 nt)

```
                ..CCGTTTCGC CCTTCACCTG GATATAATTT CCGAGCGAAG TGCCCCCAGG
 1   ATG ACC ACG CTG GCC GGC GCT GTG CCC AGG ATG ATG CGG CCG GGC CCG GGG
 1    M   T   T   L   A   G   A   V   P   R   M   M   R   P   G   P   G
52   CAG AAC TAC CCG CGT AGC GGG TTC CCG CTG GAA Ggtaagggagg gcctcagcgc..
18    Q   N   Y   P   R   S   G   F   P   L   E
```

Exon 2

```
                        ..tgacttttcc cttgcttctc tttttcacct tcccacag
 86    TG TCC ACT CCC CTC GGC CAG GGC CGC GTC AAC CAG CTC GGC GGC GTT TTT
 29     V   S   T   P   L   G   Q   G   R   V   N   Q   L   G   G   V   F
136   ATC AAC GGC AGG CCG CTG CCC AAC CAC ATC CGC CAC AAG ATC GTG GAG ATG
 46    I   N   G   R   P   L   P   N   H   I   R   H   K   I   V   E   M
187   GCC CAC CAC GGC ATC CGG CCC TGC GTC ATC TCG CGC CAG CTG CGC GTG TCC
 63    A   H   H   G   I   R   P   C   V   I   S   R   Q   L   R   V   S
238   CAC GGC TGC GTC TCC AAG ATC CTG TGC AGG TAC CAG GAG ACT GGC TCC ATA
 80    H   G   C   V   S   K   I   L   C   R   Y   Q   E   T   G   S   I
289   CGT CCT GGT GCC ATC GGC GGC AGC AAG CCC AAG gtgagcgggc gggccttgcc..
 97    R   P   G   A   I   G   G   S   K   P   K
```

For the following eight mutations, a short sequence is given, with the number of the first nucleotide shown. The changed nucleotide (or the first changed one if several change) is underlined. For each mutation, give the correct nomenclature (a) as a DNA change (b) (where appropriate) as a protein change.

c.15	CGGCGCTGTG<u>G</u>CCAGGATGATGC
c.43	GGCCCGGGG<u>T</u>AGAACTACCCGCG
c.78	GCTGGAAG<u>T</u>TAAGGGAGGGCCTC
c.86	TGTCCACTCC<u>A</u>CTCGGCCAGGGC
c.121	CTCGGCGGCG<u>T</u>TTTATCAACGGC
c.130	GTTTT<u>G</u>ATCAACGGCAGGCCGCT
c.180	CCACA<u>G</u>CGCCCACCACGGCATCC
c.248	TCTCC<u>G</u>AGATCCTGTGCAGGTAC
c.283	TCCATT<u>T</u>CCTGGTGCCATCGGCGG

(3) Referring to the *PAX3* sequence in *Box 6.4*, write out the mutant sequence of each of the following, formatted as in Question 2:

p.N47H
c.247_248ins(C)
c.185_202del
p.E61X

c.85+6G>T

c.86–2A>G

p.V29M

(4) Referring to the *PAX3* sequence in *Box 6.4*, for each of the following mutations, select one of the following options:

(a) Synonymous

(b) Mis-sense

(c) Nonsense

(d) Frameshift

(e) Non-frameshifting insertion / deletion

(f) Splice-site mutation

(g) Initiator codon

(h) Terminator codon

(i) Intronic

(1) c.85+1G>A

(2) c.86T>A

(3) c.86–18T>G

(4) c.101insGCC

(5) c.118C>T

(6) c.172_173delAA

(7) c.216C>G

(8) c.270C>G

(5) The effects of a mutation can be studied at the protein level as well as by DNA sequencing. If a suitable antibody is available, mutations can be classified into CRM+ and CRM-. CRM means cross-reacting material. Classify each of the types of mutation in *Box 6.1* in this way, commenting on cases where the result is hard to predict.

(6) A student wrote the following answer to a question about the genetics of cystic fibrosis:

'The gene for cystic fibrosis is recessive. If you have two copies of the gene you have cystic fibrosis, but if you only have one copy you are just the same as somebody who doesn't have any copy'.

Comment on this.

Chapter 7

What is epigenetics?

Learning points for this chapter

After working through this chapter you should be able to:

- Define epigenetic, imprinting, uniparental disomy, CpG island
- Explain how DNA is methylated, and how the methylation patterns can be heritable
- Describe two methods by which methylation patterns can be studied
- Explain the roles of CpG sequences in gene control and mutation
- Describe X-inactivation and its consequences for carriers of X-linked recessive conditions and balanced X-autosome translocations
- Give examples of pedigree patterns and sporadic syndromes dependent on imprinting

7.1. **Case studies**

CASE 16	Portillo family	**173**	183	214	376

- Sickly boy, Pablo
- Family history of similar symptoms
- Blood tests suggest X-linked severe combined immunodeficiency

Pilar and Pedro Portillo come from very close families and three generations live in the same part of town. When Pablo was born in 1989 Pilar and Pedro were happy that they had three children, but Pablo was a much more sickly baby than his siblings. He always seemed to have a cough, an ear infection or diarrhea and he failed to gain weight. Pilar's maternal grandmother encouraged Pilar to get an appointment for Pedro at the specialist children's hospital because Pablo's problems were very similar to those of her own two sons who had both died before they were one year old. She hoped there might be treatment available to stop Pablo deteriorating further. At the hospital Pablo was admitted immediately for investigations.

The blood tests showed that Pablo had a very low lymphocyte count. T cells and NK (natural killer) cells were absent; B cells were present but non-functional. *Box 7.1* gives some basic details about these cells. These findings, together with the family history, suggested a diagnosis of X-linked severe combined immuno-deficiency (X-SCID). This was very bad news because without successful treatment the prognosis is very poor. The doctors suggested bone marrow transplantation was Pablo's best hope (see *Chapter 8*).

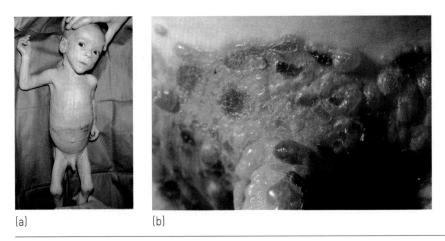

(a)   (b)

Figure 7.1 – Problems with immunodeficiency.
(a) Failure to thrive and skin problems. (b) Herpes simplex developing over an area with eczema (Koebner phenomenon). Photo. (a) courtesy of Dept of Medical Illustration, Manchester Royal Infirmary and (b) courtesy of Dr Andrew Will, Royal Manchester Children's Hospital.

Types and functions of lymphocytes

All three types of lymphocyte are derived from bone marrow. B cells and NK cells mature in the marrow but T cells undergo a process of maturation in the thymus gland. B cells give rise to plasma cells that secrete immunoglobulins. NK cells are large granular lymphocytes with a characteristic morphology; they account for up to 15% of blood lymphocytes and provide a first line of defense against virally infected cells. **T lymphocytes** are involved in the regulation of the immune response and in cell-mediated immunity, and they help B cells to produce antibody. Mature T cells express antigen-specific T cell receptors plus the CD3 molecule. In addition, mature T cells express either CD4 or CD8 cell surface molecules that enable them to play a role in cell and antibody-mediated immunity (CD4+) or to become cytotoxic (CD8+).

Box 7.1

| CASE 17 | Qian family | **174** | 185 | 376 |

- Girl, Kai, aged 2 years, showing slow development
- Seizure
- ? Angelman syndrome

Chu-Li and Chan are a hard working couple who have an import business. When their first child Kai was born Chu-Li's mother moved from Hong Kong to help look after the baby. She had looked after several grandchildren before but even she found it hard to get Kai to feed well or to settle and sleep. Kai was slow to gain weight and achieve her developmental milestones. She appeared very jittery although she seemed happy and laughed a lot. By 2 years of age she wasn't showing any signs of talking and an appointment was made with a pediatrician. However, before this could happen she had a seizure and was admitted to the children's ward.

It was clear to the pediatrician that there were major problems with Kai's development. She noted that Kai, who had just learned to walk, did so with

Figure 7.2 – A 10-year-old girl with Angelman syndrome.
She has a mutation in the *UBE3A* gene. Photo. courtesy of Dr Jill Clayton-Smith, St Mary's Hospital, Manchester.

rather stiff legs held well apart. She had lots of jerky movements especially with her arms. She laughed a lot and tended to protrude her tongue and dribble. Her records showed that her head circumference at birth was normal but it was now just below the 3rd centile. She arranged for Kai to have an EEG and the result confirmed her clinical suspicions. There were generalized EEG changes with runs of high-amplitude delta activity with intermittent spike and slow wave discharges. The pediatrician told the parents that she was sure Kai had a condition called Angelman syndrome. The family were shocked because they said no one else in the family had problems. They wanted to know what had caused the condition and if it might happen again. The pediatrician said that she needed to refer them to the genetics clinic because there were different ways that Angelman syndrome could occur and sometimes another child in a family could be affected.

CASE 18	Rogers family	**175**	185	376

- Baby boy, Robert, born to older parents
- Floppy at birth; failed to suck
- Genetic tests in pregnancy showed normal male karyotype
- ? Prader–Willi syndrome

Figure 7.3 – A baby with Prader-Willi syndrome.
Note the marked hypotonia.

Ralph and Rowena Rogers had both been married before and each had a child by their first partners. Although Rowena was 38 years old when they married, they decided to try for a baby and were delighted when, after a few months, a pregnancy was confirmed. They wanted as many tests as possible to ensure a healthy baby. An amniocentesis test (see *Chapter 14*) showed a normal male karyotype and scans didn't show any problems. Rowena did mention that she didn't feel many fetal movements but put that down to the fact that she was very busy. Labor occurred on her due date and was a rather long affair but a baby boy was born weighing 3.2 kg. The family decided to call him Robert. When he was put to the breast he didn't try to suck at all and the doctor noticed he was very floppy. The doctor mentioned his concerns to Ralph and Rowena and said he was going to ask for an urgent chromosome test to rule out Down syndrome. Rowena reminded him that the amniocentesis test had shown a normal chromosome pattern and so the doctor decided to wait and see how Robert progressed. He needed feeding by tube because he couldn't suck well and had marked truncal hypotonia. The pediatrician talked to the geneticist on the telephone and described Robert's problems. Suspecting Prader–Willi syndrome, the geneticist said he would see the family urgently in his next clinic. In the genetics department the Rogers family were seen at the same clinic as the Qian family (Case 17), which was an informative coincidence, especially for the medical student who attended because he was doing a special module in genetics.

7.2. **Background**

Epigenetic changes are genetic changes that are heritable but that do not depend on DNA sequence changes. They do depend on modification of the DNA, but on modifications that leave the basic sequence of A, G, C and T nucleotides unchanged. Such modifications are more difficult to study than the classical mutations defined by DNA sequencing, and the study of human epigenetics is still at an early stage. Some people believe that there is a whole world of epigenetically determined phenotypes waiting to be discovered. Others guess that while epigenetic mechanisms are known to be important in cancer, they will have only a limited role in hereditary disease. Epigenetic changes in cancer are discussed in *Chapter 12*. Here we will describe DNA methylation, which is the principal mechanism of epigenetic modification, and use the three cases to illustrate X-inactivation and imprinting, which are the major types of epigenetic event outside of cancer.

X chromosome dosage compensation

The fact that entirely normal people can have either one or two X chromosomes requires explanation. Having an extra or missing copy of an autosome that contained that many genes would be lethal (see below for further discussion of gene dosage). The explanation lies in a mechanism of dosage compensation called **X-inactivation** or **Lyonization** (named after its discoverer, Dr Mary Lyon).

Early in the life of every human (and other mammalian) embryo, at the blastocyst stage, each cell somehow counts its number of X chromosomes. All Xs except one are then permanently inactivated. The inactivated chromosome remains intact but most of its genes are not expressed (some X-linked genes do escape the general inactivation; why and how they do so is the subject of current research). Which X remains active is a random choice in each cell. However, once the choice is made, it is remembered by all the daughters of that cell (*Figure 7.4*). X-inactivation is an epigenetic process: the genetic change does not change the DNA sequence, but is heritable from cell to daughter cell. It is not heritable through a pedigree. In the female germ-line the inactive X is re-activated and regardless which of the mother's X chromosomes a conceptus inherits, initially that X is active.

X-inactivation is controlled by a gene called *XIST* located on the proximal long arm of the X chromosome at Xq13. *XIST* is expressed only by the inactive X. It produces a large non-coding RNA that physically coats the inactive X – how the XIST RNA spreads along the inactive X without ever jumping on to the active X is not known. This triggers a change in the chromatin conformation to make the chromosome heterochromatic and silence its genes. On a female karyotype such as *Figure 2.9* the two X chromosomes are indistinguishable – but this is because the chromosomes are being seen during mitosis when all chromosomes are highly condensed and largely inactive. On completion of cell division, while the other chromosomes of a female cell decondense, the inactive X remains condensed. In female cells it can be seen as a spot of densely staining chromatin at the edge of the nucleus, the Barr body. Counting Barr bodies was used in the past as a way of counting the number of X chromosomes (for sex tests on athletes, for example). Normal females and XXY males have one Barr body per cell; normal males and 45,X females have none, and 47,XXX females have two.

The 2.6 Mb of sequence immediately adjacent to the tip of the X chromosome short arm has special properties. A homologous sequence is present at the short

Figure 7.4 – X-inactivation is an epigenetic process.
Because of X-inactivation every female is a mosaic of cell lines with different active X chromosomes.

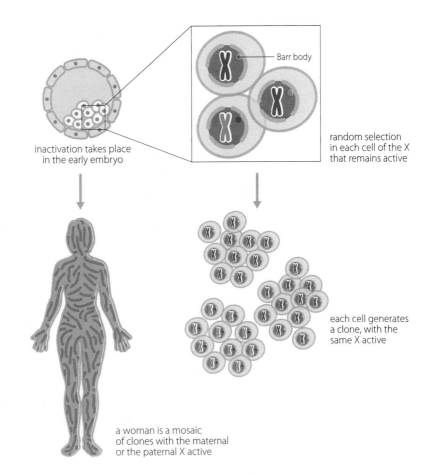

inactivation takes place in the early embryo

Barr body

random selection in each cell of the X that remains active

each cell generates a clone, with the same X active

a woman is a mosaic of clones with the maternal or the paternal X active

Figure 7.5 – Electron micrograph showing the X and Y chromosomes paired in prophase I of meiosis through the pseudoautosomal regions at the tips of their short arms. Reproduced from Connor and Ferguson Smith (1991) *Essential Medical Genetics*, 3rd edn., with permission from Blackwell Publishing, Oxford.

arm tip of the Y chromosome; the two pair in meiosis (*Figure 7.5*) and have an obligatory crossover in this region. Genes in this region escape X-inactivation. Men and women each have two active copies of these genes, and the pattern of inheritance of variants appears autosomal. For this reason the region is called the **pseudoautosomal region**. There is another small pseudoautosomal region, 300 kb long, at the tip of the long arm – but this does not usually pair or cross-over with its counterpart on the Y chromosome in meiosis.

X-inactivation has implications for female carriers of X-linked diseases, as shown below in the cases of the Davies and Portillo families (Cases 4 and 16), and for female carriers of X:autosome translocations, as described in the final section of this chapter. See the case of the Ingram family (Case 9) in the next section for further discussion of X-inactivation.

Imprinting – why you need a mother and a father

For a heterozygous person, the parental origin of each allele is not normally relevant when thinking about their phenotype. However, some observations suggest that there may be some functional differences between the maternal and paternal components of somebody's genome. Occasional accidents of fertilization produce 46,XX conceptuses that have either two maternal or two paternal

Figure 7.6 – Conceptuses that have two maternal or two paternal genomes cannot develop normally.

OVARIAN TERATOMA: disorganized fetal body parts; no membranes

HYDATIDIFORM MOLE: vigorously growing membranes; no embryo

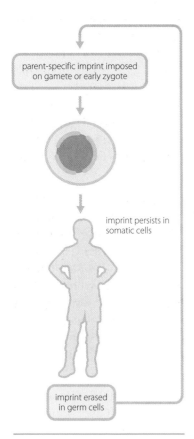

parent-specific imprint imposed on gamete or early zygote

imprint persists in somatic cells

imprint erased in germ cells

Figure 7.7 – Imprinting is epigenetic and reversible.

genomes. Despite being ostensibly chromosomally normal, such conceptuses always develop very abnormally, and quite differently from each other (*Figure 7.6*). Experiments in mice demonstrate the same effects. Evidently there is some difference between maternal and paternal genomes, and normal development requires one of each.

More refined experiments in mice allowed the contribution of each individual chromosome to this effect to be studied. Ingenious manipulations allow mice to be generated that have correct chromosome numbers, but both homologs of one particular pair are derived from just one parent. This is called **uniparental disomy** (UPD). For some chromosomes the resulting mice are normal, but for others they are abnormal, and the particular abnormalities seen depend on whether the mice have two maternal or two paternal copies of the chromosome in question. Rare human cases of UPD were also discovered by chance. Later it became apparent that certain human syndromes could be caused by UPD, as described below.

These and other observations suggest that there are human (and mouse) genes that behave differently depending on their parental origin. They must carry some sort of *imprint* that marks their origin. It is important to remember that genes are not intrinsically paternal or maternal. If a man passes on to his child an imprinted gene that he inherited from his mother, he received it with a maternal imprint but passes it on with a paternal imprint. Thus imprinting must be reversible, so that it can be erased and re-imposed with each generation (*Figure 7.7*). In fact imprinting is a major epigenetic mechanism: the expression of imprinted genes is modified, and the modification persists through all the cell divisions that lead from a fertilized egg to an adult person, but the DNA sequence is not changed. Our understanding of imprinting in humans has been greatly enhanced by the study of certain rare syndromes, in particular the two conditions described in Cases 17 and 18, Angelman and Prader-Willi syndromes.

The toolbox for X-inactivation and imprinting: DNA methylation

In *Disease box 2* and *Section 3.4* we saw how transcription of a gene is controlled by the local chromatin structure. The two major variants are the repressive heterochromatin and the permissive euchromatin. Within euchromatic regions gene expression is controlled by finer-scale modifications of chromatin structure, governed by the repertoire of proteins bound to the basic chromatin fiber. This in turn depends on two interacting and mutually reinforcing signals: modification of histones and methylation of the DNA. Histones (the small basic proteins that make up the core of nucleosomes) are subject to a wide range of modifications of amino acids in the tails that protrude from the nucleosome core. Methylation and acetylation of lysine residues are the main signals, but phosphorylation, attachment of ubiquitin (a small protein) and other modifications are also seen. Together these constitute a 'histone code' that converts the apparently uniform basic chromatin fiber into highly differentiated structures (Hendrich and Bickmore, 2001).

Interacting with the histone modifications is DNA methylation. In humans and other mammals this takes the form of adding methyl groups to the 5-position of cytosines to form 5-methyl cytosine (5MeC, *Figure 7.8*). Methylation is almost entirely restricted to cytosines that lie immediately 5′ of guanines in so-called **CpG dinucleotides** (the 'p' represents the phosphate group that links the two together). The processes of DNA methylation and histone modification are interdependent. Modified histones act as docking sites for DNA-modifying proteins, and methylated DNA binds chromatin remodeling proteins. Rett syndrome (see *Disease Box 7*) is the result of loss of function in the *MECP2* gene that encodes a 5MeC-binding protein. The protein binds to methylated regions of DNA, where it represses gene activity, either directly or by recruiting histone deacetylases and other transcriptional repressors. Jones and Baylin (2002) give details and illustrations of the process.

The methyl group of 5-methyl cytosine lies in the major groove on the outside of the double helix, where it is accessible to DNA-binding proteins but does not interfere with the base-pairing in the interior. 5MeC base-pairs with guanine in just the same way as unmodified cytosine (*Figure 7.8*), and so CpG methylation does not alter the coding properties of the DNA. Not every CpG is methylated, and the pattern of methylation differs according to the type of cell and its current metabolic state. Methylation of CpG dinucleotides upstream of a gene is a key signal for controlling gene expression. In general, methylation suppresses gene expression, but there are counter-examples.

Figure 7.8 – 5-methyl cytosine base-pairs with guanine in exactly the same way as unmodified cytosine.

CpG methylation is also the key mediator of X-inactivation and other epigenetic effects. Its importance for epigenetics stems from the fact that methylation patterns can be inherited. CpG is a palindromic sequence. That is, when read in the 5′→3′ direction, a CpG in one strand of the double helix is partnered by a CpG in the opposite strand. When DNA is replicated, a maintenance methylase enzyme methylates any CpG on the newly synthesized strand that that lies opposite a methylated CpG on the parental strand (*Figure 7.9*). Thus CpG methylation provides a mechanism for producing heritable changes in gene expression that do not depend on DNA sequence changes.

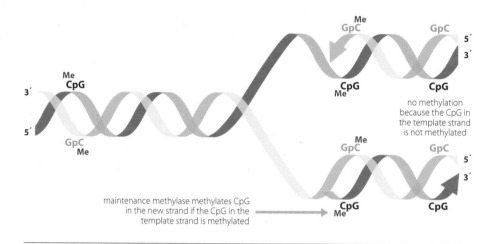

Figure 7.9 – The role of 5-methyl cytosine in epigenetics.
When the DNA is replicated a maintenance methylase specifically methylates CpG sequences in the newly synthesized strand whenever they occur opposite a methylated CpG in the template strand. As a result, patterns of CpG methylation are heritable.

Studying DNA methylation

Methylation patterns in DNA are much more difficult to study than sequence changes. As shown in *Figure 7.8*, 5MeC base-pairs with G indistinguishably from unmethylated cytosine, and so behaves identically to C in most laboratory tests. The hybridization properties of a DNA strand are unaffected by its methylation status, so hybridization-based tests cannot be used to investigate methylation. PCR and sequencing both depend on making copies of the sequence under investigation, and regardless of the state of methylation of the original DNA, the copies will be unmethylated. Thus none of the methods described in *Chapters 4* and *5* can be used to check the methylation pattern of a DNA sequence. Methylation studies mostly use two techniques:

- *Digestion by methylation-sensitive restriction enzymes.* Certain restriction enzymes whose recognition site includes a CpG sequence, will cut the site only if it is unmethylated. For example the restriction enzyme *Hpa*II cuts CCGG sequences, but will not cut C^MeCGG. Other enzymes are unaffected by methylation – for example *Msp*I cuts CCGG regardless of methylation. This difference can be exploited in various ways to reveal whether or not a particular CpG is methylated. In the investigation of Pablo Portillo (Case 16, see below) a sequence that included a CpG site was PCR amplified from DNA that had previously been digested with *Hpa*II. If the site was unmethylated, the template would have been cut in two, and no PCR product could be formed.

- *Bisulfite sequencing.* When DNA is treated with sodium bisulfite under carefully controlled conditions, cytosine is converted by deamination into uracil, but 5MeC is resistant to the reagent. Uracil is not a natural base in DNA, but it base-pairs with adenine in just the same way as thymine does. If a bisulfite-treated template is copied by PCR or used in a sequencing reaction, every unmethylated C in the original sequence appears as a T, while methylated Cs remain as C. Comparing the untreated and bisulfite-treated sequence reveals the pattern of methylation (*Figure 7.10*).

A variant of this method uses allele-specific PCR (*Figure 5.5*) to check the methylation status of one specific C. Primers are designed with 3′ terminal nucleotides G or A to match the C or U in the bisulfite-treated template. The G primer will amplify only the methylated template; the A primer amplifies only the unmethylated sequence. This method works best if the rest of the sequence to which the primer must hybridize is free of variably methylated cytosines, otherwise these too may be modified by the bisulfite treatment and prevent the primer hybridizing efficiently.

Figure 7.10 – The bisulfite method for analyzing DNA methylation.
Bisulfite treatment converts C to U. 5MeC remains unchanged. After PCR amplification, cytosines that were methylated are represented by thymines in the PCR product.

7.3. **Investigations of patients**

CASE 4	Davies family	4	10	66	102	151	**181**	279	376

- Boy (Martin) aged 24 months, parents Judith and Robert
- Clumsy and slow to walk
- Family history of muscular dystrophy
- Pedigree shows X-linked recessive inheritance
- Order diagnostic DNA test
- Frameshift mutation in the dystrophin gene

Several of Martin's female relatives are obligate or possible carriers of this X-linked recessive disease. As a result of lyonization, a normal adult XX female is a mosaic of clones, some of which have the paternal X active while others have the maternal X active. A carrier of an X-linked disease is a mosaic of normal and abnormal clones. The consequence depends on what the affected gene does, and where the cells are.

- Where the gene product is diffusible, there is an averaging effect. Carriers of X-linked hemophilia have half the normal level of the affected clotting factor (subject to the usual individual variation). The clotting time is noticeably increased above normal, but the blood still clots sufficiently well to avoid disease.

- Where the gene product is fixed, there are patches of normal and affected tissue. These may be demonstrable, for example, in anhidrotic ectodermal dysplasia (OMIM 305100), where the affected skin lacks sweat glands. The size of the patches depends on whether the tissue consists of many small clones or a few large ones, and on how much cell mixing occurs during development of that particular tissue.

- In Duchenne muscular dystrophy the picture is complicated by the fact that muscle cells are multinucleate, being formed by fusion of myoblasts. Staining a muscle biopsy with a dystrophin antibody shows a patchy distribution in muscles of heterozygous females, reflecting the random nature of X-inactivation (*Figure 7.11*). Occasional carriers have significant muscle weakness, presumably because by bad luck they inactivated mainly the normal X in their muscle cells. They are known as **manifesting heterozygotes**. Most carriers show biochemical evidence of subclinical muscle damage in the form of elevated levels of creatine kinase in their serum. As mentioned in *Chapter 4* the CK level can be used to give an estimate of a woman's risk of being a carrier, but the estimate is rarely sufficiently close to 0% or 100% to be a useful guide for reproductive decisions. Only DNA analysis can do that.

Figure 7.11 – A muscle biopsy from a female carrier of Duchenne muscular dystrophy stained with an antibody against dystrophin.
Note the patchy distribution of staining around the outer membranes of cells (compare with the sections from an affected boy and a normal control in *Figure 1.4*). Photo. courtesy of Dr Richard Charlton, Newcastle upon Tyne.

| CASE 9 | Ingram family | 26 | 41 | 68 | 101 | **182** | 376 |

- Isabel – first daughter of Irene and Ian
- Small stature despite tall parents
- ? Turner syndrome
- Diagnosis confirmed by karyotyping

Isabel Ingram has a single X chromosome, 45,X and has Turner syndrome. Given that the X-inactivation mechanism exists in order to allow normal development in people with differing numbers of X chromosomes, one might ask why there is anything wrong with her. The answer is that, even discounting the pseudoautosomal regions, not all genes on the X chromosome are subject to X-inactivation. A recent investigation of global transcription levels (Carrel and Willard, 2005) showed surprising deviations from the conventional picture of blanket X-inactivation. Even outside the pseudoautosomal regions, about 15%

of X-linked genes escape inactivation partially or totally, and a further 10% show differences between different inactive X chromosomes in the degree of inactivation.

Thus up to 25% of X-linked genes may have higher expression levels in normal females than in women with Turner syndrome. Those without functional Y-linked counterparts will also have Turner levels of expression in males – but maybe the higher expression of these genes in XX females is responsible for some of the differences between males and females. Intriguingly, it has been claimed that Turner women whose X is of maternal origin may have behavioral problems of the sort that are mainly seen in boys (whose X chromosome, of course, is of maternal origin), while Turner women with a paternal X are free of such problems. If true, this would be evidence of imprinting.

| CASE 16 | Portillo family | 173 | **183** | 214 | 376 |

- Sickly boy, Pablo
- Family history of similar symptoms
- Blood tests suggest X-linked severe combined immunodeficiency

Severe combined immunodeficiency can be either an autosomal recessive or an X-linked condition. At first it may seem surprising that an immunodeficiency should be X-linked – one might expect immunodeficiencies to be caused by mutations in the immunoglobulin genes, which are located on chromosomes 2, 14 and 22. But production of antibodies requires not only intact structural genes for those proteins, but also properly functioning B cells, whose successful development must require numerous other genetically controlled steps. In *Chapter 8* we will see some of the complicated processing that is needed to enable these cells to produce an effectively infinite repertoire of antibody molecules. Moreover, in combined immunodeficiency there is an absence of T cells as well as a functional defect in the B cells that produce antibodies. Its cause must be a failure of a much earlier stage of cell differentiation.

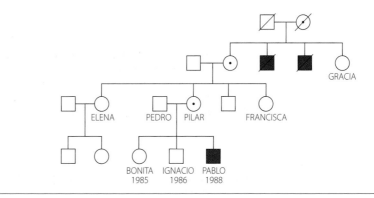

Figure 7.12 – Pedigree of severe combined immunodeficiency in the Portillo family.
The pattern shows that this is the X-linked form of this rare disease. The mother, grandmother and great-grandmother of the proband are obligate carriers. His sister, two aunts and cousin are at risk of being carriers.

When the pedigree (*Figure 7.12*) was taken it seemed clear that baby Pablo has the X-linked form of SCID. One immediate consequence for the family is to clarify the risks for relatives. Had the disease been the autosomal form, any relatives who were carriers would not be at risk of having affected children unless their partner was also a carrier. Because SCID is very rare, this risk is low provided they marry outside the family. However, now we know the condition is X-linked, Pilar's sisters, aunt and daughter are at substantial risk, although for her brother and normal son the risk is negligibly low.

At the time the family came to attention, it was not known what gene defect was responsible for X-SCID. However, it was possible to do carrier testing by looking at the pattern of X-inactivation in at-risk females. The X-SCID defect prevents development of B and T lymphocytes, therefore all lymphocytes in a carrier woman must be cells that happened to inactivate the defective X chromosome. Carriers will therefore show completely non-random inactivation in their lymphocytes, although in all their other tissues the normal random X-inactivation may be seen.

The methylation-sensitive restriction enzyme *Hpa*II was used to check the randomness of X-inactivation. The androgen receptor gene on the X chromosome contains a variable length $(CAG)_n$ trinucleotide repeat (see *Disease box 6*). The test will only work in women whose two X chromosomes have different sized repeats – but fortunately these are the majority of women because the repeat is highly polymorphic. Near the repeat are two CCGG sequences that are methylated in females on the inactive X, but unmethylated on the active X (and on the only X in males). A DNA segment containing both the $(CAG)_n$ repeat and the two CCGG sites is PCR-amplified from the person's DNA, with or without prior digestion with *Hpa*II (*Figure 7.13*).

- When the PCR is performed on a straightforward DNA sample from a woman, it amplifies the sequences from both the active and inactive X chromosomes. PCR is not affected in any way by methylation of the DNA. Assuming the woman is heterozygous for two different sized $(CAG)_n$ repeats, when the PCR product is run on a sequencer we see two equal sized peaks (*Figure 7.13b*).
- A second PCR reaction is performed on DNA that has been digested with *Hpa*II. On inactive X chromosomes, *Hpa*II fails to cut the methylated sites. The PCR target sequence remains intact and can be amplified. On active X chromosomes, the restriction enzyme cleaves the PCR target sequence. The PCR primers therefore end up hybridized to different restriction fragments, and the PCR reaction will not work. Thus the PCR product from *Hpa*II-digested DNA shows just the product from the inactive X.
- A conventional DNA sample contains DNA from a large number of lymphocytes. If X-inactivation is random, about half the cells will have had one X inactivated and about half will have had the other one inactivated. When the PCR product from the *Hpa*II-digested sample is run on a sequencer, we see the same peaks as when we amplified undigested DNA, just each peak is about half size.
- If X-inactivation is non-random, one of the peaks will be selectively lost in the PCR product from the pre-digested DNA. The sequencer can quantitate the relative peak areas, and so give a precise figure for the proportion of cells that have each X active. Any female who is a carrier of X-SCID will show completely skewed X-inactivation in her lymphocytes.

This test showed that Pilar, her sister Elena and their mother had non-random X-inactivation in their lymphocytes. A chromosome giving a 270 bp PCR product was always inactivated. This was the one that Pilar and Elena had inherited from their mother. Pilar and Elena's other X gave a 273 bp PCR product (presumably the $(CAG)_n$ repeat had one more unit) and was fully digested by the *Hpa*II enzyme, showing that it was active in every lymphocyte. This came from their father. Francisca had the paternal 273 bp allele but she had inherited her mother's 285 bp allele. The *Hpa*II digest amplified both her chromosomes to approximately equal degrees, showing that in Francisca X-inactivation was random. Thus Pilar and Elena (and their mother) were carriers of the immunodeficiency, while Francisca was not. At the time this testing was done the defective gene had not been identified and though the gene had been mapped there was some uncertainty about the data. Their story is taken further in *Chapter 8*.

(a)

(b)

Figure 7.13 – A test for randomness of X-inactivation.
(a) The region of the androgen receptor gene on the X chromosome used in the test. The positions of the PCR primers, the trinucleotide repeat and the *Hpa*II sites are shown. (b) Results of the tests. The PCR products were sized and quantitated on a DNA sequencer.

| CASE 17 & 18 | Qian family | 174 | **185** | 376 |
| | Rogers family | 175 | **185** | 376 |

Qian family
- Girl, Kai, aged 2 years, showing slow development
- Seizure
- ? Angelman syndrome
- Check for causative mutation with FISH

These two cases are considered together because although the symptoms of PWS and Angelman syndrome are completely different, the causes of both conditions have a great deal in common. Three-quarters of cases of each condition are caused by a deletion of chromosome 15q11-q13. It was natural to suppose that since the two syndromes are so different, the deletions causing them must also be different at the molecular level – but they are not. The deletions are caused

Rogers family
- Baby boy, Robert, born to older parents
- Floppy at birth; failed to suck
- Genetic tests in pregnancy showed normal male karyotype
- ? Prader–Willi syndrome
- Check for causative mutation with PCR

Figure 7.14 – The 15q11q13 deletion in Prader–Willi or Angelman syndrome patients is sometimes just visible under the microscope in a standard cytogenetic preparation. In most cases a molecular test (FISH or PCR) is needed to make the diagnosis.

by recombination between misaligned repeats – the same mechanism as we saw in Williams syndrome and the Di George-VCFS syndrome. The same 4 Mb stretch of DNA is normally deleted in each condition.

The breakthrough in understanding these conditions came when it was realized that the difference between them was due not to different sized deletions, but to different parental origins of the deleted chromosome. In PWS it is always the paternal chromosome 15 that is deleted, while in Angelman syndrome it is always the maternal copy. Thus imprinted genes at 15q11-q13 lie at the heart of the pathology. The cases of each syndrome that do not have a deletion have other disturbances affecting this chromosomal region (see below).

A FISH test for deletions. The deletion is sometimes just visible under the microscope (*Figure 7.14*) but it can readily be checked using FISH (see *Section 4.2*) or MLPA (*Section 5.2*). The array-CGH data shown in *Figure 4.8* are from a patient with PWS. This would be an expensive technique to use simply to check for the standard PWS deletion, but would be appropriate for an atypical case where there was doubt about the location or size of any deletion. In the present two cases a FISH probe for 15q11 identified a deletion in Kai Qian, confirming the diagnosis of Angelman syndrome. However, no deletion was seen in Robert Rogers, and so the provisional diagnosis of PWS still needed confirming.

A PCR test for the presence of maternal and paternal imprints. PWS is always caused by lack of a paternally imprinted copy of the 15q11q13 region, but this can arise in various ways other than by deletion. A PCR test can be used to check directly for PWS arising through any of the possible causes (and similarly for Angelman syndrome). Certain CpG sequences within the critical region are differentially methylated on chromosomes carrying a paternal or a maternal imprint. This difference may constitute the actual functional imprint or may be a consequence of the imprints – either way it allows a reliable test for the imprinting status. DNA is treated with bisulfite to convert unmethylated cytosines into uracil. The different methylation patterns in paternally and maternally imprinted DNA protect different cytosines from attack by the bisulfite. Thus the paternally and maternally imprinted copies of the same sequence are converted by the bisulfite reaction into different DNA sequences. These are then PCR-amplified using primers specific for the maternal or paternal bisulfited sequence. The two reactions give different sized products, and so can be run together in a single tube (*Figure 7.15*).

Using DNA polymorphisms to test for uniparental disomy. The PCR test showed that Robert Rogers only had the maternal imprint, which confirmed the diagnosis of PWS even though no deletion had been seen with FISH. Since FISH tests for the presence of only the one particular sequence within 15q11q13 that was used as the probe, array-CGH could have been used for further investigation of Robert, to check sequences all across the PWS candidate region in case he had an unusual deletion. In the present case, however, the next step was to check for uniparental disomy.

About 30% of PWS patients have two intact copies of chromosome 15, but both inherited from the mother. Uniparental disomy (UPD) can be detected by looking at the inheritance patterns of polymorphisms in the DNA of chromosome 15.

Figure 7.15 – Using methylation-sensitive PCR to diagnose the state of imprinting of chromosome 15q11q13.
Chromosomes carrying a maternal imprint give a 313 bp product; those carrying a paternal imprint give a 221 bp product. Normal people show both bands (lanes 3–6); Angelman patients lack the 313 bp product (lane 1) and Prader–Willi patients lack the 221 bp product (lane 2). Lane M contains size markers. See Zeschnigk *et al.* (1997) for full details of the method. Photo. courtesy of Dr Simon Ramsden, St Mary's Hospital, Manchester.

Scattered in non-coding DNA all over the genome are short runs of tandemly repeated $(CA)_n$ nucleotides. The number of CA units present in one of these so-called microsatellites often varies between normal people. This number can be checked by PCR-amplifying a DNA fragment that includes the repeat and sizing it on a gel, in the same way as we checked the number of units in the $(CAG)_n$ repeat in the Huntington disease family (Ashton family, Case 1, see *Section 4.3*). The repeats used in the present investigation are not pathogenic, but serve as markers to identify the parental origin of the chromosomes. See *Chapter 9* for a fuller discussion of these DNA polymorphisms.

Figure 7.16 shows the results for two of the polymorphisms. In the first case (*Figure 7.16a*) it happens that the particular alleles in the three samples are such that we can't work out which of Robert's two alleles came from which parent. Remember that these are non-pathogenic polymorphisms that have no role in causing PWS or any other disease, so it is purely a chance matter which alleles a person happens to have. The result does show that Robert has two copies of this particular sequence, and since this is a sequence from within the PWS critical region, it confirms the FISH test, showing that he does not have a deletion. The second marker (*Figure 7.16b*) is more informative. We see that Robert has no paternal alleles. He might be homozygous or hemizygous (having only a single copy) for the maternal allele; by itself this result is compatible with either a deletion or UPD. Knowing there is no deletion, it demonstrates UPD. This is isodisomy, in which he has two copies of the same maternal chromosome. UPD could be confirmed by finding a similar pattern with a second chromosome 15 marker (microsatellite alleles occasionally mutate, so it is prudent to confirm any finding using a second independent microsatellite).

Robert has inherited no copy of chromosome 15 from his father. Under the microscope Robert's karyotype looks completely normal, but the microsatellite analysis shows that both his copies of chromosome 15 come from his mother. The phenotype of PWS is identical in patients with UPD or those with the more common paternal deletion, showing that PWS is caused by lack of a paternal copy

Figure 7.16 – **Segregation of chromosome 15 markers in a child with Prader–Willi syndrome.**
M, mother; F, father; C, child. (a) For this marker it is not possible to say which of the child's alleles are inherited from which parent. (b) For this marker the child does not inherit either of his father's alleles. Photo. courtesy of Dr Simon Ramsden, St Mary's Hospital, Manchester.

of the 15q11q13 sequence, and that lack of paternal copies of genes elsewhere on chromosome 15 has no additional effect. A few cases of non-deletion Angelman syndrome also are caused by UPD – in that case, having two paternal and no maternal copy of chromosome 15.

The origins of uniparental disomy. The UPD explains why Robert has PWS – but how does UPD arise? When the first example was reported (a child with cystic fibrosis in 1988) it was supposed that an egg that happened, through non-disjunction, to contain two copies of the relevant chromosome had, by extraordinary good luck, been fertilized by a sperm that happened, by non-disjunction, to lack any copy of that chromosome. If such a lucky coincidence were its sole cause, UPD would be vanishingly rare. In fact, though uncommon, it is seen far too frequently to be explained by such rare coincidences. A much more likely origin is through **trisomy rescue** (*Figure 7.17*). We know that every possible trisomy occurs at conception, but nearly all are incompatible with survival to term and miscarry spontaneously. But as *Figure 7.17* shows, a chance non-disjunction in an early mitotic division of a trisomic conceptus might generate one cell with a normal chromosome count. If that happened early enough in embryogenesis, that one cell may be able to develop into a complete person. Assuming the mitotic non-disjunction is random, one time in three the result would be UPD. Supporting this view, UPD accounts for 29% of PWS cases but only 1% of Angelman syndrome. We know that the non-disjunctions that produce trisomies usually occur in the maternal meiosis, so we would expect most trisomic conceptuses to have two maternal and one paternal contribution. Therefore trisomy rescue is far more likely to generate maternal UPD than paternal UPD. It may be significant that Robert's mother Rowena was 38 years old when Robert was conceived.

Other causes of PWS and Angelman syndrome. Deletion or UPD account for nearly all cases of PWS and most cases of Angelman syndrome (*Table 7.1*) but some have other causes. If either PWS or Angelman syndrome were the result of loss of function of one gene in the candidate region, then loss-of-function point mutations in the gene (on the appropriate parental chromosome) should have the same effect. The deleted region contains a number of genes, several

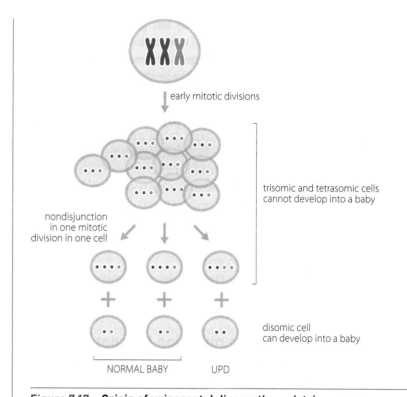

Figure 7.17 – Origin of uniparental disomy through trisomy rescue.
The initial conceptus is trisomic. A non-disjunction event in one mitotic division generates one disomic cell. If this happens very early in development that one cell is able to form the whole baby. By chance, one time in three the two copies will both be from the same parent.

of which show imprinted expression (*Figure 7.18*). As is usually the case with imprinted regions, some genes are expressed only from the paternal, and others only from the maternal chromosome. Checking each gene for mutations revealed point mutations in the *UBE3A* gene in around half of the non-deletion, non-UPD Angelman cases. Interestingly, this gene shows imprinted expression in brain but not in other tissues – thus imprinting can be tissue-specific. No point mutations of a single gene have been found in PWS – presumably the phenotype is caused by loss of more than one gene.

In a few otherwise unexplained cases of either syndrome, there seems to be a fault in the imprinting mechanism. Marker studies (as in *Figure 7.16*) show that chromosomes from both parents are present and complete, but methylation-specific PCR (as in *Figure 7.15*) shows that both carry the same parental imprint.

Figure 7.18 – Genes in the Prader–Willi / Angelman syndrome region.

Figure 7.20 – Effect of X-inactivation in an embryo with a balanced X:autosome translocation.

these cells are the only ones that form the baby

X   X/A   A   A/X

inactivation may spread into the autosomal sequence

remains active, result is a severe imbalance, cell is non-viable

Other imprinting-related disorders

The study of imprinting-related disorders takes us into some of the most intricate and poorly understood areas of human genetics, and full accounts are well beyond the scope of this book. Apart from 15q11q13, a number of other chromosomal regions are known to contain imprinted genes (*Table 7.2*). Like the Prader–Willi/Angelman region, these usually contain clusters of imprinted genes, some expressed only from the maternal and some only from the paternal chromosome. In PWS and Angelman syndrome loss of either the maternal or the paternal chromosome causes a specific syndrome, while having two copies of either seems to make no difference (because UPD cases are phenotypically identical to deletion cases). Other imprinted regions may only show effects with loss from one parent, or may show specific dosage effects from having two copies of one parental chromosome. In all cases, various different events can cause the same disorder, as in *Table 7.1*.

Table 7.2 – Some diseases that may involve imprinting-related mechanisms

Syndrome	OMIM #	Chromosomal location	Affected gene
Prader–Willi syndrome	176270 (PWS)	15q11q13	*SNRPN* (PWS);
Angelman syndrome	105830 (AS)		*UBE3A* (AS)
Beckwith–Wiedemann syndrome	130650	11p15.5	*H19, IGF2, KCNQ1OT1*
Silver–Russell syndrome	180860	7p11.2 11p15.5	*GRB10*? *H19, IGF2*?
Carotid body tumors	168000	11q23	*SDHD*
Pseudohypoparathyroidism	103580	20q13.2	*GNAS1*
Transient neonatal diabetes mellitus	601410	6q24	*ZAC/HYMAI*

What is the purpose of imprinting?

Several theories have been proposed to explain why imprinting should have evolved (see Wilkins and Haig, 2003). The conflict theory of imprinting suggests that, seen in 'selfish gene' terms, parents have conflicting interests. A father's genes are best propagated by his having plenty of children. If his partner dies from exhaustion, he can always grab another woman from the next cave. A woman's genes are best propagated if she takes care of herself and doesn't devote too many resources to any one child. Thus paternal genes promote fetal growth, even at the expense of the mother, while maternal genes limit the resources a fetus can take from her. This fits with the observations on hydatidiform moles and ovarian teratomas: the paternal genes promote proliferation of the placenta and membranes, which extract nutrients from the mother; maternal genes do the opposite. However, not every imprinted phenotype fits this theory – for example, we might expect babies with PWS to be small, and those with Angelman syndrome to be big, which is not the case. Imprinting of the *IGF2* (insulin-related growth factor 2) gene varies between healthy individuals, suggesting that not all imprinting has a function. In some cases it may be a chance side effect of gene control mechanisms.

How important are epigenetic effects?

Within a cell DNA methylation and concomitant changes in the histone code and in chromatin structure are central to gene regulation. Given the heritable nature of CpG methylation it is reasonable to suppose that epigenetic changes based on DNA methylation are important for establishing and maintaining cell and tissue identity. Support for this comes from cancer research. As we will see in *Chapter 12*, epigenetic changes are widespread and important in cancer. However, imprinting seems to be limited to a small number of genes - currently just a few dozen.

One area where epigenetic programming is important is in reproductive technology (Horsthemke and Ludwig, 2005). It is common experience that cloned mammals are often abnormal. Quite apart from the low success rate of cloning (few of the manipulated eggs develop to term), when a cloned animal is born it is often oversized and there are high rates of neonatal death. It is thought that the somatic cell nucleus used for cloning has undergone epigenetic changes during development of the animal from which it was taken; in order for it to function as the nucleus of a fertilized egg these changes must be reversed. It is supposed that this epigenetic reprogramming is effected by the cytoplasm of the egg into which the nucleus is transplanted, but that the reprogramming is incomplete and imperfect. Similar effects on a smaller scale are seen with human-assisted conception. There is an increased risk of Beckwith–Wiedemann syndrome among babies born by *in vitro* fertilization. The risk is not large (about 1 in 5000), but it is definitely larger than for naturally conceived babies. The abnormal circumstances of IVF conceptions are thought to somehow interfere with epigenetic programming, resulting in an increased risk of epigenetic disease.

Rett syndrome

Rett syndrome (OMIM 312750) is a childhood onset disorder, affecting almost exclusively females. Dr Andreas Rett, an Austrian physician, first described the disorder in 1966. Usually there is a period of normal early development followed, between 6 and 18 months, by apparent regression with loss of purposeful use of the hands and the onset of characteristic hand-wringing or other stereotypic movements. Head growth slows and over 50% develop seizures. Breathing irregularities including hyperventilation and apnea are common and eye contact is difficult to achieve. The course, severity and age of onset of the condition vary from child to child. Some girls never learn to walk or talk whilst others retain these skills to a certain extent. The condition can remain stationary for many years although complications like scoliosis occur. In later years further deterioration may lead to loss of muscle bulk, limitation of mobility and liability to chest infections.

The majority of cases of Rett syndrome are female and the only case in a family. However, there were a few reported families of affected sisters, or half-sisters with the same mother, which supported the hypothesis that Rett syndrome was caused by a mutation in a gene on the X chromosome, and that it was likely to be lethal in males. Mutations in methyl-CpG-binding protein 2 (*MECP2*) were found in these rare families and in a large majority of girls with classic Rett syndrome. *MECP2* mutations were also found in some males with a severe neonatal encephalopathy and indeed in occasional families with a girl with Rett syndrome, a male sibling with such a history of encephalopathy had been reported.

A girl with Rett syndrome, showing the characteristic hand-wringing.

The function of the MeCP2 protein in transcriptional silencing and epigenetic regulation of methylated DNA has been described above. There is a suggestion of genotype–phenotype correlation in that milder disease is observed in those with mis-sense mutations than in those with truncating mutations and in those with mutations that do not affect DNA binding. However, several individuals have been reported who have the same mutation but different phenotypes. Thus other factors such as X chromosome inactivation may influence severity. The genes regulated by MeCP2 activity are not yet all identified. It is also not understood why a period of normal development should occur.

Atypical phenotypes are described with earlier or later onset, or with milder or more severe effects and only a third of these carry an *MECP2* mutation. Some of those with early onset infantile spasms and severe phenotypes do not have *MECP2* mutations; instead they have *de novo* mis-sense mutations in another gene on the X chromosome, *CDKL5*. It has been speculated that the CDKL5 protein may be involved in regulating the phosphorylation of MeCP2. This is an example of using a phenotype to start unraveling a developmental pathway (see *Chapter 6*).

Some people believe that epigenetic changes have a fundamental role in human adaptation to a changing environment. A controversial theory (the 'Barker hypothesis', see Barker, 1995) holds that the general balance of a person's metabolism (their tendency to obesity, hypertension, etc.) is largely determined by their nutritional status in intrauterine and early neonatal life. This adaptation might well depend on epigenetic mechanisms. The *IGF2* gene might be a key player in this process, as it has important roles in the regulation of metabolism and is known to be subject to imprinting effects.

Still more controversially, a number of epidemiological observations support the idea of *transgenerational* epigenetic effects. This is a difficult area to study. Understandably, the hypotheses being tested are novel and not very precise, and the datasets include large numbers of variables. This raises considerable problems of interpretation. Transgenerational effects down the female line are anyhow difficult to interpret because transmission of metabolic signals across the placenta could be the explanation. For effects transmitted down the male line, epigenetic transmission is a strong candidate. Examples of possible male-line transgenerational effects include:

- Historical studies from northern Sweden that show an association between the childhood food supply of the father and/or the paternal grandparents and the proband's longevity or risk of diabetic / cardiovascular mortality (Kaati *et al.*, 2002, Pembrey *et al.*, 2006).
- A contemporary UK cohort study that shows an association between paternal *onset* of smoking in mid-childhood and increased body mass index in their future sons at 9 years (Pembrey *et al.*, 2006).
- A contemporary population from Taiwan that shows an association between paternal betel nut chewing and early onset of the 'metabolic syndrome' in his offspring (Chen *et al.*, 2006). The 'metabolic syndrome' includes obesity, insulin resistance, raised blood pressure and increased risk of diabetes and cardiovascular disease (see *Section 13.1*), so there is some overlap in the outcomes of these three transgenerational responses.

One has to ask why, given that it is desirable to be adapted to one's environment, the proposed transgenerational epigenetic effects appear to adapt us to our grandparents' environment rather than our own. Supporters of epigenetic programming might reply that transgenerational effects are only a very small part of the general epigenetic programming, but because they are counter-intuitive they force us to take epigenetic explanations seriously.

7.5. **References**

Barker DJP (1995) Fetal origins of coronary heart disease. *Br. Med. J.* 311: 171–174. For a hostile comment see Paneth N and Susser M (1995) Early origin of coronary heart disease (the 'Barker hypothesis') *Br. Med. J.* 310: 411–412. *Full text of both articles is freely available at* http://bmj.bmjjournals.com.

Carrel L and Willard HF (2005) X-inactivation profile reveals extensive variability in X-linked gene expression in females. *Nature,* 434: 400–404.

Chen TH-H, Chiu YH and Boucher BJ (2006) Transgenerational effects of betel-quid chewing on the development of the metabolic syndrome in the Keelung Community-based Integrated Screening Program. *Am. J. Clin. Nutr.* **83**: 688–692.

Hendrich D and Bickmore W (2001) Human diseases with underlying defects in chromatin structure and modification. *Hum. Mol. Genet.* **10**: 2233–2242.

Horsthemke B and Ludwig M (2005) Assisted reproduction: the epigenetic perspective. *Hum. Reprod. Update,* **11**: 473–482

Jones PA and Baylin SB (2003) The fundamental role of epigenetic events in cancer. *Nature Rev. Cancer,* **3**: 415–428. *This review is about cancer but the mechanisms they describe are general.*

Kaati G, Bygren LO and Edvinsson S (2002) Cardiovascular and diabetes mortality determined by nutrition during parents' and grandparents' slow growth period. *Eur. J. Hum. Genet.* **10**: 682–688.

Pembrey ME, Bygren LO, Kaati G, *et al.* (2006) Sex-specific male-line transgenerational responses in humans. *Eur. J. Hum. Genet.* **14**: 159–166.

Wilkins DF and Haig D (2003) What good is genomic imprinting: the function of parent-specific gene expression. *Nat. Rev. Genet.* **4**: 359–368.

Zeschnigk M, Lich C, Buiting K, Doerfler W and Horsthemke B (1997) A single-tube PCR test for the diagnosis of Angelman and Prader-Willi syndrome based on allelic methylation differences at the *SNRPN* locus. *Eur. J. Hum. Genet.* **5**: 94–98.

7.6. **Self-assessment questions**

(1) Suppose a gene on chromosome 6 is imprinted so that it is expressed only when it is inherited from the father. Complete absence of gene expression causes an unusual facial appearance. Draw a possible pedigree that you might see if a loss of function mutation in the gene is segregating in a large family.

(2) Repeat the exercise in SAQ1 assuming that imprinting is such that the gene is expressed only from the maternal chromosome.

(3) In the X-inactivation test, as performed on Pilar Portillo and her sisters (Case 16), after *Hpa*II digestion the product was boiled for 10 min so as to thoroughly destroy all traces of the restriction enzyme before adding the reagents for the PCR reaction. Why was this necessary?

(4) The diagram shows types for three DNA polymorphisms on chromosome 15 in the parents of a child. Marker A maps within the PWS / Angelman syndrome critical region; the other two markers map distal to this region. Write possible marker genotypes for their child if he has:

(a) PWS due to a deletion
(b) Angelman syndrome due to a deletion
(c) PWS due to uniparental disomy

(d) Angelman syndrome due to uniparental disomy

(e) PWS due to an imprinting error

(f) Angelman syndrome due to a mutation in the *UBE3A* gene

(5) Repeat exercise 4 assuming that in the paternal meiosis there was a crossover between the positions of markers A and B, and in the maternal meiosis between the positions of markers B and C. (NB this is not unrealistic – there is normally at least one crossover in each chromosome arm in each meiotic division.)

(6) Part of a DNA sequence is as follows:

```
          m                    m       m m      m
5′    CACTGCGGCAAACAAGCACGCCTGCGCGGCCGCAGAGGCAG    3′
```

The cytosines indicated are either all methylated or all unmethylated, depending on the parental origin. The DNA is treated with sodium bisulfite and then a PCR primer is used to make a complementary strand. The primer used is off the diagram to the right. Design 10-nucleotide primers to specifically amplify the methylated and unmethylated versions of this sequence in conjunction with the downstream primer, and write out the sequence of this part of the PCR product. (Real primers would be 20–40 nucleotides long – they might need to be longer than normal PCR primers because it might be impossible to avoid some mismatches depending on which cytosines were methylated).

(7) The pedigree shows genotypes for a polymorphic DNA marker that is located in the Xp–Yp pseudoautosomal region. Mark in possible genotypes for all the people in the pedigree.

Chapter 8

How do our genes affect our metabolism, drug responses and immune system?

Learning points for this chapter

After working through this chapter you should be able to:

- Describe the basic principles of inborn errors of metabolism and give examples of diseases caused by metabolic blocks
- Give examples of individual variations in response to drugs, explaining their importance
- Discuss critically the prospects for personalized medicine based on genetic testing
- Describe the general nature and function of the major histocompatibility complex and the role of HLA matching in transplantation
- Describe in outline the genetic mechanisms underpinning our ability to mount a specific immune response against virtually any foreign antigen

8.1. Case studies

CASE 19	Stott family	**199**	210	376

- Second pregnancy; scan suggests baby boy
- Baby born with ambiguous genitalia
- FISH to chromosomes
- ? Congenital adrenal hyperplasia

Sarah and Steven Stott had already had a daughter and were pleased when the scan in their second pregnancy seemed to indicate the baby was a boy. However, when the new baby was examined by the nurse soon after birth she was worried and the pediatrician was called. She explained to Sarah and Steven that the baby had ambiguous genitalia and might be a little boy with an abnormality called hypospadias, or a little girl who was virilized by an underlying hormone problem. Otherwise the baby was well, but the pediatrician arranged for urgent tests for sodium and potassium, and for chromosome analysis. Using FISH studies the cytogenetics lab. was soon able to report that the baby was chromosomally a girl, and the biochemical tests were normal. The pediatrician asked her pediatric endocrinology colleague to become involved and samples were sent off for 17-hydroxy progesterone and testosterone levels to be assessed. Samples were also sent to the molecular genetics lab. for genetic testing for congenital adrenal hyperplasia. When the results came back they indicated that this was the diagnosis, and the baby, who by then had been called Susie, had the less severe type where salt is not lost. Her levels of 17-hydroxy progesterone and testosterone were raised and mutations had been found in both copies of Susie's *CYP21* genes. Hydrocortisone treatment was started and surgery was planned for later that year. When Sarah and Steven looked back at Susie's first week they recalled how difficult it was for them because they were very worried about the baby, couldn't tell their friends and relations whether they had had a girl or boy, and couldn't choose a name for the baby.

Figure 8.1 – Ambiguous genitalia of a baby girl with the simple virilizing form of congenital adrenal hyperplasia.

| CASE 20 | Tierney family | **200** | 213 | 310 | 376 |

- 4-year-old boy, Jason
- Pale with extensive bruising and tachycardia
- ? Acute lymphocytic leukemia

Jason is a previously fit and well 4 year old boy who presented with a two-week history of extensive bruising and a pain in his back. His mother took him to the family doctor who noted that he was pale and tachycardic (a fast heart rate) without obvious fever. Blood tests revealed a low hemoglobin level (anemia), a raised white blood cell count ($90 \times 10^9 / l$, normal level 4–$11 \times 10^9 / l$) and low platelet level. Analysis of the blood count showed a high level of lymphocytes. These results raised the possibility of a diagnosis of childhood acute lymphocytic leukemia.

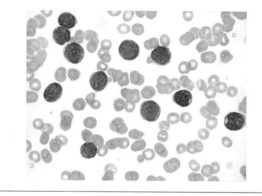

Figure 8.2 – Typical appearance of acute lymphocytic leukemia.
Small blasts with high nuclear – cytoplasmic ratio, some with prominent nucleoli. Photo courtesy of Dr John Yin, Manchester Royal Infirmary.

8.2. **Background**

In this chapter we cover three areas of genetics, all of which concern causes of genetic differences between people:

- inborn errors of metabolism
- common variation in drug responses (**pharmacogenetics**)

- the systems that enable us to mount an immune response against virtually any foreign antigen, but that also lead to transplant rejection (**immunogenetics**)

The present section and *Section 8.4* are each divided into three parts, covering these three areas.

Inborn errors of metabolism

The concept of inborn errors of metabolism was developed at the very dawn of clinical genetics (see *Box 8.1*). If a metabolic pathway requires the sequential action of several enzymes, a loss of function mutation in any one of the genes encoding those enzymes will lead to a metabolic block (*Figure 8.3*). Substrate accumulates before the block, and there is a lack of product downstream of the block.

Figure 8.3 – **Effects of a metabolic block in a simple pathway.**

- In a biosynthetic pathway the most noticeable effect is likely to be the absence of the end product. For example, tyrosinase is the key enzyme for biosynthesis of melanin, and homozygous loss of function of tyrosinase causes albinism (*Figure 8.4*).
- In a degradative pathway, it is usually the accumulation of the blocked substrate that causes problems. The lysosomal storage diseases are typical examples. Lysosomes are vesicles that contain a collection of around 40 different hydrolytic enzymes that are required to degrade a variety of large molecules. Lysosomes import high molecular weight material, but can only export the low molecular weight products of degradative reactions. A deficiency of one or other of the lysosomal enzymes therefore causes undegraded or partially degraded high molecular weight material to accumulate within the lysosome. This can lead eventually to the death of the cell. Patients with lysosomal storage diseases are normal at birth, but there is a progressive deterioration as undegraded material builds up in the lysosomes. For instance, in mucopolysaccharidoses like Hunter syndrome (OMIM 309900) and Hurler syndrome (OMIM 607014), lack of one or another enzyme required for the breakdown of glycosaminoglycans (mucopolysaccharides) leads to accumulation of undegradable and unexportable high molecular weight material. *Figure 10.1* illustrates the consequences in one lysosomal storage disease, Tay-Sachs disease.
- The high concentration of substrate upstream of a block in a degradative or synthetic pathway can also lead to the production of abnormal metabolites. For example, in phenylketonuria (see Vlasi family, Case 22 in *Chapter 11*) a block in the normal catabolic pathway for phenylalanine

leads to an accumulation of phenylalanine in the blood and tissues (*Figure 8.4*). This eventually spills over into production of phenylketones. The porphyrias (see *Disease box 8* at the end of this chapter) are caused by accumulation of pathogenic intermediates in a blocked synthetic pathway.

Figure 8.4 – Metabolism of the amino acids phenylalanine and tyrosine.
Consequences of a metabolic block can include absence of product (albinism), excretion of the material immediately upstream of the block (alkaptonuria), or excretion of alternative metabolites of a blocked substrate (phenylketonuria). PHPA = *p*-hydroxy phenylalanine.

Box 8.1

Some history

The concept of *inborn errors of metabolism* goes back to the very early days of human genetics: in 1902 Archibald Garrod published a paper entitled 'The incidence of alkaptonuria: a study in chemical individuality'. Alkaptonuria (OMIM 203500 – see *Figure 8.4*) is a rare recessive condition in which affected individuals lack homogentisate 1,2-dioxygenase (also called homogentisic acid oxidase) and accordingly excrete in their urine large amounts of homogentisic acid, an intermediate in the catabolism of phenylalanine and tyrosine. This readily darkens on exposure to air, hence the name. Garrod noted that parents of patients were often first cousins, and that brothers and sisters were sometimes affected. He speculated that alkaptonuria might be a mendelian recessive condition – a remarkable insight, given that Mendel's work had only been rediscovered two years previously. In a series of lectures in 1908, Garrod coined the term 'inborn error of metabolism' and suggested cystinuria and pentosuria as further examples.

Rather like Mendel, Garrod was perhaps ahead of his time. Geneticists at the time were more concerned with understanding the basic mechanisms of heredity, and biochemists with understanding basic biological chemistry. Patients with exceedingly rare diseases were not amenable to experimental investigation. It was over 30 years later that Beadle and Tatum developed a suitable experimental system, X-ray mutagenesis and biochemical analysis of the fungus *Neurospora crassa*. Their 1941 paper 'Genetic control of biochemical reactions in *Neurospora*' does not contain the phrase associated with their names, 'one gene – one enzyme' but does say:

> *It should be possible, by finding a number of mutants unable to carry out a particular step in a given synthesis, to determine whether only one gene is ordinarily concerned with the immediate regulation of a given specific chemical reaction.*

Within five years, Beadle had clearly enunciated the one gene – one enzyme hypothesis and placed it at the centre of contemporary understanding of gene action. At that time neither the structure of proteins nor that of genes was known. A further seminal development was the demonstration by Ingram in 1956 of the difference between normal hemoglobin and hemoglobin S. By the early 1960s all the basic concepts of biochemical genetics were in place.

Biochemical genetics is defined more by its methods and practitioners than by anything else. During the period 1960–1990, before PCR became routine, possibilities for clinical genetic testing by DNA analysis were limited. Biochemists, however, had a sophisticated knowledge of metabolic pathways and enzymology, and they applied this to any suitable genetic condition. They used specialized tools, such as gas chromatography coupled to mass spectrometry (GC–MS), to identify abnormal metabolites in blood or urine. They ran large-scale newborn screening programs, and were closely involved in managing children in whom they diagnosed inborn errors. All this set them a little apart from mainstream clinical genetics. Nowadays the two have very much come together. The biochemists have not abandoned their GC–MS and other special technologies, but the use of DNA methods and of concepts from biochemistry and cell biology is now universal across all of clinical genetics.

Congenital adrenal hyperplasia (CAH), the condition affecting Susie Stott (Case 19), illustrates a rather more complex situation. CAH is a result of a metabolic block that prevents the production of the glucocorticoid and mineralocorticoid hormones. *Figure 8.5* shows the main synthetic pathways. All steroid synthesis starts from cholesterol. The enzymes involved are mostly members of the cytochrome P450 family of oxidative enzymes. P450 enzymes are also involved in the metabolism of many drugs, as we shall see below. Several of the enzymes act on multiple, closely related substrates and some of them catalyze more than one reaction. The result is more of a meshwork than the simple linear pathway of *Figure 8.3*.

CAH could result from failure of any of five enzymes highlighted in the figure, although 95% of cases are due to deficiency of 21-hydroxylase. In the most severe form (salt-wasting CAH) the lack of aldosterone causes episodes of life-threatening loss of salt through the kidneys. Susie is an example of the milder 'simple virilizing' form. The absence of the glucocorticoid and mineralocorticoid hormones causes increased secretion of adrenocorticotrophic hormone (ACTH) via a feedback loop, and this in turn leads to increased production of androgens. Females are virilized *in utero* to varying degrees by the excess androgens. The internal anatomy is normal female, but the external genitalia may be ambiguous, requiring plastic surgery soon after birth. A mild or attenuated form of CAH is a cause of infertility in adult females. The different pathologies are partly due to different mutations in the 21-hydroxylase gene (gene deletion or truncating mutations causing complete loss of function versus mis-sense mutations causing partial loss), or to different numbers of gene copies (see below).

As described in *Box 8.2*, mutations at the 21-hydroxylase locus often occur through interaction with an adjacent pseudogene. A practical consequence of this interesting genetic mechanism is that the mutations it produces are limited to those already present in the pseudogene. Around 75% of all mutations can be found by checking for a few specific variants already present in the pseudogene, without having to sequence all 10 exons of the gene. This was the procedure followed in the case of the Stott family (Case 19).

Pharmacogenetics

It has been known for years that many drugs work in only a proportion of the people taking them, and may produce unwanted or dangerous effects in some people (*Table 8.1*). Variation in drug response is a serious clinical problem. It has been estimated that adverse drug reactions are responsible for around 100000 deaths each year in the US, while in the UK 1 in 15 hospital admissions have been attributed to this cause. Much of this individual variation in response is genetically determined. Genetic factors affect both the pharmacokinetics (the absorption, distribution, metabolism and excretion of the drug) and the pharmacodynamics (the actual effect of the drug). There is now serious interest in using genetic tests to determine what drug would be best for a patient. Many of the compounds in the development pipelines of pharmaceutical companies are likely to be offered in conjunction with a genetic test. A cynic may argue that drug companies have no interest in limiting the market for a drug – but they have an overwhelming interest in avoiding serious adverse reactions. The total cost of developing a new drug and bringing it to the market can be as high as $1 billion, and all this can be wasted if a drug has to be withdrawn soon after launch because of unanticipated adverse effects. Thus drug companies have a huge incentive to understand the basis of idiosyncratic adverse reactions

Figure 8.5 – Biosynthetic pathways for steroid hormones.
Except for 3-β-hydroxysteroid dehydrogenase, all the
enzymes shown here are members of the cytochrome P450
family. Several catalyze more than one reaction (CYPA11,
CYP17A1). Most act on several related substrates. CAH is
usually caused by deficiency of 21-hydroxylase, but can be
the result of deficiency of other enzymes in the pathway.

Box 8.2

Deletions and gene conversions in 21-hydroxylase deficiency

Research into the genetics of 21-hydroxylase deficiency has revealed an interesting mutational mechanism. The *CYP21* gene is part of a tandemly duplicated sequence lying within the major histocompatibility complex (MHC) on chromosome 6p21. We will consider the primary functions of the MHC below, when discussing immunogenetics. There is a 30 kb tandem duplication (see the figure). The *C4A* and *C4B* genes both encode complement factor 4, but only one of the duplicated *CYP21* genes is functional. *CYP21P* is an inactive pseudogene. Compared to its functional counterpart it has acquired several mis-sense mutations plus splicing, frameshifting and nonsense mutations, any one of which would make it non-functional. As mentioned in *Chapter 3*, duplicate copies of genes often degenerate into pseudogenes because there is no selection against random mutations.

We have already seen how such repeated sequences are hotspots for duplication and deletion mutations through recombination between misaligned repeats (*Disease Box 3*). The non-functional product has a 30 kb deletion of one C4–21OH unit. This mechanism is responsible for about 20–25% of 21-hydroxylase mutations, and also for the existence of a complex range of haplotypes in the general population, containing one or three copies of the repeat, with varying numbers of functional genes and pseudogenes. In the majority of CAH patients, however, the normal duplicated structure is still present, but the functional gene has acquired inactivating mutations identical to one or more of those present in the pseudogene. Analysis of flanking sequence variants showed that they are not recombinant. This is evidence of **gene conversion**, a process in which a short DNA sequence is replaced by one copied from, in the vast majority of cases, a highly homologous sequence in the immediate vicinity, but without recombination. Analysis of 21-hydroxylase mutations provided the first evidence that gene conversion, a mechanism well known in fungi, also occurred in mammals.

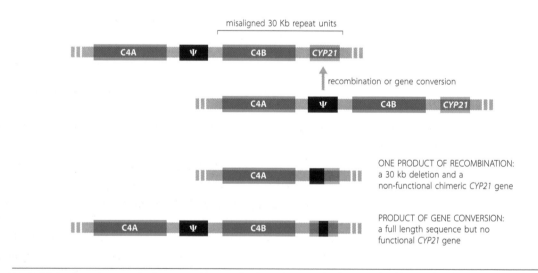

Most 21-hydroxylase mutations are the result of crossovers between misaligned C4-21OH repeats. 20–25% of mutant alleles have the 30 kb deletion; the rest are full-length with part of the functional gene sequence replaced by sequence from the pseudogene (ψ).

Although the end result is different, gene conversion is in fact a product of the recombination mechanism. As explained in *Chapter 2*, recombination does not involve two clean cuts being made the in recombining chromosomes at precisely identical places. Rather, a loose strand from the first cut invades the other partner. Subsequent events can lead either to full

Box 8.2 – continued

recombination or to replacement of a short stretch of the invaded receptor sequence by the invading donor sequence. Mismatch repair enzymes may then 'correct' any mismatches in the recipient sequence to match the donor sequence; alternatively the heteroduplex may persist until the next round of DNA replication produces one daughter cell with the full duplex donor sequence. Gene conversion is difficult to prove. It usually replaces only a very short stretch of sequence, 100 bp or so. If all the products of the conversion can be recovered and characterized, as in some fungi, the non-reciprocal nature of the exchange is apparent; otherwise the effect cannot be distinguished from close double recombination.

Table 8.1 – Examples of drugs that produce serious side effects in some people

Drug	Effect
Azathioprine	Life-threatening bone marrow suppression from normal dose in people with low activity thiopurine methyl transferase
Fluorouracil	Fatal nervous system toxicity from standard doses in people with deficiency of dihydropyrimidine dehydrogenase (1%)
Hydralazine	Risk of systemic lupus erythematosus in slow acetylators
Isoniazid	Risk of polyneuropathy in slow acetylators
Succinylcholine	Prolonged apnea in people with pseudocholinesterase deficiency
Warfarin	Excessive bleeding in people with low-activity *CYP2C9* or *VKORC1*

so that they can modify the dosage regime or the prescription guidelines to minimize the risk.

Many of the most striking individual differences in response are due to large individual variations in the rate of metabolism of drugs. For a substantial proportion of all prescription drugs (maybe 25–30%) their elimination starts with an enzymic oxidation catalyzed by one of three enzymes, CYP2C9, CYP2C19 and CYP2D6. These are members of the large P450 family of enzymes, that we encoutered when considering steroid biosynthesis. For each of these enzymes, common polymorphisms affect their activity. People can be classified as poor, intermediate, extensive and ultra-rapid metabolizers (*Figure 8.6*). The clinical effect of a given dose of drug is greater in a poor metabolizer, and much less in an ultra-rapid metabolizer because of the different rates of elimination of the drug. If a standard dose is used, ultra-rapid metabolizers may get no benefit from the drug, while poor metabolizers may suffer effects of an overdose.

Some drugs require P450 action to produce the active form. Codeine is converted by CYP2D6 to its active form, morphine. Poor metabolizers get no pain relief

● poor metabolizer
● intermediate metabolizer
● extensive metabolizer
● ultrametabolizer

Figure 8.6 – Polymorphisms in the CYP2D6, CYP2C9 and CYP2C19 genes cause common variations in enzyme activity. Variation is present in all populations but at different frequencies; these figures are for white people of Northern European origin and are redrawn from the data of Service (2005).

from standard doses of codeine, while ultra-rapid metabolizers are at increased risk of adverse effects such as breathing problems and sedation.

Many other enzyme systems are involved in pharmacokinetic variations. A long-standing example is the risk of prolonged apnea as an adverse effect of the surgical muscle relaxant suxamethonium. This occurs in patients homozygous for a variant form of butyrylcholinesterase (*CHE1* gene, OMIM 177400). Other drugs are metabolized via acetylation, and people can be divided into fast and slow acetylators depending on the activity of *N*-acetyl transferase.

The case of the Tierney family (Case 20) concerns a variant of thiopurine methyl transferase (TPMT). This enzyme catalyzes the first step in the breakdown of the immunosuppressant drugs azathioprine and mercaptopurine. These are widely used in transplantation, for treating inflammatory bowel disease and inflammatory arthritis, and for acute lymphocytic leukemia. In 1980, cases were first described of TPMT deficiency in red blood cells, and subsequent studies established that reduced red blood cell TPMT activity was associated with adverse effects of thiopurine drugs, including azathioprine and 6-mercaptopurine. About 10% of the UK population are heterozygous for a low activity allele, and 0.3% are homozygous. These people are much more sensitive than normal homozygotes to the effects of these powerful drugs. In low-activity homozygotes, normal doses can cause life-threatening bone marrow toxicity and collapse of the hemopoietic system. TPMT status can be tested either by measuring the enzyme activity or by DNA analysis of the gene.

TPMT tests do not predict all cases of neutropenia or the other side effects associated with use of these drugs. However, in 2004, the Food and Drug Administration (FDA) in the US directed that 6-mercaptopurine should include labeling information outlining the availability of genetic and phenotypic tests to determine TPMT status. Currently a large randomized controlled trial is being undertaken in the UK to determine the clinical utility and cost effectiveness of using TPMT testing as standard prior to thiopurine treatment. See McLeod and Siva (2002) for further discussion.

For further discussion of genetic effects on drug performance, see the reviews by Evans and McLeod (2003), and Weinshilboum (2003).

Immunogenetics

Immunogenetics involves two main aspects:

- understanding how we can produce an apparently infinite number of different specific antibodies, in a clear exception to the one gene – one polypeptide hypothesis
- understanding how we can distinguish self from non-self, and mount an immune response against almost any foreign cell or antigen

Here we outline the genetics behind the recognition problem; the mechanisms for generating antibody diversity are outlined in *Section 8.4*. Immunogenetics is a large subject, and the treatment here is necessarily introductory. Any recent immunology textbook will go much more deeply into this fascinating area of genetics. For background and much further detail on the recognition problem as described below, a good source is Chapter 5 of *Immunobiology* by Janeway *et al.* (2001), which is available on the NCBI Bookshelf (see *References*).

As is well known, transplanted organs are rejected unless they are tissue-matched. This will turn out to be a problem for Pablo Portillo (Case 16) who needs a bone marrow transplant (see *Section 8.3*). The major determinants of rejection are antigens encoded by genes in the MHC on chromosome 6p21.3. Transplants that are fully matched at the MHC will not normally be rejected. Unfortunately, full MHC matching is seldom achievable, except between identical twins, because the MHC is the most polymorphic and variable region in the human genome.

Genes are densely packed within the MHC – the 'classical MHC' contains around 200 genes in a 4.1 Mb region; the 'extended MHC' (*Figure 8.7*) is 7.6 Mb long and contains over 400 genes – though nearly half of these are non-expressed pseudogenes. Unusually, many of the genes are functionally related. In higher organisms functionally related genes are usually scattered apparently randomly over the genome, except for some clusters of recently duplicated and diverged genes. In the MHC, however, most of the genes play some part in the immune process – although there are exceptions, such as the 21-hydroxylase gene mentioned above. Within the MHC, the key determinants of self versus non-self recognition are cell surface molecules encoded by a series of structurally related genes, the Human Leukocyte Antigen (HLA) genes.

HLA molecules are divided into Class I and Class II.

- Class I molecules are present on the surface of most nucleated cells. They consist of a heavy chain, encoded by an HLA gene, and a constant light chain, β2-microglobulin, encoded on chromosome 15. There are 26 Class I genes in the MHC, but only nine are functional. The HLA-A and HLA-B molecules are the most important Class I antigens for tissue matching. Both loci are highly polymorphic: with 511 recorded alleles, the HLA-B locus is the most polymorphic in the human genome.
- Class II antigens are found mainly on B-lymphocytes and macrophages. They consist of alpha and beta chains, both encoded within the MHC. Of the 24 Class II loci, 15 are functional. The main Class II molecules are DR, DP and DQ, and again these are highly polymorphic (in 2001 a World Health Organization committee listed 323 DRβ alleles).

Clearly there has been selection in favor of this very extensive variability. Alleles frequently differ by substantial blocks of amino acid residues, suggesting that recombination and gene conversion have both been important in generating the diversity.

HLA molecules present peptides derived from foreign proteins to T-lymphocytes. Class I molecules present endogenous antigens to CD8+ T cells, while Class II molecules present exogenous antigens to CD4+ T cells. T cells initiate an immune response to either non-self peptides presented by self-HLA molecules, or cells carrying non-self-HLA molecules. T cells that respond to self peptides presented by self-HLA molecules occur but are eliminated during early development ('clonal deletion'). The response to cells carrying non-self-HLA molecules is the

Figure 8.7 – The human MHC locus at 6p21.3 is conventionally divided into Class I, II and III regions, with extensions at either end.
The figure shows the most important genes for tissue matching, together with the C4 / 21-hydroxylase cluster. Data from Horton *et al.* (2004).

cause of transplant rejection. Ideally a transplant donor and recipient should be matched for both alleles at the HLA-A, –B and –DR loci (i.e. six matches). With modern immunosuppressive treatments, transplantation across mismatches is often successful, but immunosuppression brings problems of its own.

8.3 Investigations of patients

| CASE 19 | Stott family | 199 | **210** | 376 |

- Second pregnancy; scan suggests baby boy
- Baby born with ambiguous genitalia
- FISH to chromosomes
- ? Congenital adrenal hyperplasia
- PCR testing for mutations

The 98% sequence homology between the *CYP21P* pseudogene and the active gene, and the variable number of copies of either gene, make molecular investigation of CAH quite challenging. Large deletions can only be characterized by Southern blotting, normally by comparing the positions and intensities of hybridizing bands in each parent and in the affected child. Mutations due to gene conversions can be identified using a battery of PCR tests. The protocol used here checks for six specific point mutations, for an 8 bp deletion in exon 3, and for chimeric genes comprising 5′ pseudogene and 3′ functional gene sequences. Between them these comprise 70% of all mutations. Again, defining the mutations involves comparing the results in the child and in both parents across a range of PCR tests. The tests depend on the fact that a PCR primer will only work if the 3′ end nucleotide is correctly base-paired to the template sequence (see *Figure 5.5*).

A two-stage PCR protocol is used. The functional gene (*CYP21*) and pseudogene (*CYP21P*) differ by numerous point mutations, and these can be exploited to design gene-specific PCR primers. Thus the first stage PCR is designed to amplify just the functional gene. The product from this reaction (if any) is not checked, but is used as starting material for a second round of PCR that uses allele-specific primers to detect each individual point mutation. In this second stage two alternative PCR reactions are performed, one with primers specific for the mutant sequence and the other with primers specific for the corresponding normal sequence. An absence of any product in both secondary PCR reactions would imply that there was no starting material. This would mean that the primary PCR reaction gave no product, which must be because only *CYP21P* sequence was present in the original sample. It is crucial to include PCR primers for a control sequence in each reaction, to confirm that an absence of product is specific and not due to a total failure of the PCR reaction. *Table 8.2* shows the results.

Table 8.2 – Results of 21-hydroxylase mutation testing in Susie Stott

1st round PCR to specifically amplify:	2nd round PCR to check for:	Result on child
(1) Exons 1–3 of *CYP21* only	89C>T mutation 655A/C/G mutation	Normal (C) Normal
(2) Exons 3–10 of *CYP21* only	999T>A mutation 1683G>T mutation 1994C>T mutation 2108C>T mutation	Mutant only (A) Normal (G) Normal (C) Normal (C)
(3) Exons 3–6 of either *CYP21* or 5′-*CYP21P* – 3′-*CYP21* chimeric gene	8 bp deletion	Heterozygous
(4) Exons 3–6 of *CYP21* only	8 bp deletion	Normal

The results of the specific mutation tests using the products of the first two primary PCR reactions would be compatible with several possibilities:

- homozygosity for the 999T>A mutation
- compound heterozygosity, one allele of *CYP21* having acquired just the single 999T>A point mutation, the other being a chimeric gene that would not amplify in the primary PCR
- compound heterozygosity, one allele of *CYP21* having acquired just the single 999T>A point mutation, the other being a large deletion (seen in about 25% of cases)

The third reaction shows the presence of the 8 bp deletion characteristic of the pseudogene. The possibilities are now:

- compound heterozygosity for the 999T>A mutation and 8 bp deletion, both introduced into otherwise normal *CYP21* genes by gene conversion
- compound heterozygosity; one allele of *CYP21* having acquired just the single 999T>A point mutation, the other being a chimeric gene carrying the 8 bp deletion, and probably other pseudogene-specific changes
- the presence of both mutations on the same chromosome, containing more than one mutated *CYP21* gene (*CYP21* gene duplications, *CYP21P* gene duplications and *CYP21P* gene deletions are non-pathogenic and common in the general population); the other chromosome containing no *CYP21* gene

The fourth PCR reaction shows that the 8 bp deletion must be present on a chimeric gene. The test results are shown in lane 1 of each gel in *Figure 8.8*. It is still necessary to check whether both detected changes might be on the same chromosome. This is done by checking the parents with the same primary PCR reactions and the appropriate mutation-specific secondary PCR (*Table 8.3*).

Table 8.3 – Results of 21-hydroxylase mutation testing in parents of Susie Stott

1st round PCR to specifically amplify:	2nd round PCR to check for:	Result on father	Result on mother
(1) Exons 1–3 of *CYP21* only	89C>T mutation	Normal	Normal
(2) Exons 3–10 of *CYP21* only	999T>A mutation	Normal	Heterozygous
(3) Exons 3–6 of either *CYP21* or 5'-*CYP21P* – 3'-*CYP21* chimeric gene	8 bp deletion	Heterozygous	Normal
(4) Exons 3–6 of *CYP21* only	8 bp deletion	Normal	Normal

Figure 8.8 – Identifying the 21-hydroxylase genotype.
(a) Testing for the 999T>A mutation (test 2 in *Table 8.2*) by allele-specific amplification of the T (left track) or A (right track) allele. Samples 1, 2 and 3 are A/A, A/T and T/T respectively. (b) Testing for the 8 bp deletion in either the *CYP21* or the chimeric gene. The left track of each pair amplifies only the non-deleted allele, the right track amplifies only the deleted allele (which runs a little faster because it is smaller). For each sample the upper part of the gel amplifies the sequence from either *CYP21* or the chimeric gene (test 3 in *Table 8.2*) and the lower part of the gel amplifies specifically from *CYP21* only (test 4 in *Table 8.2*). All bands marked C are PCR controls. Photos courtesy of Dr Simon Tobi, St Mary's Hospital, Manchester.

The two mutations are seen to come one from each parent, so they are confirmed to be on two different copies of chromosome 6 in the child. The results on the father confirm that he has a chimeric gene including the 8 bp deletion, and also a normal *CYP21* gene.

The overall result is that we now know that Susie is a compound heterozygote for two loss of function changes. One is a gene conversion that introduced a T>A change at nucleotide 999 from the pseudogene, resulting in the amino acid substitution I172V. This mutant allele retains a low level of residual 21-hydroxylase activity. The other is the result of mispaired recombination creating a completely non-functional chimeric gene, the 5′ part of which (at least up to exon 3) is derived from the pseudogene, while the 3′ part (at least from exon 6) comes from the *CYP21* gene. Susie probably has enough residual 21-hydroxylase activity to escape the severe salt-wasting phenotype, but not enough to avoid *in utero* virilization.

| **CASE 20** | Tierney family | 200 | **213** | 310 | 376 |

- 4 year old boy, Jason
- Pale with extensive bruising and tachycardia
- ? Acute lymphocytic leukemia
- Bone marrow test and check diagnosis
- TPMT enzyme analysis prior to 6-mercaptopurine treatment

The blood counts on Jason raised the possibility of a diagnosis of childhood acute lymphocytic leukemia (ALL). The diagnosis of ALL was confirmed by the pediatrician at the local hospital who performed a bone marrow test, which revealed a large number of blast cells (immature lymphocytes, see *Figure 8.2*). Jason was admitted to hospital and treated with induction chemotherapy including prednisolone, vincristine, daunomycin and L-asparaginase. He responded well to this treatment and progressed to consolidation treatment with methotrexate. He was then started on maintenance treatment of 6-mercaptopurine and methotrexate, which was planned to continue for 3 years.

Prior to treatment with 6-mercaptopurine a blood sample was taken for TPMT enzyme analysis. As mentioned above, this drug causes severe adverse effects in people with low TPMT activity. Three variant alleles account for 80–95% of intermediate or low activity cases (*Table 8.4* and *Figure 8.9*).

Table 8.4 – Common low-activity thiopurine *S*-methyl transferase alleles

Allele	Frequency in Caucasians
TPMT*2	0.5%
TPMT*3A	5%
TPMT*3C	0.5%

Figure 8.9 – Sequence of normal and low-activity alleles of thiopurine *S*-methyl transferase.
Note that the *TPMT**3A sequence includes two mis-sense changes.

The TPMT test on Jason revealed a normal level of enzyme activity. However, after treatment started Jason suffered severe neutropenic sepsis, an infection associated with a very low neutrophil count. He was given intravenous antibiotics and supportive treatment and recovered well. The doctors noted that before he had the TPMT test he had been given a blood transfusion to correct his anemia. Because the TPMT enzyme test is performed on red blood cells, this may have provided an inaccurate measure of his TPMT status. A blood sample was therefore sent for TPMT genotyping. This revealed that Jason was homozygous for the *TPMT**3A allele, predicting absent TPMT activity. He was recommended on the maintenance treatment with a reduced dose of 6-mercaptopurine and remained disease free.

CASE 16	Portillo family	173	183	**214**	376

- Sickly boy, Pablo
- Family history of similar symptoms
- Blood tests suggest X-linked severe combined immunodeficiency
- Check that bone marrow transplantation is appropriate

In the previous chapter we saw the pedigree of this family (*Figure 7.10*). Baby Pablo has been diagnosed with SCIDX1. Bone marrow transplantation is the treatment of choice for severe immunodeficiencies such as Pablo has. At first sight an immunodeficient patient would seem an ideal choice as a transplant recipient. Pablo lacks all T-cell function and therefore cannot reject a graft. However, a problem with bone marrow transplants is graft-versus-host (GvH) disease. If the grafted bone marrow successfully reconstitutes an immune system it will recognize the host tissue as foreign and initiate an immune response that could be fatal. Good matching should reduce the risk of this. Pablo and other family members were typed for HLA-A, -B and -DR with the results shown in *Figure 8.10*.

Sibs have a 1 in 4 chance of sharing both MHC haplotypes. Unfortunately neither of Pablo's sibs Ignacio or Bonita turned out to be a perfect match. His parents, of course, each shared one haplotype with him. Transplant donor registries were searched in the hope of finding a well-matched unrelated donor, but not surprisingly no perfect or even good match could be found. *Table 8.5* shows the frequencies in Spaniards from Murcia of each of the alleles and of the whole haplotypes carried by Portillo family members. Even though these are among the commonest haplotypes in that population, the chance a randomly selected member of the population would have the same two haplotypes as Pablo is 1 in 1500.

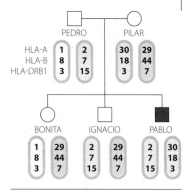

Figure 8.10 – Results of HLA typing in the Portillo family. Because the *HLA-A*, -*B* and -*DR* loci are close together on chromosome 6, they are normally inherited as a block (haplotype).

Time passed, and eventually it was decided to act on his mother Pilar's offer to donate some of her own marrow. A new technique gave hope that GvH disease could be minimized. The problem is caused by T cells in the donor marrow, and in the 1980s techniques were developed to deplete human marrow of T cells. This made it, in principle, possible to restore immune function by bone marrow transplantation in patients with any form of SCID. Some T cells are inevitably present, so it is still preferable to match the transplant as well as possible, but mismatches are no longer a major problem. The method had recently become available in her regional transplant center, and so bone marrow was taken from Pilar, depleted of T cells, and infused into Pablo. However, the results were disappointing. The child acquired only low levels of T-cell function. Evidently the marrow had engrafted poorly. Despite receiving a booster transplant, again

Table 8.5 – Frequencies of Portillo family alleles and haplotypes in a Spanish population

Locus	Allele	Frequency	
HLA-A	1	0.095	
	2	0.230	
	29	0.083	
	30	0.107	
HLA-B	7	0.056	
	8	0.052	
	18	0.071	
	44	0.179	
HLA-DRB1	3	0.123	
	7	0.179	
	15	0.052	

Haplotype	Observed frequency	Calculated frequency
A1-B8-DR3	0.023	0.00011
A2-B7-DR15	0.019	0.00067
A29-B44-DR7	0.051	0.00266
A30-B18-DR3	0.035	0.00093

Note that HLA genes tend to occur in particular combinations. The observed frequency of each haplotype is much greater than the product of the individual allele frequencies (shown in the Calculated frequency column). This is an example of linkage disequilibrium. See *Chapter 13* for more discussion. Data from www.allelefrequencies.net; note that the nomenclature has been simplified.

from his mother, he succumbed to a cytomegalovirus infection and died at the age of 14 months. Experience suggests that the success rate is much lower in transplants performed after about 3.5 months of age. Buckley (2004) gives an authoritative and readable review of bone marrow transplantation in SCID.

Pablo died in 1989. At that time the gene causing the family disease had not been identified. The options open to his parents, if they wanted more children and wished for prenatal testing, were limited. They could opt for fetal sexing and terminate any pregnancy where the fetus was male. Given that in half those cases the fetus would have been unaffected, this was not acceptable to Pilar or Pedro. The geneticists could use genetic markers to try to identify whether a male fetus had inherited Pilar's normal or abnormal X chromosome, as described in *Chapter 9*. A DNA sample had been banked from Pablo to help with this, or with mutation analysis once the gene had been identified. The problem was that genetic mapping of X-SCID at that time had not provided an unambiguous localization. Probably the defective gene mapped to the proximal long arm, at Xq12-q13, but there was some question over whether this was true of all cases. Thus there was a risk that an inappropriate genetic marker would be used, and a false negative result obtained. Pedro and Pilar were unwilling to take this risk, and in any case they already had two healthy children and decided not to have more; Pedro had a vasectomy.

In 1993 the faulty gene in X-SCID was identified as *IL2RG*. This encodes the gamma subunit that is part of the receptors for several different cytokines (interleukins 2, 4, 7, 9 and 15). Lack of cytokine signaling prevents development of T cells and NK cells; B cells are present but do not produce antibodies. The gene is quite small, consisting of eight exons covering 4.2 kb at location Xq13. A variety of loss of function mutations have now been described in affected males.

The DNA sample from Pablo Portillo was retrieved from the freezer and tested. A C>T substitution was found in exon 7 that converted a CGA codon for arginine 293 into a TGA stop codon (*Figure 8.11*). Note that this mutation is of a CpG sequence and is likely a result of demethylation of a 5-methyl cytosine. It has been reported several times in unrelated cases, confirming that this particular CpG sequence is a mutational hotspot. Previously Pilar's sisters Francisca and Elena had been carrier-tested by checking for non-random X-inactivation (*Chapter 7*). Now they were re-contacted and offered a definitive mutation test. Both accepted. PCR-amplifying and sequencing exon 7 of the gene confirmed the X-inactivation pattern, showing that Elena was a carrier but Francisca was not. A note was made to contact Pilar's daughter Bonita and Elena's daughter when they were about 16 and could make an informed decision about carrier testing.

NORMAL SEQUENCE	C G G A C G A T G C C C C G A A T T C C C A C C C T G A A G
	R T M P R I P T L K
MUTANT SEQUENCE	C G G A C G A T G C C C T G A A T T C C C A C C C T G A A G
	R T M P X

Figure 8.11 – The mutation in the *IL2RG* gene that produced X-SCID in Pablo Portillo.
X in the mutant sequence means a stop codon.

Years later another affected baby was born in a different branch of the family, and by that time there were more possibilities for treatment. This story will be taken up again in *Chapter 14*.

8.4. Summary and extension

Inborn errors of metabolism

One gene – many enzymes?
The one gene – one enzyme hypothesis, though not true in all circumstances, is the essential guiding idea in biochemical genetics. How then can we explain diseases where a single gene defect results in defects in multiple enzymes? Two examples illustrate how defects in post-translational modification can cause loss of activity of multiple enzymes:

- Mucolipidosis II (OMIM 252500) patients have disproportionate dwarfism, a coarse face and mental retardation, similar to those with Hurler syndrome (OMIM 607014). Both diseases involve lysosomal enzyme defects, but whereas Hurler syndrome is caused by loss of function of one specific lysosomal enzyme, α-L-iduronidase, lysosomes

Figure 8.12 – The active site of several sulfatases requires post-translational modification of cysteine to formyl glycine by the SUMF enzyme. Loss of SUMF function produces multiple sulfatase deficiency.

in patients with ML II (also known as I-cell disease) have deficiencies of a whole range of enzymes. ML II is one of the family of carbohydrate-deficient glycoprotein diseases. Lysosomal enzymes require a specific attached carbohydrate as a signal that they should be transported to lysosomes after they are synthesized in the cell cytoplasm. In ML II this signal is defective. There is almost complete absence of lysosomal targeting, and instead most lysosomal enzymes are secreted into the bloodstream. The signal consists of *N*-acetylglucosamine-1-phosphate attached to mannose sugars that are in turn attached to the polypeptide chains of many lysosomal enzymes. The underlying defect in ML II is in a single enzyme, the transferase needed to produce the signal molecule (*GNPTAB* gene).

- **Multiple sulfatase deficiency (OMIM 272200)** combines the features of six mendelian diseases that are each caused by deficiency of one specific sulfatase enzyme. mRNAs for each individual enzyme appear to be produced normally. This is again a defect in post-translational processing. All the affected enzymes have an unusual amino acid, formylglycine, as part of their active site. This is produced by modifying a cysteine residue in the protein after it has been synthesized (*Figure 8.12*). Multiple sulfatase deficiency is the result of loss of function mutations in the gene encoding sulfatase-modifying factor (SUMF) I, the enzyme responsible for the modification.

One enzyme – one disease?

There is no neat one-to-one correspondence between enzymes and diseases. You cannot take a metabolic pathways chart and write in beside each reaction the disease that results from an inborn error in that step. To begin with, any disease that is the result of failure of a multi-step pathway could be produced by a block at any step in the pathway. Thus several inborn errors might produce the same

---

Box 8.3

Inability to make vitamin C – a universal inborn error in humans

If you lived on the diet that your dog or cat eats, you would develop scurvy because of lack of vitamin C. How do they stay healthy despite never eating lemons? It turns out that almost all animals have the enzymes necessary to synthesize ascorbic acid, and so are not dependent on an external supply. Exceptions to this include humans and other higher primates, guinea pigs, fruit-eating bats and the red-vented bulbul bird. All these species lack the enzyme L-gulono-gamma-lactone oxidase (GULO), which catalyzes the last step of ascorbic acid biosynthesis. The human version of this gene, on chromosome 8p21, is a defective pseudogene with missing exons and other mutations, relative to the functional mouse *gulo* gene. Human cells transfected with the mouse *gulo* gene make their own ascorbic acid. Presumably the defective species all had such a fruit-rich diet that there was no selective pressure against *GULO* loss of function mutations.

D-glucuronic acid → L-gulonic acid → L-gulonolactone —**X**→ 2-keto L-gulonoloactone → L-ascorbic acid

Biosynthesis of ascorbic acid.
The final reaction is non-enzymic and occurs spontaneously. **X** indicates the metabolic block in humans.

disease. This is similar to the way that defects in many different genes can produce inherited hearing loss. Also, many enzymes are dispensable – perhaps lack of the reaction product has no obvious adverse effect, or maybe there are other ways of achieving the same function. Thus some enzyme defects would not produce a disease. Vitamin C biosynthesis provides an interesting example of this – an inborn error that all humans have, and that only manifests as disease in exceptional environments (*Box 8.3*). In other cases the result is a distinct phenotype, but one that we would not classify as a disease. Lactose intolerance is an example (*Box 8.4*). Finally, different degrees of deficiency in one enzyme may produce phenotypes that are sufficiently different to be classed as different diseases – see the example of DTDST deficiency below.

Genotype–phenotype correlations

Most inborn errors involve loss of function mutations, and as is usually the case with loss of function mutations, there is often extensive allelic heterogeneity (see *Chapter 6*). Because biochemists can measure enzyme activity quantitatively, inborn errors are a promising field for establishing genotype–phenotype correlations. We might expect a mutation that causes a partial loss of activity of an enzyme to cause a milder disease than one causing total loss.

Box 8.4

Lactose intolerance – a common metabolic polymorphism

Most adults of Northern European origin have a dominant trait: hereditary persistence of intestinal lactase. This makes them able to tolerate a diet rich in milk. Conversely, most people in East Asia and in tropical and subtropical regions of the world shut off production of intestinal lactase in early childhood. It is quite common for people who lack intestinal lactase to suffer abdominal distension, pain, and diarrhea if they drink fresh milk. Dairy products such as cheese and yoghurt contain less lactose and cause fewer problems. Across the world the correlation with milk drinking is close – for example, certain nomadic tribes in Africa (e.g. the Bedouin, and the Beja people of Sudan) who drink fresh milk have high levels of persistence of intestinal lactase, whereas most African populations are non-persistent.

Persistence or non-persistence of lactase is not an inborn error but a common polymorphism: both states are common among normal people. The ancestral state is undoubtedly non-persistence, as found in most mammals. Evidently there has been powerful selection for the persistence variant among populations who have taken up dairy farming. This must all have happened within the last 9000 years, making it one of the strongest selective changes in recent human history.

The causative DNA variant has proved hard to identify. Recent data point to a C/T polymorphism 14 kb upstream of the start codon of the lactase gene on chromosome 2q21. In a survey of 236 individuals from four populations (Finnish, French, European American and African–American), every individual with one or more T alleles had persistent lactase, while every individual homozygous for the C allele had non-persistence. This variant is typical of the sort of variants that are likely to surface as susceptibility factors for common diseases (*Chapter 13*). Mendelian diseases are usually the result of mutations that cause major loss or gain of function of a gene, but here we have an example of a change that modifies the timing of expression of a gene without affecting the integrity of the gene product.

In many cases this expectation is fulfilled. CAH illustrates this. In one study (see OMIM 201910) a complete lack of enzyme activity usually produced the salt-wasting form; a 2% residual activity produced the simple virilizing form, and 10–20% activity produced the non-classical forms. However, as in many other examples, the correlation between enzyme activity and phenotype was far from perfect. Mutations in a sulfate transporter enzyme provide another example. High molecular weight sulfated polysaccharides are important components of connective tissue, and loss of function mutations in the Diastrophic Dystrophy Sulfate Transporter (*DTDST*) enzyme cause skeletal dysplasias. Four different autosomal recessive skeletal dysplasia syndromes, which were distinguished on clinical grounds, turned out all to be caused by defects in DTDST. In ascending order of severity they are:

- multiple epiphyseal dysplasia 4 (MED4, OMIM 226900),
- diastrophic dysplasia (DTD, OMIM 222600).
- atelosteogenesis type II (AOII, OMIM 256050)
- achondrogenesis type 1B (ACG1B, OMIM 600972).

Many different mutations have been reported in the *DTDST* gene. An interesting paper by Karniski (2001) explores the relationship between enzyme activity and clinical phenotype.

Enzyme activity was measured for a series of reported mutant alleles (*Figure 8.13*). Most patients are compound heterozygotes, and it is important to remember that what matters in physiology is the overall level of activity provided by the two alleles of the gene. Grouping the mutations into zero (0), low (L) and medium (M) activity, Karniski reported the following genotypes in patients:

Disease	Observed genotypes of individual cases
MED, DTD	M/M, L/L, L/L, M/0
AOII	L/0, L/0, L/0, M/0
ACG1B	0/0, 0/0, L/L, M/0

The general conclusion is that genotype–phenotype correlations exist, but they are usually rather loose. A paper by Scriver and Waters (1999) describes why this might be so.

LEVEL OF RESIDUAL *DTDST* GENE FUNCTION

Figure 8.13 – Genotype–phenotype correlations in skeletal dysplasias caused by loss of function of the DTD sulfate transporter. Data from Karniski (2001).

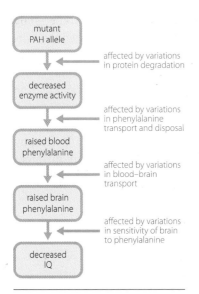

Figure 8.14 – In phenylketonuria many factors weaken the correlation between genotype and phenotype.
PAH: phenylalanine hydroxylase; This figure summarizes the arguments of Scriver and Waters (1999).

Phenylketonuria (PKU, OMIM 261600) is an inborn error caused by lack of phenylalanine hydroxylase (we will meet an example in *Chapter 11*, *Case 22*). Phenylalanine accumulates upstream of the block, and high levels of phenylalanine damage the developing brain. Thus the major clinical problem of PKU is mental retardation. Many different mutations have been described, leading to varying degrees of loss of function. The question Scriver and Waters ask is how far a patient's IQ can be predicted from a knowledge of the mutation. The answer is, not very far, and *Figure 8.14* summarizes their arguments why this is so (their paper is recommended reading).

Pharmacogenetics

Case 20 (Tierney family) and the examples discussed in *Section 8.2* have all concerned individual differences in drug metabolism (pharmacokinetics). Another aspect of pharmacogenetics concerns variations in the primary action of a drug because of genetic variation in the targets with which it interacts (pharmacodynamics). Natural polymorphisms in drug targets can also cause individual differences in drug response. Drugs are now becoming available that are designed to treat specific genotypes. Well-known examples are Herceptin and Gleevec.

- Herceptin (trastuzumab) is a monoclonal antibody against the HER2 (ERBB2) protein. Many breast cancers over-express this cell surface receptor because one of the genetic changes occurring during tumorigenesis has been an amplification of the gene. These cancers respond to Herceptin, but breast cancers that do not over-express HER2 do not.
- Gleevec (imitanib) is a small molecule that inhibits an abnormal protein kinase, the Bcr–Abl fusion protein. This protein is specifically produced in chronic myeloid leukemia following a chromosomal rearrangement that creates the *Bcr–Abl* fusion gene (see *Chapter 12*). Because the action of the Bcr–Abl protein is central to the development of the disease, Gleevec is a remarkably effective drug, inducing complete remission in the great majority of patients.

It is likely that other genotype-specific drugs will be developed over the coming years. This could be controversial. In June 2005 the US FDA approved the marketing of the combination drug BiDil as a treatment for severe heart failure specifically in African–Americans. The drug combination is appropriate for people with low vascular levels of nitric oxide. That condition is commoner in African–Americans than in Caucasians; self-identified ethnicity is here being used as a crude indicator of genotype. The BiDil archive (see *References*) gives access to much of the debate surrounding this decision.

Despite all the talk about personalized medicine, it is striking that there has so far been very little practical application of genetic tests for prescribing. One reason for this is that pharmaceutical companies now try to design drugs so that they are not metabolized by the P450 system, and are not affected by other well-known common causes of variations in pharmacokinetics. Thus the main targets for pharmacogenetic testing would be established drugs, most of which are now out of patent protection. The industry has little incentive to develop and market tests for drugs that are not bringing in much money.

A second problem is imperfect understanding of the genetic factors underlying many variations. We can illustrate this by two examples.

- Malignant hyperthermia (MH) is an autosomal dominant condition (see OMIM 145600) that involves a very serious life-threatening abnormal response to anesthetics. Many MH patients have mutations in the ryanodine receptor gene, but others do not. Linkage analysis has suggested the existence of at least a further five MH loci. Thus where somebody has a family history of MH, before risking a general anesthetic a phenotypic test (*in vitro* contraction test using a biopsied muscle sample) is usually performed, rather than a genetic test.
- The P450 enzyme CYP3A4 is the most abundant P450 enzyme in liver and is involved in the metabolism of around half of all prescribed drugs (see OMIM 124010). Liver enzyme activity can vary 30-fold between individuals. However, very little of this variability can be ascribed to coding-sequence variants of the *CYP3A4* gene. Much of the variation may well be genetic, but must lie in unidentified factors that control the expression of CYP3A4.

Even when there is reasonable understanding of the genetics, genotypes may not be sufficiently predictive. The anti-coagulant warfarin illustrates some of the complexities. Warfarin is very widely prescribed to people who have coronary artery disease or venous thrombosis, especially after surgery. Its target is a vitamin K epoxide reductase encoded by the *VKORC1* gene, and it is metabolized by the CYP2C9 P450 enzyme (see *Figure 8.6*). Individuals with low-activity variants of CYP2C9 and/or some variants of *VKORC1* are at risk of serious bleeding episodes when given a standard dose of warfarin. However, many other factors also affect a person's response. These include the age of the patient, the presence of other illnesses and the concurrent use of other drugs. Thus normal practice is to start the patient on a low dose of warfarin and gradually increase it until the desired degree of anti-coagulation is obtained. Even if patients were pre-screened for their *CYP2C9* and *VKORC1* genotypes, it would probably still be prudent to follow this protocol.

A final problem has been the logistics of incorporating genetic testing into routine clinical practice. All these problems may change with the introduction of microarrays that can rapidly characterize a large number of relevant genetic factors. If that can be achieved in a cheap and convenient form, personalized medicine may finally become a reality of day-to-day clinical practice. Ultimately, it might be possible to perform a single once-in-a-lifetime microarray analysis that would be usefully predictive of a person's reaction to a whole series of drugs. Data from such an analysis might become part of a person's standard medical record.

Immunogenetics

In *Section 8.2* we mentioned two challenging aspects of immunogenetics: how antigens are recognized as self or non-self, and how the effectively infinite diversity of antibody molecules is produced. The role of the MHC in recognition was described above; here we discuss the remarkable genetic mechanisms that underlie antibody diversity.

Antibodies are proteins (immunoglobulins, Ig) composed of heavy and light polypeptide chains. These can be assembled in various ways to produce the different classes of antibody – IgA, IgD, IgE, IgG and IgM. Each class has a specific heavy chain and a choice of κ or λ light chains. The five types of heavy chain are all encoded at the *IGH* locus on chromosome 14, and the light chains at the *IGK* or *IGL* loci on chromosomes 2 and 22, respectively. Each of these loci, however, contains a large pool of possible coding sequences (*Figure 8.15*). The C-terminal part of each Ig chain of a given class is constant, but the N-terminal part, that carries the antigen binding site, is highly variable. Mature immunoglobulin genes have a conventional multi-exon structure, with a single exon encoding the N-terminal variable region and several exons encoding the constant region. However, the exon encoding the variable region is the product of highly variable DNA rearrangements during B cell maturation.

As explained in the caption to *Figure 8.15*, the sequence encoding each variable region is made by joining a V (variable), J (joining) and (for heavy chains) D (diversity) segment, each chosen from a range of alternatives. Do not confuse this process with the splicing of exons and introns. Exons and introns are spliced in the RNA transcript by the spliceosome (*Chapter 3*). Ig genes are spliced at the DNA level specifically in B lymphocytes. The product is a multi-exon gene whose primary transcript is spliced in the usual way.

The total diversity of antibodies depends on several additional mechanisms.

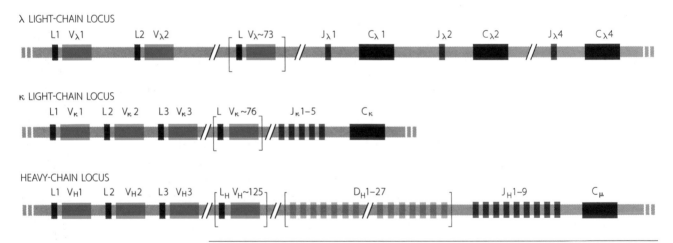

Figure 8.15 – Each type of immunoglobulin gene is assembled by DNA rearrangements that occur specifically in B lymphocytes.
In light chains one of 73 (λ) or 76 (κ) V regions is joined to one of 5–11 J regions, giving 365–836 combinations. In heavy chains one of 27 D regions is joined to one of nine J regions, and the new sequence is then joined to one of about 125 V regions, giving about 30 000 combinations. This combinatorial diversity is only one of the ways in which B cells are enabled to produce an almost infinite diversity of immunoglobulins. Redrawn from Janeway *et al.* (2001) with permission from Garland Science.

- Unlike conventional genetic recombination, the specialized mechanism joining V, D and J segments adds or removes random small numbers of nucleotides at the junctions. Where the result produces a frameshift, the rearranged gene is non-functional, but in the one-third of cases where the reading frame is conserved, a whole extra layer of diversity is created.
- After gene rearrangement is complete, a process of somatic hypermutation introduces random point mutations at high frequency into the variable region of the genes in activated B cells.
- The different classes of heavy chain in IgA, IgD, IgE, IgG and IgM are made by yet another specialized recombination mechanism. Each rearranged IgH gene has at its 3′ end sequences encoding each of the five types of constant region (only the C_μ is shown in *Figure 8.15*; the others are downstream of this). Only the C sequence closest to the VDJ exon is used. Class switching occurs by an intramolecular recombination event that physically excises one or more C sequences, so that a different one lies adjacent to the VDJ sequence.
- Finally, the combination of a heavy chain and a light chain in an antibody molecule provides yet another source of combinatorial diversity.

It remains only to add that a similar generator of diversity operates on the T cell receptor genes. For more detail of all of these processes, consult an immunology textbook, such as Janeway *et al.* (2001, see *References*).

The porphyrias

The porphyrias are a family of diseases caused by disorders of heme biosynthesis. A complete absence of heme would undoubtedly be lethal, and all the porphyrias are caused by disturbances of biosynthesis that fall short of total failure. The first specific step in the biosynthesis of heme is synthesis of δ-amino levulinic acid from glycine and succinyl CoA (see figure), catalyzed by δ-amino levulinic acid synthase (ALAS). This is the rate-determining step for the whole pathway. Specific enzyme defects causing porphyria are known for each of the six subsequent steps.

All the porphyrias result in circulation and excretion of various abnormal porphyrins due to the accumulation of synthetic intermediates before the metabolic block. It is these intermediates rather than a deficiency of heme that cause the clinical problems. All porphyrias are marked by cutaneous and/or neuro-visceral symptoms. Cutaneous problems are caused by deposition of the non-physiological porphyrin, uroporphyrin I, which is a photosensitizing compound. Patients with acute intermittent porphyria, variegate porphyria or coproporphyria are normally healthy, but various environmental, hormonal or metabolic factors can precipitate an attack of the disease. Anything that induces hepatic ALAS activity can lead to overload of the compromised synthetic pathway and release of pathogenic intermediates. Precipitants include alcohol and many drugs. During an attack the patient suffers severe gastric pain and sometimes psychological disturbances, but between attacks she (the sex ratio is 5F:1M for attacks) is healthy. It may be significant that porphyrins have been reported to act as ligands for some benzodiazepine receptors. It has been suggested that various famously 'mad' historical figures, including Vincent van Gogh and the British King George III, may have suffered from porphyria.

Disease box 8

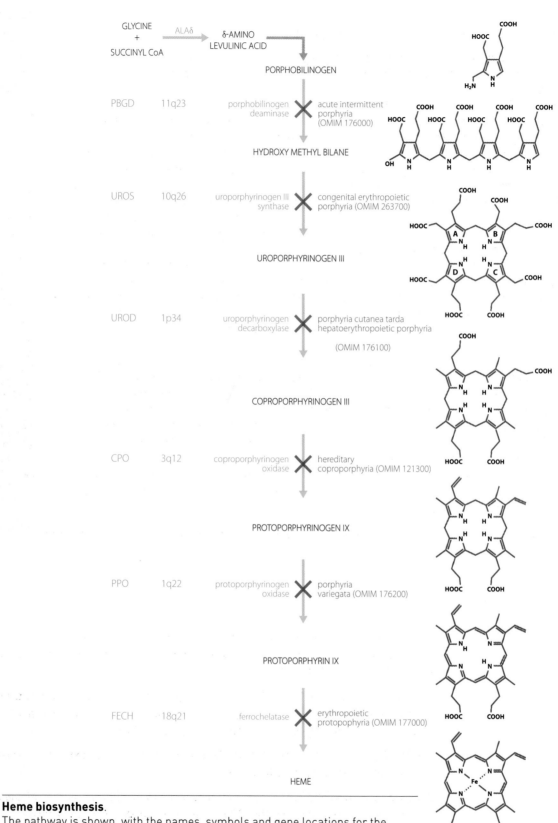

GLYCINE + SUCCINYL CoA

ALAδ

δ-AMINO LEVULINIC ACID

PORPHOBILINOGEN

PBGD   11q23   porphobilinogen deaminase   ✕   acute intermittent porphyria (OMIM 176000)

HYDROXY METHYL BILANE

UROS   10q26   uroporphyrinogen III synthase   ✕   congenital erythropoietic porphyria (OMIM 263700)

UROPORPHYRINOGEN III

UROD   1p34   uroporphyrinogen decarboxylase   ✕   porphyria cutanea tarda hepatoerythropoietic porphyria (OMIM 176100)

COPROPORPHYRINOGEN III

CPO   3q12   coproporphyrinogen oxidase   ✕   hereditary coproporphyria (OMIM 121300)

PROTOPORPHYRINOGEN IX

PPO   1q22   protoporphyrinogen oxidase   ✕   porphyria variegata (OMIM 176200)

PROTOPORPHYRIN IX

FECH   18q21   ferrochelatase   ✕   erythropoietic protopophyria (OMIM 177000)

HEME

Heme biosynthesis.
The pathway is shown, with the names, symbols and gene locations for the enzymes, and the names and OMIM numbers of the diseases caused by an inborn error at each step.

Disease box 8 – *continued*

There are several points of genetic interest in the porphyrias.

- As usual in higher organisms, the genes encoding these functionally related enzymes are not organized into an operon, like in bacteria, but are scattered over different chromosomes.
- Most porphyrias are dominant, but the variety and nature of the mutations described (see the relevant OMIM entries) make clear that these are loss of function changes and therefore the pathology is due to haplo-insufficiency. The one recessive condition, congenital erythropoietic porphyria, is associated with a partial loss of function of the affected enzyme. Clinical severity of congenital erythropoietic porphyria correlates quite well with residual enzyme activity; very low levels cause hydrops fetalis.
- Porphyria cutanea tarda is the most common form of porphyria but only 20% of cases are genetic in origin. There are many environmental precipitants, especially alcohol, and susceptibility is also greater in people who carry one of the *HFE* gene mutations associated with hemochromatosis (see OMIM 235200).
- Erythropoietic protoporphyria appears to be dominant, but many carriers of a single non-functional *FECH* allele remain perfectly healthy. Just 35% of the normal enzyme activity is sufficient to avoid disease – so why do people affected by this dominant condition have less than 50% of normal ferrochelatase activity? One explanation would be a dominant negative effect (see *Section 6.4*). However, people with the same *FECH* mutation may be either healthy or affected, so this cannot be the explanation.

  It turns out that almost all affected patients are in fact compound heterozygotes for a rare non-functional allele and a common partially functional allele. A single T>C nucleotide substitution 48 nucleotides from the 3′ end of intron 3 of the *FECH* gene (SNP rs2272783) is widespread in several populations (Japanese 43%, South-East Asian 31%, white French 11%) but rare in others (black West Africans <1%). The frequency of the SNP in different populations correlates with the frequency of erythropoietic protoporphyria. This polymorphism affects the efficiency of splicing. Much of the RNA produced by the C allele is aberrantly spliced and broken down by nonsense-mediated decay (see *Chapter 6*). Such a mechanism might perhaps explain some of the variability of other dominant phenotypes.

8.5. **References**

Buckley RH (2004) Molecular defects in human severe combined immunodeficiency disease and approaches to immune reconstitution. *Ann. Rev. Immunol.* **22**: 625–655.

Evans WE and McLeod HL (2003) Pharmacogenomics: drug disposition, drug targets and side effects. *New Engl. J. Med.* **348**: 538–549. *Free text available at* http://content.nejm.org/cgi/content/extract/348/6/538.

Horton R, Wilming L, Rand V, *et al.* (2004) Gene map of the extended human MHC. *Nat. Rev. Genet.* **5**: 889–899.

Janeway CA, Travers P, Walport M and Shlomchik M (2001) *Immunobiology*, 5th edn. Garland Science, New York. *Available on the NCBI Bookshelf* http://www.ncbi.nlm.nih.gov/books.

Karniski LP (2001) Mutations in the diastrophic dysplasia sulfate transporter (DTDST) gene: correlation between sulfate transport activity and chondrodysplasia phenotype. *Hum. Molec. Genet.* **10**: 1485–1490.

McLeod HL and Siva C (2002) The thiopurine S-methyltransferase gene locus – implications for clinical pharmacogenomics. *Pharmacogenomics*, **3**: 89–98.

Scriver C and Waters PJ (1999) Monogenic traits are not simple: lessons from phenylketonuria. *Trends Genet.* **15**: 267–272. *This is highly recommended reading.*

Service RF (2005) Going from genome to pill. *Science*, **308**: 1858–1860.

Weinshilboum R (2005) Inheritance and drug response. *New Engl. J. Med.* **348**: 529–537. *Free text available at* http://content.nejm.org/cgi/content/extract/348/6/529.

Useful websites

BiDil archive: http://www.nottingham.ac.uk/igbis/reg/bidil.htm

Personalised medicines: hopes and realities – a report by the Royal Society 2005: http://www.royalsoc.ac.uk/displaypagedoc.asp?id=17570

8.6 **Self-assessment questions**

(1) The diagram shows the biosynthetic pathways leading from precursor A to products E and G. Enzymes E1-E5 catalyze the reactions. E1 converts 90% of A to B and 10% to

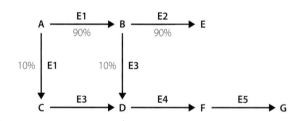

C. 90% of B is normally converted to E by E2, but 10% is converted to D by E3. Which enzyme(s) might be deficient in a condition marked by (a) deficiency of E and G, (b) deficiency of G only, and (c) deficiency of E together with a raised amount of G?

(2) Describe ways in which a mendelian condition might be the result of loss of function of several enzymes if, (a) each of several unrelated patients shows a loss of function of just one of the enzymes, different in each patient and, (b) if each patient shows loss of function of all of the enzymes.

(3) Acute intermittent porphyria is a dominant condition, yet it is estimated that 80% of people heterozygous for a pathogenic *PBGD* mutation go through their lives completely unaware of the fact, and never suffer an episode of the disease. Discuss possible reasons for this low penetrance.

(4) Discuss the case for regarding scurvy as a genetic disease. Can similar arguments be applied to other examples?

(5) Arthur, Bridget and their three children Charles, Daniel and Eliza were typed for the HLA-A, -B and -DR loci. The results (using a simplified nomenclature) were:

Arthur	A3,23;	B7,27;	DR3,4
Bridget	A2,23;	B15,27;	DR3,4
Charles	A3,23;	B15,27;	DR3,4
Daniel	A2,23;	B7,27;	DR3,4
Eliza	A2,3;	B27;	DR4

Assuming there is no recombination, so that a person's A, B and DR alleles are passed on as an unbroken haplotype, work out the haplotypes in this family.

(6) What features of the gene locus or mutational spectrum in a disease would lead you to suspect that gene conversion might be a major mutational mechanism?

(7) What are possible genotypes for the samples shown in tracks 6, 8 and 9 of the two gels in *Figure 8.8*?

Chapter 9

How do researchers identify genes for mendelian diseases?

Learning points for this chapter

After working through this chapter you should be able to:

- Describe the principle of genetic mapping in humans
- Identify recombinants and non-recombinants in a simple pedigree
- Describe the use of microsatellites and SNPs as genetic markers
- Describe in outline different routes by which human disease genes have been identified
- Show how the Human Genome Project databases can be used to address clinical problems
- Show how linked markers can be used to track a disease gene through a pedigree

9.1. **Case studies**

| Dyschromatosis symmetrica hereditaria | **229** | 238 |

Although this condition (OMIM 127400) is rare and is not particularly troublesome clinically, we chose it because all the steps in the standard route for gene identification are described in a single paper in a source that is likely to be accessible to most readers (Miyamura *et al.*, 2003). Because these are real families, we have not tried to invent a clinical story.

Figure 9.1 – Dyschromatosis symmetrica hereditaria
Patients with DSH have small hyperpigmented and hypopigmented macules on the backs of their hands and the dorsal surface of their feet. The abnormalities are otherwise asymptomatic and do not affect the general health of the person. The condition is autosomal dominant. Photos courtesy of Drs Tamio Suzuki and Yasushi Tomita, Nagoya University.

9.2. **Background**

Genes can be defined in two very different ways:

- as determinants of mendelian characters ('the Huntington disease gene', etc.)
- as functional units of DNA

Ultimately the two must correspond, and in this chapter we will see how corresponding pairs are identified. The Human Genome Project and related initiatives are giving us a good catalog of genes as functional DNA units. For each gene we know its exact physical location, measured in base pairs of DNA from the end of a chromosome. The catalog is not yet complete – genes whose product is a non-translated RNA are under-represented, and details of many protein-coding genes are incomplete. Nevertheless the current list and the associated physical map are a tremendous resource, at least for protein-coding genes.

However, knowing the human genome sequence does not in itself tell us anything about the Huntington disease gene – neither its DNA sequence nor its chromosomal location. Genes that are defined through phenotypes have to be identified using different methods. Once identified, they will almost always nowadays turn out to be genes that have already been defined as DNA units – but it is usually impossible to say in advance which functional DNA unit will be the right one. The major achievement of clinical genetics during the years 1985–2000 has been to identify the genes underlying the great majority of mendelian diseases and to make the connection between characters and DNA sequences.

There are several possible ways to identify the gene responsible for a mendelian character, including the following.

- If the sequence of the protein product is known, a cDNA sequence can be worked out by reading the genetic code table. An oligonucleotide probe can be synthesized corresponding to the sequence, and used to screen a cDNA library to isolate a clone containing the cDNA (see *Box 9.1*).
- If one member of a gene family has been shown to cause a certain disease, other members of the same family are candidates for related diseases. For example, after the fibrillin gene was shown to be mutated in Marfan syndrome (see Case 10, Johnson family) a related gene, fibrillin 2, was a good candidate for a related condition, congenital contractural arachnodactyly (OMIM 121050).
- If a gene causes a phenotype in an animal, its human homolog is a candidate for a similar human condition. *Sox10* was shown to cause the *Dominant megacolon* mutation in mice. Its human homolog *SOX10* therefore became a candidate for the similar Type IV Waardenburg syndrome (OMIM 277580) in humans.
- If a gene product is part of a developmental, regulatory or metabolic pathway, and that gene is mutated in some but not all people with a certain disease, other genes in the same pathway are candidates for the remaining cases. The example of *CDKL5* in Rett syndrome was given in *Disease box 7*.

- If a disease shows genuine anticipation (that is, it becomes more severe or has earlier onset in each succeeding generation – see *Disease box 4*) then it may well be caused by an unstable expanding DNA repeat. There are techniques for checking a patient's DNA directly for such repeat expansions. If an expansion in a particular gene is found, DNA from other patients can be checked for the same expansion.

However, none of these methods is generally applicable to *any* mendelian condition. In any case, because genotype–phenotype correlations are generally poor and hard to predict, the chance of phenotype-based predictions hitting on the correct gene is not high. Before investing much effort in mutation screening, most researchers would want some extra confirmation that they are looking in the right place. This confirmation comes from mapping the character.

Thus the standard route, by which the great majority of genes underlying mendelian characters have been identified, starts with mapping the character to reveal its chromosomal location. In pre-genomic days, once the location was known it was then necessary to clone all the DNA from the candidate region, identify every gene in the region, and screen each for mutations in affected people. That approach is called **positional cloning** and was an heroic undertaking. Nowadays, in the post-genome era, everything is much easier. Having mapped the gene, a list of genes at that location is downloaded from the

---

Box 9.1

Identifying genes through their protein product

This was the route used in some early successes at identifying disease genes. Until the late 1970s, techniques for isolating and characterizing proteins outstripped those for isolating and characterizing human DNA. Examples include:

- *The α- and β-globin genes* – these were among the earliest human genes to be cloned, based on the knowledge that most of the protein synthesis in red cell precursors was of the two globin chains. RNA isolated from these cells therefore constituted an impure preparation of globin mRNA, and could be used to screen libraries to identify matching DNA clones.

- *Factor VIII* – this gene was identified in 1984 from information about the protein it encoded. It was known that hemophilia A was caused by a lack of blood clotting Factor VIII. A sufficient quantity of Factor VIII protein was isolated from pig blood to allow a partial amino acid sequence to be obtained. This was used to predict the sequence of the mRNA encoding those parts of the protein, by reading the genetic code table in reverse. The prediction contained many ambiguities – for example, the amino acid serine could be encoded by any of six codons. At the other extreme, tryptophan and methionine each have only a single codon. A run of 15 amino acids was chosen that minimized the ambiguities, and a mix of oligonucleotides was synthesized, including all possible sequences encoding the 15 amino acids. This mix was used as a probe to find a matching sequence in a pig genomic DNA library. Having isolated the pig *F8* gene, a pig clone was used to identify the human *F8* gene by screening a human library.

Modern techniques of proteomics may once again make it practicable to identify the gene defect underlying a disease through the study of changes in the protein repertoire.

databases, and suitable candidates picked for mutation screening. This is often called the **positional candidate** approach.

Below we consider how the genes causing human phenotypes can be mapped, and then how the correct gene can be identified within the candidate region. In *Section 9.3* we go through the stages of a real example of the positional candidate method: the identification of the gene causing DSH.

Fundamentals of gene mapping

All genetic mapping depends on the behavior of chromosomes at meiosis (*Figure 2.7*). Non-homologous chromosomes assort independently. This means that alleles at loci on different chromosomes have a 50% chance of ending up in the same gamete (non-recombinant) and a 50% chance of ending up in different gametes (recombinant). Loci that are on the same chromosome will travel together unless a crossover between the paired homologous chromosomes separates them (*Figure 9.2*). They will be separated if a crossover occurs at a position between the two loci. This will happen often to widely separated loci, but only rarely to those close together. Thus the chance of recombination between two loci is a measure of the distance between them. Loci that are separated by recombination in 1% of meioses are defined as being 1 centiMorgan (cM) apart.

Genetic distances, defined in this way and measured in centiMorgans, are not the same as physical distances, measured in bp, kb or Mb of DNA. The two would correspond exactly only if the chance of a crossover were identical in every stretch of a chromosome. In fact, some regions have a higher frequency of crossovers than others. The order of loci should still be the same on genetic and physical maps, but the spacing may be different. As a rule of thumb, 1 cM corresponds to 1 Mb – but there are considerable local variations.

RECOMBINATION				
between A and B:	NR	R	R	NR
between B and C:	NR	NR	R	R
between A and C:	NR	R	NR	R

Figure 9.2 – Crossing over between paired homologous chromosomes in the first division of meiosis produces recombination between genetic loci.
This example shows the effects on three loci, A, B and C, of two crossovers that happen to involve three of the four chromatids. Double crossovers can involve two, three or all four strands. NR, non-recombinant for this pair of loci; R, recombinant for this pair of loci.

Genetic mapping depends on studying two (or more) loci in a set of independent meioses and estimating the proportion of meioses where there was recombination between them. If the recombination fraction is significantly below 50%, the loci are said to be linked, and will be on the same chromosome. Unlinked loci may be on different chromosomes or may be on the same chromosome but distant from each other. Studying a series of linked loci and estimating the pairwise recombination fractions allows the loci to be arranged in order along a genetic map (*Figure 9.3*). The figure shows a breeding experiment in fruit flies, the organism in which the concepts of genetic mapping were developed by TH Morgan around 1910–1920. Experiments such as this established the methodology of genetic mapping; applying similar concepts to humans requires elaborate statistical methods.

Three recessive characters were studied:

Vermilion (v)	vs. normal (red, v^+) eyes
Crossveinless (cv)	vs. normal (cv^+) wings
Cut (ct)	vs. normal (ct^+) wing border

The available fly stocks were:
red eyes, crossveinless and cut wings (v^+/v^+, cv/cv, ct/ct)
vermilion eyes, normal wings (v/v, cv^+cv^+, ct^+/ct^+)

(a) *Two lines were produced for the mapping experiment:*
Triply recessive v/v, cv/cv, ct/ct with vermilion eyes, crossveinless and cut wings
Triply heterozygous, v/v^+, cv/cv^+, ct/ct^+ with an all normal phenotype

(b) *Triple heterozygotes are crossed with flies homozygous for all three recessive characters and the offspring phenotyped:*
The male parent contributed the three recessive alleles, so the phenotype of each progeny fly gives a direct readout of the genotype of the maternal gamete that produced it.

(c) *For each pair of loci recombinants are identified and the recombination fraction calculated*
Gametes are recombinant if they contain a combination of alleles different from the parental combinations (v^+, cv, ct) and (v, cv^+, ct^+) – see the way the triply heterozygous females were obtained.
Results were:

| v | v^+ | ct^+ | 580 | } non-recombinant ($n = 1172$) |
| v^+ | cv | ct | 592 | |

| v | cv | ct^+ | 45 | } recombinant between (v, ct) and cv loci ($n = 85$) |
| v^+ | cv^+ | ct | 40 | |

| v | cv | ct | 89 | } recombinant between v and (cv, ct) loci ($n = 183$) |
| v^+ | cv^+ | ct^+ | 94 | |

| v | cv^+ | ct | 3 | } recombinant between (v, cv) and ct loci ($n = 8$) |
| v^+ | cv | ct | 5 | |

1488

Note that only 316 of the 1488 gametes (21%) are recombinant. Clearly the three loci are linked.

(d) *Combining the data establishes the order and genetic distances of the loci*
The rarest class must be those that require a double recombination to produce them. This establishes that the gene order must be v – ct – cv.

Next, we count recombinants in each interval:

Between v and ct:	183 + 8	= 191/1488	= 13.2%
Between ct and cv:	85 + 8	= 93/1488	= 6.4%
Between v and cv:	183 + 85 + (2 × 8)	= 284/1488	= 19.6%

The map established by this experiment is: v – 13.2 cM – ct – 6.4 cM – cv.

Figure 9.3 – Genetic mapping in the *Drosophila* fruit fly.
Distances are genetic distances, measured in centimorgans (cM). Data from Griffiths *et al.* (1999)

Special problems of genetic mapping in humans

The need to use genetic markers

Human genetic mapping asks exactly the same questions as mapping in fruit flies, but the methods used have to be adapted to handle typical human families. Mapping always looks at pairs (or larger numbers) of loci. Although any meiosis may in fact involve a crossover between the two loci, we can only tell whether or not that has occurred if the person in whom the meiosis takes place is heterozygous at both loci. With the flies in *Figure 9.3* the experimenter could set up an appropriate cross. With humans we have to take families as we find them. The chance of finding families in which two diseases are segregating, so that there are double heterozygotes, is very low. Instead, we look for families in which the disease of interest is segregating, and then type them for genetic markers. Markers, for these purposes, need to have four properties:

- they must be inherited in a clean mendelian manner
- they must be sufficiently polymorphic that there is a good chance that a person, picked because they are heterozygous for the disease we are studying, is also heterozygous for the marker
- they must be reasonably easy to type, using material that family members are reasonably likely to be willing to provide
- markers must be available across the whole genome at reasonably close intervals. How close is 'reasonably close' depends on the family material available. If very large numbers of meioses can be studied, the whole genome could be tested using markers 40 cM apart. Realistic pedigree collections require markers no more than 10 cM apart. That translates to 300–500 markers, spread across the genome.

In the past, attempts were made to use blood groups, protein electrophoretic variants and tissue types as markers, but each failed one or more of the criteria listed. Only DNA polymorphisms can satisfy the requirements. Two types of polymorphisms are generally used (*Figure 9.4*).

- **Microsatellites** are short tandem repeats (for example, $(CA)_n$ sequences) that are present in everybody at the same specific chromosomal locations, but where the number of repeat units varies from person to person. The early phases of the Human Genome Project were largely devoted to identifying suitable microsatellites. Over 20 000 are now cataloged. They are genotyped by PCR-amplifying a segment of DNA containing the microsatellite and determining its size by gel electrophoresis (often using fluorescent labeling and a DNA sequencing machine). They have the advantage of having many possible alleles (that is, people might have 5, 6, 7 …, etc. repeats), increasing the likelihood that a meiosis will be informative.
- **Single nucleotide polymorphisms** are less informative, because there are almost always only two alternative nucleotides at a polymorphic site. However, they are abundant (about 10 million are cataloged in the dbSNP database, see *References*) and they can be typed by techniques that avoid gel electrophoresis. This is important because it allows various very high throughput techniques to be used, such as

Figure 9.4 – Common types of DNA polymorphism.
(a) A (CA)$_n$ microsatellite, (b) an A/C SNP, (c) a C/T SNP that causes an RFLP (in this case loss of an *Eco*RI site by a CpG→TpG change). *Eco*RI recognizes the sequence GAATTC.

(a)
```
ctctcacagt agccacacac acaccgctgc acagcggcct              n=5
ctctcacagt agccacacac acacaccgct gcacagcggc ct           n=6
ctctcacagt agccacacac acacacaccg ctgcacagcg gcct         n=7
```

(b)
```
tttttttg tttcccttcc atgggtgata ttgcttcttg aaatacggac     A
tttttttg tttcccttcc atgggtgatc ttgcttcttg aaatacggac     C
```

(c)
```
tgcacagtga tgtggaattc gaaagctgac tgca        EcoRI site present
tgcacagtga tgtggaattt gaaagctgac tgca        EcoRI site absent
```

microarrays ('SNP-chips') or methods based on flow-sorting microscopic beads. Some SNPs create or abolish a recognition site for a restriction enzyme, thus creating a **restriction fragment length polymorphism (RFLP)**. RFLPs were the original DNA markers, superseded by microsatellites for general mapping, but still useful because they are easy and convenient to type in a small laboratory.

All DNA polymorphisms have one big advantage as genetic markers: they can easily be located to a specific chromosomal region. Originally this was done by FISH (see *Section 4.2*) or related methods; now it can be done simply by searching the genome database for the location of adjacent unique sequences. Thus genetic mapping now has available a dense framework of markers, all mapped relative to one another and in defined chromosomal locations.

Recognizing recombinants

Figure 9.5 shows a pedigree where recombinants and non-recombinants can be counted unambiguously. A dominant disease is segregating in this family, and individuals have been typed for a DNA polymorphism that has alleles 1, 2, 3 and 4. Recombination between the disease and marker loci might have occurred in any meiosis in the pedigree, but we can only detect it in the offspring of the doubly heterozygous individual II–2. She received marker allele 2 with the disease gene from her mother and marker allele 4 with the normal allele at the disease locus from her father. Offspring who inherit either of those combinations are non-recombinant; those who inherit disease + 4, or normal + 2, are recombinant. There are two recombinants in ten meioses.

If we had DNA from only the lower two generations of the family in *Figure 9.5* (the grandparents were dead, or declined to give DNA) we could not tell which of the offspring in the bottom generation were recombinant and which were

Figure 9.5 – Identifying recombinants and non-recombinants in a human pedigree.
NR, Non-recombinant. **R**, recombinant. See text for full details.

non-recombinant. We would know there were two of one type and eight of the other, and we might guess that the two were probably recombinant, but we would not know. Individual II–2 might have inherited marker allele 4 with the disease, in which case there would be eight recombinants and only two non-recombinants. If we are collecting families with an uncommon genetic disease, we cannot restrict ourselves to families with the ideal structure of *Figure 9.5*. We will probably end up relying on families whose structure does not allow recombinants to be identified unambiguously.

To get round this problem, human gene mapping relies on computer programs that don't try to identify individual recombinants, but instead calculate the likelihood of the overall pedigree data, on the alternative assumptions that the two loci are linked (with a specified recombination fraction) or not linked. The ratio of the two likelihoods provides evidence for or against linkage. If the likelihood ratio supports linkage, the most likely recombination fraction is the one that gives the most favorable likelihood ratio. The output statistic from this analysis is the logarithm of the likelihood ratio, which is known as the **lod score**. The reasons for using this statistic, and its properties, are explained briefly in Strachan and Read (2003), or in detail in Ott (1999).

Getting enough meioses

Even in the most favorable circumstances – an ideally structured pedigree with no recombinants – a minimum of ten meioses is needed to provide statistically significant evidence of linkage. If we want to map a disease, we have to take the families as we find them. The structure is seldom ideal; vital people may be homozygous for the marker (remember we can only score doubly heterozygous meioses) and there will probably be some recombinants. Because of these factors, linkage analysis will seldom be successful with fewer than 20 meioses. This usually means that several families must be combined. It is then very important to be sure that they really do all have the same disease, caused by mutation at the same locus. Locus heterogeneity is a serious obstacle.

Protocol for a linkage trawl

A typical mapping project would start with collecting families where the disease of interest is segregating. Excellent clinical input at this stage is crucial to success. It is imperative to get the diagnosis right, to be confident that all the families really do have the same disease and that people are correctly classified as affected or unaffected. When diseases show variable expression (see *Disease box 1*), this can be a demanding task. Having ascertained the families, affected and unaffected family members must be persuaded to give a sample, usually blood, for the research. Fortunately, many people in families where a genetic disease is segregating are keen to help research, but there is no place for compulsion. Unlike fruit flies, individuals have every right to refuse.

DNA is extracted in the laboratory, and then the samples are genotyped for a series of markers. Over the years this has become much easier. Once it was a massive undertaking using Southern blots and taking years; now it can be automated and done in weeks. Markers are typed by PCR, either using panels of commercially available primers for microsatellites, or using chips that allow large panels of SNPs to be genotyped in a single operation. For each marker, the genotypes must be aligned to the pedigrees and checked for co-segregation with the disease under study. This is done using computer programs to calculate the lod scores.

As mentioned above, the statistical test of linkage is the lod score. This is the *log*arithm of the *od*ds of linkage (at a stated recombination fraction) compared to non-linkage. The essential points about lod scores are:

- each lod score refers to a specific recombination fraction; for each marker it is usual for the computer to calculate a table of lod scores for a series of possible recombination fractions (see *Table 9.1*)
- a lod score of +3 is the threshold of statistical significance ($P=0.05$).
- higher lod scores are stronger evidence of linkage; the lod score is logarithmic, so a lod score of 4 is ten times as good as a lod score of 3
- a lod score below –2 is significant evidence against linkage at the stated recombination fraction

The linkage trawl is continued, testing marker after marker, until a convincingly positive lod score is obtained. *Table 9.1* shows a real example.

The next step is to narrow down the candidate region. The initial analysis may have located the disease gene to a 10 cM interval between adjacent markers. Averaged across the whole genome, loci 10 cM apart on the genetic map are separated by 10 Mb of DNA, though the exact relation varies from location to location. Before the work can proceed to testing candidate genes for mutations, it is highly desirable to narrow down the candidate region to less than 1 Mb – otherwise the number of possible candidate genes will probably be excessive. To narrow down the candidate region, the Genome Project or dbSNP databases are used to select a series of new markers (microsatellites or SNPs) that cover the region at high density. At this stage it is often best to review the results by eye, rather than relying on the computer. *Figure 9.7* shows a real example.

The endgame: testing candidate genes for mutations

Once a reasonably small candidate region has been defined by linkage analysis, a list is drawn up of all the genes within the region. Once, this meant several years of work by a team of skilled postdoctoral researchers to discover the genes; now a suitable list can be downloaded from the Human Genome Project database (though it must be borne in mind that the list may be incomplete). Genes are prioritized for mutation testing on several criteria.

- **Function** – does available information on the gene function make it seem a likely candidate for this particular disease? Bear in mind, though, that the relation between biochemical function and disease symptoms is often very far from obvious. For example, the *FMR1* gene encodes an RNA-binding protein; loss of function mutations cause Fragile-X syndrome (OMIM 309550, see *Disease box 4*), the main features of which are mental retardation, a characteristic face and macro-orchidism.
- **Pattern of expression** – is the gene expressed in the tissues that are affected by the disease? Data on expression are available from analyses

of cDNA libraries. A cDNA library prepared from a given tissue will contain only cDNAs of genes that are expressed in that tissue.

- **Other related genes** – are there related genes elsewhere in the genome, and if so, are any of them known to be mutated in a similar disease?
- **Animal models** – is there an animal mutant known for this gene, and if so is the phenotype appropriate? We would not look for an exact correspondence, but there should at least be points of resemblance.
- **Size and complexity** – all other things being equal, it is much easier to test a gene with two exons than one with 67.

Having established a prioritized list, each gene in turn is scanned for mutations in a panel of unrelated affected individuals – preferably those whose disease is known to map to the candidate location. Any of the techniques described in *Section 5.2* (*Methods for scanning a gene for any sequence change*) could be used. This is still not a completely routine task – not every exon of every gene is correctly represented in the databases, and some mutations are deep within introns, or otherwise hard to spot. However, barring ill luck, the whole process might take one scientist a few months. Nowadays collecting the necessary families and samples is the most difficult part of the work.

For loss of function diseases, it is reasonable to hope to find a diversity of nonsense, splicing and frameshift mutations in different unrelated people. Such a finding would unambiguously identify the gene as the correct one. If only one change is found, but in several unrelated affected people (which might often be the case for a gain of function disease), it will be important to check that this is not a common non-pathogenic polymorphism. That is done by typing a suitably large number of healthy controls from the same ethnic background. Final confirmation that the correct gene has been identified might come from constructing an animal model, using the techniques of targeted knockouts or RNA interference (Bantounas *et al.*, 2004; Iredale, 1999).

9.3 **Investigations of patients**

| Dyschromatosis symmetrica hereditaria | 229 | **238** |

Several Japanese families were ascertained in which this condition was segregating, and many family members donated blood for DNA extraction (*Figure 9.6*). DNA samples from three families were typed for 343 microsatellite markers spaced across the genome and lod scores calculated. Most of the markers gave negative lod scores, but a series of adjacent markers on chromosome 1 gave the lod scores shown in *Table 9.1*.

Things to note about this table.

- Some of the lod scores are well above 3, showing strong evidence of linkage.
- The fact that the lod score at zero recombination is minus infinity for every marker, means that with every marker there are some recombinants between the marker and the disease. In other words, none of the markers is extremely close to the disease locus.

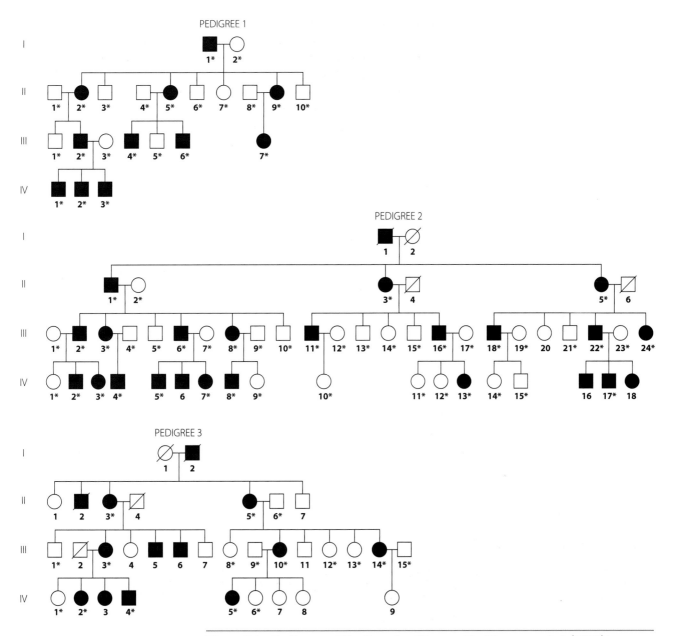

Figure 9.6 – Pedigrees of the three families used by Miyamura *et al.* (2003) to map the dyschromatosis gene.
Individuals marked with asterisks provided DNA samples. Adapted from Miyamura *et al.* (2003) with permission from University of Chicago Press.

- The markers are shown in chromosomal order. The lod scores are much stronger for markers in the center of the table than those at the top and bottom. This implies that the disease locus is somewhere in the middle part of the region covered by these markers.
- Don't try to read too much into the exact value of a strongly positive lod score. The lod score for one marker may be lower than that for an adjacent marker because one or two individuals happened to be homozygous for one marker and not for the other. Homozygous individuals contribute

Table 9.1 – Linkage analysis in the families shown in *Figure 9.6*

Marker	LOD at θ =:						
	0	**0.05**	**0.1**	**0.15**	**0.2**	**0.3**	**0.4**
D1S424	–inf.	0.17	1.15	1.51	1.59	1.30	0.66
D1S206	–inf.	–1.21	0.56	1.29	1.59	1.51	0.90
D1S502	–inf.	3.81	4.88	5.02	4.75	3.51	1.68
D1S252	–inf.	5.46	5.96	5.78	5.29	3.77	1.79
D1S498	–inf.	4.49	4.43	4.09	3.62	2.42	1.06
D1S484	–inf.	1.80	2.99	3.34	3.31	2.62	1.42
D1S196	–inf.	–0.76	0.46	0.99	1.21	1.17	0.72
D1S218	–inf.	–7.17	–4.03	–2.40	–1.41	–0.36	0.02

The table shows lod scores calculated by computer for a series of microsatellite markers from the long arm of chromosome 1. θ symbolizes the recombination fraction. See text for discussion.

The microsatellites are named according to a standard scheme (D = DNA segment, 1 = on chromosome 1; S = single copy; the number just records the order in which each marker was first described).

Adapted from Miyamura *et al.* (2003) with permission from University of Chicago Press.

no information to the mapping process, so the lod score is lower. But the overall pattern shows strong support for linkage to markers in the central part of the region covered.

The markers shown in *Table 9.1* span a genetic distance of just over 60 cM on the long arm of chromosome 1. To narrow this down, the families were genotyped for a new set of closely spaced microsatellites across the candidate region. *Figure 9.7* shows the crucial parts of the data for *D1S498* and 11 new microsatellites that map in the 13 cM gap between *D1S498* and *D1S484*. For the 12 microsatellite markers in the figure, the different alleles are given arbitrary numbers, and the genotypes of seven individuals are shown, each as two haplotypes. The haplotypes are deduced by typing the parents. Rather than calculate lod scores (irrelevant since at this stage they knew that this region was linked to the disease locus), the researchers used the haplotypes to pinpoint individual recombinations.

In a given family, most affected people had inherited the same complete haplotype of markers with the disease gene – that is, in the meiosis in the parent who transmitted the disease gene to that individual, that region of chromosome had not been disrupted by any crossover. Most affected people in Family 1 had the haplotype shown in green in individual 1-I1 on his disease-related chromosome. Similarly in Family 2 most had the blue haplotype, and in Family 3 most had the yellow haplotype on their disease–bearing chromosome. However, several individuals had recombinant haplotypes, indicated in *Figure 9.7* by the part-colored boxes. Because these individuals

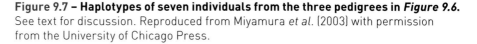

INDIVIDUAL	1-I1		1-IV3		2-II1		2-IV4		2-IV5		3-III3		3-IV4	
D1S498	5	2	5	4	2	3	2	2	2	5	3	2	2	4
D1S2347	1	4	1	1	4	1	4	1	4	1	1	3	3	1
D1S2345	4	4	4	8	7	2	7	1	2	1	2	2	2	1
D1S2858	2	1	2	2	1	1	1	2	1	2	2	2	2	2
D1S305	6	6	6	7	6	5	6	1	6	6	6	8	8	2
D1S2715	5	6	5	5	1	1	1	5	1	3	6	3	3	1
D1S2777	1	4	4	3	3	3	3	3	3	3	5	3	5	3
D1S2624	3	3	3	3	5	1	4	3	5	1	4	2	4	4
D1S506	6	6	5	4	5	5	5	4	5	5	5	2	5	5
D1S2635	7	8	8	8	7	8	8	7	7	7	7	7	7	8
D1S2771	3	1	1	1	1	1	1	3	1	1	1	1	1	3
D1S2707	6	2	2	6	4	6	2	6	4	6	5	6	5	2

Figure 9.7 – Haplotypes of seven individuals from the three pedigrees in *Figure 9.6.*
See text for discussion. Reproduced from Miyamura *et al.* (2003) with permission from the University of Chicago Press.

were affected, they must have inherited the disease gene. This therefore had to be located within the colored segment of their recombinant haplotype, or in the immediately adjacent gap. Thus individual IV–3 in Family 1 tells us that the disease locus must lie above marker *D1S2777*. (Although *D1S2715* is the lowermost marker in the colored part of the haplotype, the disease gene might lie between this and the next marker down – but not at or below *D1S2777*.) Individual IV–4 in Family 3 tells us it must lie below marker *D1S2715* (in the yellow segment of the chromosome). Therefore it must actually lie between these two markers. The other recombinant individuals are consistent with this localization.

This analysis narrowed down the candidate region to just 500 kb at chromosomal location 1q21.3. A genome browser program was used to check this region in the Human Genome Project database. Only seven genes were listed in the region. DNA from affected individuals in each pedigree (and another unrelated individual with the same disease) was then scanned for mutations in each gene. Single strand conformation polymorphisms (SSCP, see *Figures 5.7b* and *5.10*) were used to check each exon of each gene. Changes were found in each sample in one of the genes, *DSRAD* (double-stranded RNA-specific adenosine deaminase). Within a family, each affected person had the same change, but they were different between families, and not all in the same exon (exons 2, 10, 10 and 15 in the four unrelated cases).

It remained to be proven that the changes detected were the true pathogenic mutations. Pointers to this were as follows.

- Two of the four mutations were nonsense mutations, which are unlikely to be common polymorphic variants.
- The other two mutations were both mis-sense mutations involving amino acids that were completely conserved in the corresponding protein in 11 different animal species surveyed. Such conservation implies that these amino acids have important functions, so the mutations are unlikely to be common polymorphisms.

- DNA from 116 unrelated normally pigmented Japanese adults was tested for each mutation; none was found. Again, this argues against them being non-pathogenic polymorphisms.

Surprisingly, when the *DSRAD* gene was knocked out in mice, the result was an embryonic lethal, even in heterozygotes. Although unexpected, this does not disprove the identification of *DSRAD* as the dyschromatosis gene. Although the similarities between mice and humans greatly outweigh the differences, there are differences. These are especially likely to be seen where an effect is due to haplo-insufficiency (where a 50% level of gene activity is not enough for normal function), as here. Note also that none of the research described shows why a 50% reduction in the activity of this gene should cause pigmentary abnormalities of the skin of just the hands and feet. Often identifying the gene is just the start of research into what it does.

| CASE 3 | Choudhary family | 3 | 9 | 66 | **242** | 260 | 376 |

- Girl (Nasreen) aged 8 months, parents Aadnan and Mumtaz
- Deaf
- Parents are first cousins
- Pedigree suggests autosomal recessive deafness

When we last met this family (*Chapter 3*), it was still only a hypothesis that Nasreen's deafness was autosomal recessive, or even that it was genetic at all, since there are so many different causes of hearing impairment. The fact that she had two affected uncles, and that all were offspring of consanguineous marriages, strengthened the case for it being autosomal recessive, but the only way to prove it would be to demonstrate a mutation. As described in *Chapter 3*, this is very difficult because mutations in at least 50 different genes can cause autosomal recessive hearing impairment.

Although any one of over 50 genes might be responsible, in most populations mutations in one gene, *GJB2*, are by far the most common cause. This gene encodes the connexin 26 protein that forms gap junctions between cells in the inner ear. These are important for recycling potassium ions, which enter the hair cells when they fire in response to sound. *GJB2* is a very simple gene, having just two exons, and all the coding sequence is in exon 2. In specific populations particular mutations are common, for example, c.35delG in Europeans (see *Figure 6.2*) and c.235delC in Chinese. It is simple to test for the commonest mutations in the patient's ethnic group, and reasonably simple to sequence the whole small gene, so this test is often performed. It provides a definite answer in up to half of all cases. However, a negative result leaves the investigation no further forward.

The whole *GJB2* coding sequence was sequenced in Nasreen's DNA, but no mutation was found in either copy. Normally this would be the end of the story, but in this case the geneticist decided to try harder. Partly this was because the family were particularly keen to know the cause of Nasreen's hearing loss. Partly it was because she wanted to be able to give better recurrence risks to Nasreen's uncle Waleed and aunt Benazir (see *Figure 1.9* for the pedigree) who, as explained in *Chapter 1*, were planning to marry. Partly it was because the family structure allowed further investigation.

On the assumption that Nasreen, Waleed and his brother Mohammed all had the same autosomal recessive hearing loss, it was likely that one or other of

Nasreen's great-great-grandparents had carried a mutation in heterozygous form, and that the three deaf individuals had each inherited two copies of that original mutant gene as a result of the consanguinity in the family. If they did indeed all have two copies of that ancestral chromosome segment, they should all be homozygous for the same set of marker alleles on the chromosomal region immediately surrounding the mutant gene. That would be something quite unlikely to happen just by chance. It was therefore decided to type the three of them for highly polymorphic microsatellite markers from the immediate vicinity of as many deafness loci as possible. The Hereditary Hearing Loss Homepage (see *Section 9.5*) provides lists of microsatellites that are closely linked to deafness loci. Using this and the Human Genome Project database, the geneticist drew up a list of markers and asked the laboratory to genotype the three samples for each marker. This procedure, used in inbred families, is known as **autozygosity mapping**. Autozygosity means homozygosity by descent from a defined common ancestor.

Two markers, *D2S174* and *D2S158*, that are tightly linked to the *DFNB9* deafness locus, showed a pattern consistent with linkage (*Figure 9.8*). This was confirmed by typing for a further series of closely linked markers on chromosome 2p22. This showed that Nasreen, Waleed and Mohammed were all homozygous for an extended haplotype of markers surrounding the *DFNB9* locus. The relevant gene, *OTOF* (Otoferlin), has 48 exons. Without the high index of suspicion provided by the linkage analysis, it would not be worth searching such a large gene for mutations. At this stage it was justified, and the search revealed that the three deaf individuals were all homozygous for an A > G transition at the intron 8 – exon 9 junction of the *OTOF* gene. This alters the invariant AG acceptor splice site, and is virtually certain to make the gene non-functional. Interestingly, although there is extensive allelic heterogeneity in *OTOF* mutations, as is usual for loss of function conditions, the same mutation had been previously described, this time in an affected family in India. It would be possible to work out whether both families had inherited the mutation from an unknown common ancestor, if DNA could be

GENOTYPES FOR:			
D10S537	2-4	4-4	4-1
D10S1432	2-1	2-1	4-2
D2S174	6-6	6-6	6-6
D2S158	2-2	2-2	2-2

Figure 9.8 – Autozygosity mapping.
The three deaf individuals in the Choudhary family were typed for a series of markers linked to different deafness loci. Results are shown for markers *D10S537* and *D10S1432*, which excluded the *DFNB12* locus on chromosome 10q22, and for markers *D2S174* and *D2S158* which gave results consistent with linkage to the *DFNB9* locus at 2p22–p23.

obtained from an affected member of the Indian family. If the Indian case had the same ancestral chromosome segment, they would have the same haplotype of SNPs immediately surrounding the mutation.

9.4. Summary and extension

Using chromosomal abnormalities to suggest a candidate region or candidate gene

Linkage analysis requires an absolute minimum of 10 **informative meioses** to have any possibility of the lod score reaching 3 (the threshold of significance). In reality, at least 20 meioses are needed to have a reasonable chance of success. A meiosis is informative for linkage if we can work out whether or not it is recombinant for the disease and the marker. The basic requirement is a parent who is heterozygous for both the disease and the marker, where we can work out which allele at each locus the parent received from his or her parent, and which allele was passed on to a child.

Rare individuals with a disease and a chromosome abnormality can sometimes allow an investigator to circumvent linkage analysis and go directly to testing genes in a candidate region. This is especially important for a dominant disease where affected people seldom reproduce. As mentioned in *Chapter 2*, occasionally the breakpoint of a chromosomal translocation or inversion disrupts a gene. If loss of one copy of that gene causes a disease, the person will have that disease. Thus clinicians should always keep an eye open for people who have both a mendelian disease and a chromosomal abnormality, especially if both occur *de novo* in one individual. Sometimes it will just be coincidence, but several such cases have provided the vital clue to identifying a disease gene. Rubinstein–Taybi syndrome (see *Disease box 9*) is a good example. Other examples are given in *Table 9.2*.

Gene tracking: using linked markers to predict genetic risks in a pedigree

In the dyschromatosis families, the investigators knew which individuals were affected or unaffected, and they tested many markers to find one that co-segregated with the disease. However, once research has identified a marker that reliably co-segregates with a disease, it is sometimes possible to use the marker to predict who in a family has or has not inherited the disease gene. This is known as **gene tracking**. *Figure 9.9* shows a hypothetical example. The pedigree shows an X-linked recessive disease and genotypes for a polymorphic marker that is known to be closely linked to the disease locus. Evidently the disease-bearing chromosome carries allele 1 of the marker. Individual III–2 inherited allele 3 from her carrier mother, and is therefore at very low risk of being a carrier. Her risk is not zero, because it is possible that there was a recombination between the disease and marker loci in the meiosis that produced the egg from which she developed. Note that you cannot deduce risk simply by looking at the individual marker genotypes (e.g. III–2 has the same marker genotype as her

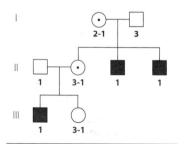

Figure 9.9 – Using gene tracking to predict genetic risk.
See text for discussion. NB, males have only one allele of any X chromosome marker.

Table 9.2 – Cases where an alert clinician provided a vital clue to identify a disease gene

Disease	Chromosomal location	Crucial clinical observation
Duchenne muscular dystrophy	Xp21.3	(a) a boy with DMD and a visible deletion at Xp21.3 (b) a woman with DMD and a balanced reciprocal X;21 translocation Both these cases pointed to Xp21.3 and gave researchers a handle on DNA from the disease region in the pioneering days of positional cloning
Type I Waardenburg syndrome	2q35	A boy with *de novo* disease and a *de novo* inversion of 2q35–q37.3 directed linkage analysis to those locations in the days when testing each marker required a week's work or more
Williams–Beuren syndrome	7q11.23	A family in which supravalvular aortic stenosis co-segregated with a balanced reciprocal translocation, t(6;7)(p21.1;q11.23) – see *Disease box 3*
Sotos syndrome	5q35	A patient with the disease and a balanced reciprocal translocation t(5;8)(q35;q24.1). The breakpoint was shown to disrupt the *NSD1* gene, which was then shown to be mutated or deleted in other cases of the syndrome

Figure 9.10 – A fetal exclusion test in Huntington disease.
Numbers are alleles of a marker closely linked to the HD locus. See text for further explanation.

carrier mother, but in her case this means that she is not a carrier). You have to follow the segregation of a chromosome through the pedigree.

In the days when the loci for major diseases had been mapped, so that linked markers were known, but the disease gene had not yet been identified, gene tracking was an important part of clinical genetics. Once a disease gene has been identified it is usually preferable to check directly for mutations. Gene tracking is still sometimes used for some large genes with many exons, where scanning the whole gene for mutations is not cost-effective. A special application is the **fetal exclusion test**. In *Figure 9.10*, II–1 is at 50% risk of developing Huntington disease because his mother is affected. He has opted against having a predictive test for himself, but he and his wife do not want any child of theirs to suffer the same life-long anxiety. A direct prenatal test for the Huntington disease mutation (expansion of a $(CAG)_n$ repeat, see *Figure 4.18*) would say definitively whether or not a fetus carried it; but if it was positive, II–1 would know that he too carried the Huntington disease mutation, and he does not wish to know this. Instead, a linked marker is used. Fetus III–1 has inherited the chromosome that II–1 received from his unaffected father. It is therefore free of risk (barring recombination in the paternal meiosis). Fetus III–2 has inherited the chromosome that came from its affected grandmother. It is at 50% risk of having inherited the Huntington disease mutation. The parents had decided that they would terminate any such pregnancy. That way, they were assured of having only unaffected children, without finding out whether or not II–1 carried the mutation. The downside is that any aborted fetus had a 50% chance of being entirely normal.

Note that in gene tracking, the marker genotype of an individual tells us nothing in itself. What matters is the pattern of segregation of the disease and marker in the family. In *Figure 9.10*, the marker genotype 2–1 that is present in the affected grandparent, indicates a low risk when it is found in the fetus, while the fact that II–1 also types 2–1 tells us nothing about his disease status. The marker is not the disease gene; it is a non-pathogenic variant that just happens to lie on the same region of a chromosome as the disease gene.

Disease box 9

Rubinstein–Taybi syndrome (OMIM 180849)

Rubinstein–Taybi syndrome (RSTS) is a well recognized clinical diagnosis. Patients are mentally retarded, have a characteristic facial appearance, and broad thumbs and big toes. For the most part cases occur sporadically; sibs of RSTS patients are almost never affected (recurrence risk *c.* 0.1%). However, a dozen cases have been reported of monozygotic twins with the syndrome, and almost always both twins are affected (that is, they are concordant). Rare cases are known where somebody with RSTS has a child, and the recurrence risk for the child is high, maybe 50%. The likely interpretation is that RSTS is an autosomal dominant condition; because affected people almost never reproduce, almost all cases are new mutations.

(a)   (b)   (c)

Clinical features of Rubinstein–Taybi syndrome.
(a) The typical face, (b) broad thumb, and (c) characteristic appearance of large toes.

Given the absence of suitable pedigrees, it was clearly impossible to map the RSTS gene(s) by linkage analysis. Two reports of patients with RSTS and balanced reciprocal chromosomal translocations provided vital clues. One patient had a 2;16 translocation, t(2;16)(p13.3;p13.3) and the other a 7;16 translocation, t(7;16)(q34;p13.3). Either individually might be just a coincidental finding, but it was surely significant that both had a breakpoint at 16p13.3. A team of Dutch investigators assembled a panel of patients, and used a series of cloned probes from 16p13.3 in fluorescence *in situ* hybridization (FISH, see *Section 4.2*) against their chromosomes. Six of 24 patients tested had a microdeletion. The deletion breakpoints all fell in a 150 kb region, from which the researchers cloned the *CREBBP* gene. When this was examined in non-deleted RSTS patients, two nonsense mutations were found. Thus the RSTS gene was identified without recourse to linkage analysis.

The protein product of the *CREBBP* gene, CREB binding protein, is a large nuclear protein with histone acetyltransferase activity, that is involved in chromatin remodeling and transcriptional activation of many target genes. This is reminiscent of the *ATRX* gene product (*Disease box 2*). Like ATRX, RSTS is a chromatin disease. Without detailed knowledge of the target genes, it is not possible to relate the clinical phenotype to the gene defect. Causative changes in *CREBBP* have been identified in only around 40% of RSTS cases (36/92 in a recent study); 3/92 had mutations in the *EP300* gene that encodes a closely related histone acetyltransferase. This is an example of the way investigation of a clinical syndrome can contribute to understanding a biochemical pathway (see *Section 6.4*). It remains to be seen whether the remainder have more subtle changes affecting CREB binding protein function, or whether they have mutations in some of the many other genes whose products interact with CREB binding protein.

RSTS is not a microdeletion syndrome in the true sense. True microdeletion syndromes, such as Williams–Beuren syndrome (*Disease box 3*), are always caused by microdeletions because the phenotype depends on haplo-insufficiency for several contiguous genes. RSTS is caused by haplo-insufficiency of a single gene, *CREBBP*. One mechanism for producing this is a microdeletion, but any change causing loss of function will produce the phenotype. A similar situation is seen in Alagille syndrome (OMIM 118450): 7% of Alagille patients have deletions at 20p12 including the *JAG1* gene; the rest have other *JAG1* mutations. The microdeletions and other chromosomal rearrangements have provided invaluable routes to identifying the disease genes, but are not essential parts of the pathogenesis.

Dominant conditions that are incompatible with reproduction pose enormous challenges for gene identification. Linkage analysis is not possible; if no chromosomal abnormalities point to a candidate location, the main alternative is to guess a candidate gene, based on analogy with diseases caused by mutations in related genes in humans or animals.

9.5. **References**

Bantounas I, Phylactou LA and Uney JB (2004) RNA interference and the use of small interfering RNA to study gene function in mammalian systems. *J. Mol. Endocrin.* **33**: 545–557. *Free full text at* http://jme.endocrinology-journals.org/cgi/content/full/33/3/545

dbSNP public database: http://www.ncbi.nlm.nih.gov/SNP/

Hereditary Hearing Loss Homepage http://webhost.ua.ac.be/hhh

Iredale JP (1999) Demystified ... gene knockouts. *Mol. Pathol.* **52**: 111–116. *Free full text at* http://mp.bmjjournals.com/cgi/reprint/52/3/111

Miyamura Y, Suzuki T, Kono M, *et al.* (2003) Mutations of the RNA-specific adenosine deaminase (DSRAD) gene are involved in dyschromatosis symmetrica hereditaria. *Am. J. Hum. Genet.* **73**: 693–699.

Griffiths AJF, Gelbart WH, Lewontin RC and Miller JH (1999) *Modern Genetic Analysis*. WH Freeman, New York.

General background

Ott J (1999) *Analysis of Human Genetic Linkage* 3rd edition. Johns Hopkins University Press, Baltimore. *A highly authoritative exposition of the basis of human genetic mapping.*

Strachan T and Read AP (2003) *Human Molecular Genetics*, 3rd edition. Garland Science, New York. *This covers the material of this chapter in somewhat greater depth. See Chapter 11 of the 2nd edition, available on the NCBI Bookshelf, or Chapter 13 of the 3rd edition.*

9.6. **Self-assessment questions**

(1) The pedigree shows a family with a fully penetrant autosomal dominant disease. Genotypes are shown for a DNA polymorphism that has alleles 1 and 2.

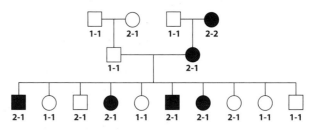

(a) Mark each meiosis as definitely non-recombinant, definitely recombinant, probably non-recombinant, probably recombinant or uninformative.

(b) What is the best estimate of the recombination rate?

(c) Test the significance of the deviation from the null hypothesis of 50% recombinants (no linkage) using χ^2. Is the result significant?

(d) In what proportion of such pedigrees would you expect to see the observed pattern of markers in generation III if there were no linkage between the marker and the disease? Call this L1.

(e) In what proportion of such pedigrees would you expect to see the observed pattern of markers in generation III if there were linkage (recombination fraction θ) between the marker and the disease? Call this L2 (L2 is a function of θ, of course).

(f) Tabulate the values of L1, L2, L2/L1 and $\log_{10}$(L2/L1) for θ = 0, 0.05, 0.1, 0.15, 0.2....0.5.

(g) $\log_{10}$(L2/L1) is the lod score. What is the maximum lod score? Is this significant? Comment.

(2) In the family below, a fully penetrant autosomal dominant disease is segregating. The disease has been mapped to chromosome 2q35 in previous studies. The pedigree shows genotypes for four DNA polymorphisms from within the candidate region, arranged in chromosomal order. Can you narrow down the disease locus using these data?

3-2   4-3   3-1   2-2

JOHN   2-1   JANET

2-1   ?
BEN, CF

(3) Janet was pregnant with their second child when her husband John and 14 year old son Ben were killed in a car crash. Ben had cystic fibrosis. Janet desperately wants to have the baby, but feels she cannot cope with a second tragedy in the form of another child with cystic fibrosis. It was only after the double funeral that she raised the issue with her physician. He pointed out that prenatal diagnosis required DNA samples from Ben and John, who had been cremated. John's elderly parents were contacted and they agreed to give small mouthwash samples for mutation testing. A week later the laboratory requested blood samples so that they could do extensive sequencing, because the initial multiplex OLA test had not revealed any mutation in the parents' samples. However, by this time they were uncontactable, having embarked on a world cruise to forget their grief. A search through old files hit on a Guthrie blood spot card that had been used for Ben's routine neonatal screening. The sample was too degraded to be used for mutation screening, but the laboratory was able to type it for a DNA polymorphism known to be tightly linked to the cystic fibrosis locus. All available DNA samples were typed for the marker, with the results shown. What are the possible genotypes and implications for the fetus if a prenatal test is carried out?

(4) Linkage studies have mapped the gene causing a mendelian disease to a 2 Mb region. Database searching shows this region contains the following genes:
- an enzyme involved in detoxification reactions in the liver
- a phosphate transporter
- a component of the large ribosomal subunit
- a nuclear-encoded component of the mitochondrial electron transport chain
- a ubiquitously expressed protein of unknown function containing a variable length run of glutamines
- an enzyme catalyzing one step in the tricarboxylic acid cycle
- a protein of unknown function expressed in the adult central nervous system and retina
- a transcription factor expressed only in restricted regions of early embryos
- a ubiquitously expressed transcription factor
- a component of the DNA damage repair pathway

What would be your first candidate for mutation testing if the disease in question was
(a) an adult-onset neurodegenerative disease showing anticipation
(b) a rickets-like skeletal malformation
(c) absence of the pituitary gland
(d) an accelerated aging syndrome
(e) a combination of deafness and diabetes

Chapter 10

Why are some conditions common and others rare?

Learning points for this chapter

After working through this chapter you should be able to:

- Define gene frequency, inbreeding, founder effect, coefficient of relationship
- Use the Hardy–Weinberg formula to calculate carrier frequencies for autosomal and X-linked recessive conditions
- Describe qualitatively the effects of inbreeding and use Sewall Wright's path coefficient method to calculate gene sharing by relatives
- Describe the consequences of heterozygote advantage and give examples
- Explain why it is difficult to change population gene frequencies by medical interventions

10.1. **Case studies**

| CASE 21 | Ulmer family | **251** | 259 | 281 | 376 |

- Hannah, a 6-month-old baby girl
- Ashkenazi Jewish origin
- Tay–Sachs disease

Rachel and Uzi Ulmer's families originally came from Eastern Europe and are of Ashkenazi Jewish origin, though neither family was religious, and Rachel and Uzi didn't attend Jewish schools or the synagogue. Hannah was their third child; they had two healthy children, aged 5 and 3 when Hannah was born. Hannah seemed very well as a young baby and smiled and held her head up at the normal time. However, at her 6 month check, the doctor noted her head control was not good and arranged a further appointment 4 weeks later. He was more concerned then because her head control was even worse and she seemed less responsive. He undertook a full neurological examination and found that she had cherry red spots in the maculae of both eyes. He felt fairly sure that Hannah had Tay–Sachs disease (OMIM 272800) and arranged for blood samples to be sent to measure levels of hexosaminidase A. Sadly the levels were extremely low and the diagnosis was confirmed. Rachel and Uzi and their families were devastated at the poor prognosis they were given for Hannah, but resolved to try to make her life as comfortable as possible. Over the next 3 years Hannah deteriorated further; her limbs became spastic and she lost her vision and hearing. She died at the age of four and a half years.

(a)

(b)   (c)   (d)

Figure 10.1 – (a) The characteristic cherry red spot on the retina of a child with Tay–Sachs disease. (b) Ballooned neurons in the central nervous system (arrows). (c) Abnormal cell bodies seen under the electron microscope. (d) Vacuolated lymphocytes. These are typical features of lysosomal storage diseases. Photos courtesy of Drs Ed Wraith and Guy Besley, Royal Manchester Children's Hospital.

10.2. **Background**

This chapter is about **gene frequencies**: what determines them, how they can change, and the way gene frequencies can be used to work out genetic risks in a variety of situations. Note that the term 'gene frequency' is a misnomer – we really mean *allele frequency* – but 'gene frequency' is too thoroughly established in genetic parlance to change now. Gene frequencies are numbers that lie between 0 and 1; traditionally they are symbolized as p and/or q.

Gene frequencies depend on the concept of a **gene pool**. This would consist of all the alleles at a particular locus in some defined population. The population might be anything from a small community to the whole of humanity. Within the gene pool, the gene frequency of allele $\underline{A}$ is the proportion of all the alleles that are $\underline{A}$. It is also the probability that a gene, picked at random from the pool, would be $\underline{A}$. Alleles can be defined in various ways for different purposes. Most discussion of gene frequencies in relation to disease classifies all alleles at a locus into just two categories, normal alleles and disease alleles. If you sequenced the DNA, you would probably find that each included quite a range of variants, and for some purposes you might wish to count each sequence variant as a separate allele. Whatever scheme you use to classify alleles, the frequencies of all the alleles in a population must add up to 1.

Clinicians are usually more interested in frequencies of genotypes than frequencies of genes. They want to know the probability that a randomly selected person is homozygous or heterozygous for a disease allele. The Hardy–Weinberg distribution (*Box 10.1*) describes the relationship of genotype frequencies to gene frequencies. The Hardy–Weinberg distribution makes it possible to calculate the frequency of carriers of recessive conditions in a population, without having to sample a large number of people and genotype them in the laboratory. Along with the basic mendelian rules, it is the central tool for assessing genetic risks.

The bean–bag model that we use in *Box 10.1* to derive the Hardy–Weinberg distribution illustrates an important precondition of the distribution. The probability that the second bean will be $\underline{A}$ or $\underline{a}$ must be entirely independent of whether the first bean was $\underline{A}$ or $\underline{a}$. In genetic terms, the genotype distribution

Box 10.1

The Hardy–Weinberg distribution

Suppose there are two alleles, A and a in a population (there may or may not be others as well; it doesn't matter). Say the gene frequency of A is p and the gene frequency of a is q. p and q will sum to 1 if A and a are the only alleles in the population; if there are other alleles $p+q$ will be less than 1. The Hardy–Weinberg distribution predicts that the frequencies of the three possible genotypes are:

$$\begin{array}{ccc} \underline{AA} & \underline{Aa} & \underline{aa} \\ p^2 & 2pq & q^2 \end{array}$$

Books sometimes state this as $p^2 + 2pq + q^2 = 1$. This is wrong. The Hardy–Weinberg distribution is not an equation. It describes the relation between gene frequencies and genotype frequencies. p^2, $2pq$ and q^2 only add up to 1 if those two alleles are the only alleles on the population, so that everybody must be either AA or Aa or aa. If there are three alleles in the population (say, A, a and a_1, with frequencies p, q and r) the frequencies of AA, Aa and aa are still p^2, $2pq$ and q^2, but there are also other genotypes in the population, The total distribution is:

$$\begin{array}{cccccc} \underline{AA} & \underline{Aa} & \underline{aa} & \underline{Aa_1} & \underline{aa_1} & \underline{a_1a_1} \\ p^2 & 2pq & q^2 & 2pr & 2qr & r^2 \end{array}$$

The basis of the Hardy–Weinberg distribution can easily be seen by doing a little thought experiment. Imagine all the genes in a gene pool as a large collection of beans in a bag. A proportion p of the beans are of type A and a proportion q are of type a. Eyes shut, reach into the bag and pick a bean. The chance it is A is p, and the chance it is a is q. Pick a second bean. Again the chance it is A is p, the chance it is a is q (we assume there are enough beans in the bag that removing the first one did not significantly change p or q). The chance both beans were A is p^2; the chance both were a is q^2. The chance the first bean was A and the second a is pq; similarly the chance you picked first a then A is pq. Overall, the chance you picked one A and one a is $2pq$.

will be Hardy–Weinberg only if there is **random mating**. Random mating does not mean free love; it just means that you don't ask your beloved's genotype before you pop the question. This is not as far-fetched as it sounds. There are many ways in which people tend to select mates based partly on genotype. There is **assortative mating** for height, intelligence, deafness and many other phenotypes that are at least partly genetic. The effect of assortative mating is to increase the proportion of homozygotes for each allele in the population, and decrease the proportion of heterozygotes, compared to the predictions of Hardy–Weinberg.

Assortative mating is mainly important in clinical genetics in the context of inbreeding. Relatives share genes, and so if you marry a relative rather than an unrelated person you increase the chance that your partner will have alleles in common with you. If you carry an allele for a recessive condition there is an increased chance that your partner will also carry it, and thus an increased risk of having a child with the condition, compared to an outbred couple. This is discussed further in *Section 10.3* in relation to the Choudhary family (Case 3).

Using Hardy–Weinberg to calculate carrier risks

Suppose the sister of a boy with cystic fibrosis is getting married. She knows the disease is genetic, and she wants to know the risk that she might have an affected child. She is healthy, but of course it is quite likely that she is a carrier of cystic fibrosis (see below for the exact probability). This has no implications for her own health, but her children would be at risk if her partner happens also to be a carrier. Calculating the risk that her partner is a carrier is the same as calculating the probability that a person, picked at random from the population, is a carrier. Hardy–Weinberg enables us to do this.

If we ignore the extensive allelic heterogeneity among cystic fibrosis mutations, and classify all alleles as $\underline{A}$ (functional) and $\underline{a}$ (non-functional), with frequencies p and q, the proportions of the genotypes are:

AA	Aa	aa
p^2	$2pq$	q^2

Cystic fibrosis affects one birth in 2000 in Americans of Northern European origin (it is less frequent among Hispanics, African–Americans and Asian Americans). Therefore q^2 is $1/2000$. Hence q is the square root of $1/2000$, which is nearly $1/45$. One allele in 45 at the *CFTR* locus is $\underline{a}$; the remaining $44/45$ must be $\underline{A}$ (we had decided to classify *all* alleles as $\underline{A}$ or $\underline{a}$, so in this case $p+q=1$). We can now calculate the carrier frequency: $2pq = 2 \times 44/45 \times 1/45 = 1/23$, approximately. Assuming random mating, there is a 1 in 23 chance the girl's partner is a carrier.

For an X-linked condition the calculation is even simpler. If hemophilia A (see Case 12, Lawton family in *Chapter 4*) affects one boy in 5000 in a certain population, what proportion of the women are carriers? Males can only be $\underline{A}$ or $\underline{a}$, so the frequency of the disease allele is simply equal to the proportion of males who are affected:

Females			Males	
AA	Aa	aa	A	a
p^2	$2pq$	q^2	p	q

The carrier frequency among women is $2 \times 4999/5000 \times 1/5000$ or 1 in 2500.

For a rare condition, the frequency of the normal allele can usually be approximated to 1, which makes the calculation easier. However, it is important to note that for rare autosomal recessive conditions, a significant proportion of cases are the offspring of consanguineous marriages. This is not a major factor with cystic fibrosis in the USA or UK, because cystic fibrosis is a relatively common disease. But the rarer a condition is, the higher is the proportion of cases where consanguinity is a factor. Ignoring this and simply assuming a Hardy–Weinberg distribution can lead to serious over-estimation of carrier frequencies for very rare diseases (see below).

Changing gene frequencies

Gene frequencies can change from generation to generation for a number of reasons:

- New mutations increase the number of disease alleles in the gene pool. There can also be back mutation, changing a disease allele into a normal allele. However, for loss of function mutations, the process is largely uni-directional. Any one of a large number of possible sequence changes can convert a functioning gene into a non-functioning one, but only a very specific back-mutation can restore the function of a non-functional allele. The ratio of forward to back mutation rates is likely to be of the order of 1000 : 1. Other mutations may well occur to non-functional alleles, but the allele remains non-functional.
- Natural selection will remove disease alleles from the gene pool if the disease is such that affected people are less likely to reproduce. Artificial selection might have a similar effect (see *Section 10.4*).
- A large influx of migrants from a population with substantially different gene frequencies could change the gene pool.
- If the reproducing population is very small, random effects can cause the gene frequency to change between generations. If only a small number of gametes contribute to the next generation, they may not be an exactly representative selection of the parental gene pool. This **genetic drift** can only make rapid large changes to gene frequencies when the reproductive population is no more than a hundred or so individuals.

Whatever the initial genotype frequencies in a population, one generation of random mating is enough to establish a Hardy–Weinberg distribution. If, when a population is surveyed, the distribution is seen to differ significantly from Hardy–Weinberg, this might mean one of several things:

- *The survey methodology is flawed.* This is seen most often when a new DNA polymorphism is being checked. A non-Hardy–Weinberg distribution of genotypes probably means that the genotyping method is producing errors and needs to be improved to make it reliable.
- *Selection has already occurred.* A genotype that causes substantial prenatal or infant mortality will be under-represented in a sample of living people.
- *There is significant assortative mating.* This might be simple inbreeding, or perhaps the population is not freely interbreeding, but consists of two or more groups that have different gene frequencies and that largely breed among themselves (population stratification).

Note that if you are using a chi-squared test to check whether genotype numbers fit Hardy–Weinberg, with two alleles there is only one degree of freedom, even though you have three observed and expected numbers. That is because once you have fixed q, everything else in the expected numbers follows.

Factors determining gene frequencies

People sometimes imagine that dominant characters should be common and recessive ones rare. Actually there is no connection between the gene frequency of an allele and whether it causes a dominant or recessive phenotype. Huntington disease is one example among many of a rare dominant; blood group O is a common recessive.

For a neutral character where selection plays no role, the gene frequencies reflect the frequencies in the founders of that population, modulated by genetic drift if, at any time, the breeding population was reduced to small numbers. Most common neutral DNA polymorphisms (SNPs or microsatellites, see *Chapter 9*) fit this category. Occasional mutations will introduce some random variation by changing one allele into another. As explained in *Chapter 7*, deamination of methylated cytosines has tended, over evolutionary time, to convert CpG sequences systematically into TpG, but this effect on gene frequencies is only noticeable on an extremely large timescale.

For diseases, the gene frequencies reflect additional factors. Recurrent mutations tend to increase the pool of loss of function alleles, while selection acts to remove disease alleles from the population. For dominant and X-linked diseases selection is very effective, because everybody (dominant), or all males (X-linked), who carry the disease allele have the disease and so are exposed to selection. For autosomal recessive conditions, selection acts much more slowly, because most of the disease alleles are in healthy heterozygotes, who are not subject to selection. For this reason, alleles for recessive diseases can persist for very many generations in a population, even if the disease is very severe. This leads to important **founder effects** in many populations. If a population, however numerous today, derives from a small number of founders, or passed through a bottleneck when only a few individuals contributed to the next generation, then any recessive allele that was present in one of the founders is likely to be present at high frequency in the modern population. Equally, if a normally common recessive condition happened to be absent from the small pool of founders, it will be rare or absent in the modern population (*Figure 10.2*).

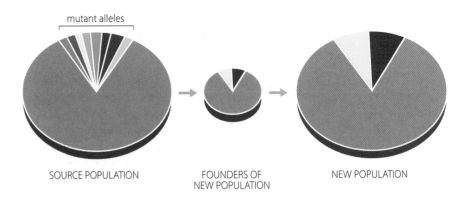

Figure 10.2 – **Founder effects.**

Founder effects are seen in many populations. For the reasons explained above, they affect the frequencies of recessive conditions but not usually of dominant or X-linked conditions. *Table 10.1* shows some examples, and *Disease box 10* describes in more detail some diseases characteristic of one such population, Ashkenazi Jews.

Table 10.1 – Diseases common in certain populations, probably because of a founder effect

Disease	OMIM	Mode of inheritance	Population	Comments
Diastrophic dysplasia	222600	AR	Finns	90% of Finnish cases have a splice donor mutation in intron 1
Aspartylglucosaminuria	208400	AR	Finns	Carrier frequency 1:30; 98% have p.Cys163Ser mutation
Neuronal ceroid lipofuscinosis	256730	AR	Finns	Single mutation, p.R122W, found in 97% of Finnish cases
Hermansky–Pudlak syndrome	203300	AR	Puerto Ricans	Carrier frequency 1:21; much rarer in most other populations
Bardet–Biedl syndrome	209900	AR	Bedouin	Two non-allelic forms, BBS2 and BBS3 both relatively frequent
Myotonic dystrophy	160900	AD	Quebec – Sanguenay	Prevalence 1:500, 30–60 × prevalence in most other populations
Butyrylcholinesterase deficiency	177400	AR	Alaskan Eskimos	Deficiency allele frequency 0.1. Three different alleles reported in this population
Usher syndrome type 1C	276904	AR	French-Acadians in Louisiana	43/44 cases homozygous for a c.216G>A mutation
Hereditary motor and sensory neuropathy, Lom type	601455	AR	Bulgarian gypsies	The OMIM entry gives an interesting commentary

Note that all diseases are autosomal recessive (AR) except for myotonic dystrophy.

Heterozygote advantage

There is a second reason why a recessive condition may be common in a population. The classic case is sickle cell disease. This is common in many populations where falciparum malaria is or was recently endemic, but is absent from populations where malaria was not frequent. The driving force is that heterozygotes are relatively resistant to malaria. Thus in historical times normal homozygotes often died of malaria, and sickle cell homozygotes died of their disease, leaving the heterozygotes to contribute disproportionately to the next generation (*Figure 10.3*).

Even a very small degree of heterozygote advantage, continued over many generations, can greatly influence the gene frequencies. If, relative to Aa heterozygotes, a proportion s_1 of aa and a proportion s_2 of AA homozygotes fail to reproduce, at equilibrium the ratio of gene frequencies, q/p, is s_2/s_1. For cystic fibrosis s_1 is effectively 1 (we are talking about conditions during the past, not today) while q/p is $1/45$ for people of Northern European origin. It follows that s_2

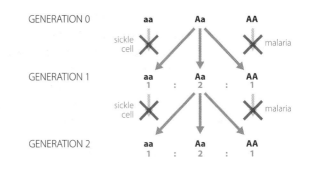

Figure 10.3 – Heterozygote advantage.
A hypothetical extreme example in which everybody with sickle cell disease (aa) fails to reproduce because of their disease, while all normal homozygotes (AA) fail to reproduce because of malaria. Only heterozygote × heterozygote matings contribute to the next generation. Regardless of how many generations the selection continues, at birth every generation always consists of 25% sickle cell homozygotes, 50% heterozygotes and 25% normal homozygotes. No real situation is this extreme.

must also be about 1/45. In other words, in order to account for the high proportion of people of Northern European origin who are carriers of cystic fibrosis, carriers must have enjoyed a 2% reproductive advantage over normal homozygotes over past centuries. Such an advantage is too small to be easily detectable in survey data, and its nature is controversial.

Heterozygote advantage or founder effect?

If a disease is common in a certain population because of a founder effect, we would expect most affected people to have exactly the same ancestral mutation. On the other hand, if heterozygote advantage has been the mechanism, a whole range of mutations might be common. A good example is β-thalassemia in Jews from Kurdistan. The carrier frequency is as high as 20%, but 13 different β-globin mutations have been described in this small group. Clearly, heterozygote advantage (presumably resistance to malaria) has been the driving force here. On the other hand, among the Amish of Lancaster County, Pennsylvania, the rare recessive Ellis–van Creveld syndrome (OMIM 225500) is relatively common, with a gene frequency of 0.07. All affected people in nine families studied had the same sequence changes in each copy of the *EVC* gene on chromosome 4. All could trace their ancestry back to one couple, Samuel King and his wife, who immigrated in 1744. This is an example of a founder effect. In this particular case the founder is relatively recent, so the shared ancestry is demonstrable genealogically. In most cases it has to be inferred by identifying a shared haplotype of non-pathogenic polymorphisms on the chromosomal segment carrying the mutant gene. As it happens, the *EVC* mutation in the Amish families is always accompanied by a second, non-pathogenic sequence change in the *EVC* gene. The change is not found on non-mutant chromosomes. This provides additional confirmation that we are looking at copies of a single ancestral chromosome.

There are several examples of isolated populations where more than one mutation causing a certain recessive disease is relatively common. Heterozygote advantage is a likely explanation, but there may also be an observational bias. Mutations are normally identified by studying affected people, not by screening a whole population. If one disease allele is fairly common, there will be plenty of people heterozygous for that allele. Whenever such a person happens to carry another disease allele they will be affected, and so both their disease alleles will be identified. Thus a common recessive disease allele provides a mechanism for bringing the rarer alleles in a population to medical attention. But as some of the Jewish diseases in *Disease box 10* illustrate, sometimes the effects of heterozygote advantage, founder effects and genetic drift are hard to disentangle.

10.3. Investigations of patients

CASE 21	Ulmer family	251	**259**	281	376

- Hannah, a 6-month-old baby girl
- Ashkenazi Jewish origin
- Tay–Sachs disease
- Test the sibs?

Tay-Sachs disease is a lysosomal storage disease (see *Chapter 8*) caused by lack of hexosaminidase A. Because of the enzyme deficiency, G_{M2} ganglioside accumulates in lysosomes in retinal ganglia and other neurons, leading to death, usually at age 2–4 years. The disease is known from all ethnic groups, but is about 100 times more common in Ashkenazi Jews compared to most other groups. About 1 in 30 North American Jews is a carrier, compared to perhaps 1 in 300 people in most other populations. This has led to carrier screening programs being set up specifically in Jewish communities in the USA and several other countries, as described in *Chapter 11*. As their families led entirely secular lives and were not part of any Jewish community, Rachel and Uzi had missed out on screening.

Having learned about Tay–Sachs disease, Rachel and Uzi were very concerned to know whether either of their healthy children was a carrier and pressed for them to be tested. The geneticist contended that it was unethical to test young children. Any test result would have no implications for the child's health or management. The time to offer a test was when the child was of an age to make an independent informed choice. They might prefer not to know, and it was wrong to close off that possibility for them when there was no compensating benefit in testing a child. The geneticist did point out that each child had a 2 in 3 risk of being a carrier (not 1 in 2 – see *Box 10.2*).

Rachel and Uzi thought they might have more children, and if so they would want prenatal diagnosis. To prepare for this possibility, mouthwash samples were taken from both of them and the *HEXA* gene checked. Three *HEXA* mutations together make up over 90% of all Tay–Sachs mutations in Ashkenazi Jews (*Table 10.2*). Rachel and Uzi each carried one of those mutations. Rachel had a mutation of the intron 12 splice site and Uzi had a 4 bp frameshifting insertion in exon 11. Hannah was a compound heterozygote for these two loss-of-function mutations.

Table 10.2 shows the results of a survey that looked just for the three major Ashkenazi mutations in Tay–Sachs carriers. In non-Jewish populations these mutations are not particularly common, and other work has demonstrated the expected wide assortment of individually rare mutant alleles. The situation in Ashkenazi Jews is interesting. As explained above, if the high frequency of

The risk a healthy sib is a carrier

If two carriers of an autosomal recessive disease have a child, the chance is 1 in 4 that it will be affected, 1 in 2 that it will be a carrier, and 1 in 4 that it will be homozygous normal. However, the chance that a healthy sib of an affected child is a carrier is not 1 in 2, but 2 in 3. As the figure shows, we know the child is not affected, so it must be one of the three in the shaded box.

This is an interesting example of how hard it can be to spot an error when the error consists of giving the right answer to the wrong question.

- The right question is, what is the risk that a healthy sib is a carrier? Answer 2 in 3.
- The wrong question is, what is the risk that any child of a carrier couple will be a carrier? Answer 1 in 2 – but this is not the question the parents asked.

Tay–Sachs disease were just a founder effect we would not expect more than one mutation to be common. This is discussed further in *Disease box 10* at the end of this chapter.

Table 10.2 – Distribution of hexosaminidase A mutations

Mutation	Percentage in Ashkenazi carriers (n = 156)	Percentage in non-Jewish carriers (n = 51)
4 bp insertion in exon 11	73	16
Intron 12 splice site mutation	15	0
p.Gly269Ser in exon 7	4	3
Unidentified	8	81

Data of Paw *et al.* (1990) cited in OMIM entry 272800.

| CASE 3 | Choudhary family | 3 | 9 | 66 | 242 | **260** | 376 |

- Girl (Nasreen) aged 8 months, parents Aadnan and Mumtaz
- Deaf
- Parents are first cousins
- Pedigree suggests autosomal recessive deafness

In this highly inbred family there had been a question whether Nasreen's deafness was autosomal recessive, and whether her two uncles, Waleed and Mohammed, were deaf from the same cause or some other cause. This question was eventually answered (*Section 9.3*) by exploiting the family structure to perform autozygosity mapping. This highlighted a candidate gene, *OTOF*, for mutation analysis. The causative mutation was identified, allowing testing and exact counseling for all the family members who wished it. This was particularly important for Waleed and his cousin Benazir, who were planning to marry.

The autozygosity mapping required considerable resources in the laboratory, and before she felt able to request it, the geneticist wished to calculate whether these extra investigations could make a substantial difference to her counseling. She decided to calculate what the likelihood was that a child of Waleed and Benazir would be deaf, assuming all the family deafness was autosomal recessive. She wanted to compare this with the low likelihood of recurrence if the cases in the family were coincidental. On the recessive hypothesis, Benazir's brother Aadnan (Nasreen's father – individual I, in *Figure 10.4*) was a carrier. Therefore, one of Benazir's and Aadnan's parents was a carrier – presumably their mother, since she was the link into the other side of the family. Thus Benazir's carrier risk would be 1 in 2, and the overall risk that a child of hers and Waleed's would be deaf was 1 in 4. This calculation showed that there was a large uncertainty in the risk – high if the family condition was genetic and recessive, much lower if not. It was therefore felt justifiable to expend some effort in the laboratory to try to resolve the uncertainty.

For more general genetic counseling of consanguineous couples, we need to calculate coefficients of relationship and of inbreeding.

- The **coefficient of relationship of two people** is the proportion of their genes that they share by virtue of having one or more definable common ancestors.
- The **coefficient of inbreeding of a person** is the proportion of loci at which the individual is expected to be homozygous because of the

---

Box 10.3

Calculating the effects of inbreeding

What proportion of their genes do relatives share?

For close relatives the answer may be intuitively obvious:

- parent and child share half their genes (always)
- full sibs (same two parents) share half their genes (on average)
- half-sibs (one parent in common) share one-quarter of their genes (on average)
- uncles / aunts and nephews / nieces share one-quarter of their genes (on average)
- first cousins share one-eighth of their genes (on average)

If these figures are not intuitively obvious, or where the relationship is more complicated, Sewall Wright's path coefficient method is easy to follow and reliable:

(1) draw the pedigree showing only the common ancestor(s) and the links to them
(2) choose one path between the two relatives, through a common ancestor and count the number of links
(3) if that path has *n* links it contributes $(½)^n$ to the coefficient of relationship
(4) if there is more than one possible path, do the same for each path
(5) add together the contribution of each path

This is illustrated below for the simple cases of full sibs and first cousins, to show that it does indeed produce the right answer. A more complicated example is shown in *Figure 10.4*.

Full sibs:

Pathway	Contribution
C–A–D	$(½)^2 = ¼$
C–B–D	$(½)^2 = ¼$
Total:	½

First cousins:

Pathway	Contribution
E–C–A–D–F	$(½)^4 = 1/16$
E–C–B–D–F	$(½)^4 = 1/16$
	⅛

consanguinity of the parents. It is half the coefficient of relationship of the parents. Equally, it is the probability that at any given locus the individual receives two genes that are identical by descent.

The easiest method for doing the calculation is Sewall Wright's path coefficient method (*Box 10.3*). *Figure 10.4* shows how Nasreen's coefficient of inbreeding could be calculated. Using the path coefficient method, the coefficient of relationship of Aadnan and his wife Mumtaz is calculated as $^{10}/_{64}$ – a bit closer than the $^1/_8$ of first cousins. The coefficient of inbreeding of Nasreen is therefore $^5/_{64}$. Note that even quite highly inbred pedigrees produce relatively moderate coefficients of inbreeding. Without resorting to incest, it is difficult to invent a pedigree where a child has a coefficient of inbreeding as high as $^1/_4$. Mouse geneticists use repeated brother–sister matings over many generations to produce highly homozygous lines. Only the pharaohs of ancient Egypt are recorded as trying the same thing in humans.

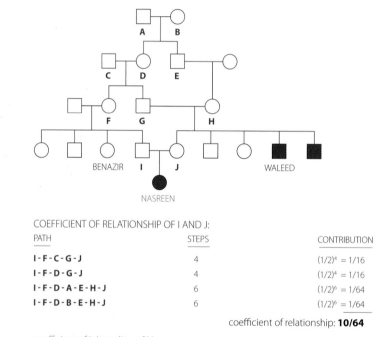

COEFFICIENT OF RELATIONSHIP OF I AND J:

PATH	STEPS	CONTRIBUTION
I-F-C-G-J	4	$(1/2)^4 = 1/16$
I-F-D-G-J	4	$(1/2)^4 = 1/16$
I-F-D-A-E-H-J	6	$(1/2)^6 = 1/64$
I-F-D-B-E-H-J	6	$(1/2)^6 = 1/64$

coefficient of relationship: **10/64**

coefficient of inbreeding of Nasreen
= 1/2 coefficient of relationship of her parents = **5/64**

Figure 10.4 – Calculation of the coefficient of inbreeding of Nasreen Choudhary (Case 3).
Because there is more than one inbreeding loop, it is not easy to do this calculation intuitively. The path coefficient method is used to calculate the coefficient of relationship of Nasreen's parents.

10.4. **Summary and extension**

The frequencies of genetic diseases in a population depend on the opposing effects of mutation and selection, working on whatever frequencies were present in the initial founder population.

For dominant and X-linked diseases mutations normally have a short half-life.

- In the extreme case of a lethal dominant condition, every case must be a new mutation. The parents would not be parents if they were themselves affected. Note that genetic lethality means inability to pass on one's genes, and not necessarily physical lethality.
- A mutation will usually persist for only one or a few generations if it causes a dominant condition that reduces a person's chance of passing on his genes, even if it does not wholly prevent reproduction. An unusual appearance or a mild disability can be quite enough to reduce a person's chances of success in the marriage market. A classic survey of achondroplasia (OMIM 100800) provided a perfect illustration. In 1941 ET Mørch surveyed 94 075 consecutive births in Denmark and noted 10 achondroplastic babies. Only two of them had an achondroplastic parent, so he assumed that 80% were new dominant mutations. He also surveyed achondroplastic adults in Denmark and found that, although achondroplastic people are perfectly fertile, they had on average only 20% the number of children that was normal in the population. Mørch's data have been questioned because he may have unwittingly included cases of similar recessive skeletal dysplasias in his newborn survey. Maybe his figures are best regarded as a thought experiment. The principle remains clear and valid. Neurofibromatosis I (*Disease box 1*) illustrates this: about 50% of cases are new mutations.
- For an X-linked recessive condition, selection is effective only against affected males. If a population has roughly equal numbers of XX females and XY males, one-third of all X chromosomes are in males (*Figure 10.5*). For a genetically lethal condition such as DMD, this means that one-third of all DMD mutant alleles are wiped out each generation. Since DMD is still with us, this loss must be roughly balanced by fresh mutations. If the rates of mutation and selection balance out, one-third of cases of DMD would be fresh mutations. This has major implications for risk estimation. We cannot assume that the mother of a DMD boy is a carrier – the chance is 2 in 3. Only if she also has an affected brother or other maternal relative is she an obligate carrier (as with Judith Davies in Case 4).

For recessive characters, selection works on mutant alleles only when they are in homozygous form. The ratio of genes in homozygotes to those in heterozygotes

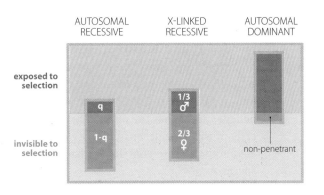

Figure 10.5 – Conditions with different modes of inheritance have different degrees of exposure to natural selection.
See text for calculations.

is $2q^2:2pq$ ($2q^2$ because there are two mutant alleles in each homozygote). Assuming p is very close to 1, the ratio simplifies to just q (*Figure 10.5*). In other words, for a typical recessive with $q = 0.01$, the mutant alleles are exposed to selection only 1% of the time. Over evolutionary time selection will be effective, but mutant alleles can easily persist over a few dozen generations.

The result of these different dynamics of selection is that serious dominant and X-linked conditions are likely to show a high proportion of new mutations and extensive allelic heterogeneity. For most recessives, mutation can be discounted when considering families and individual mutant alleles may be quite common in a population. These considerations apply best to loss of function conditions, where in principle there can be extensive allelic heterogeneity. Dominant conditions may be the result of gain of function mutations, in which only one or a few specific mutations may be able to cause the condition.

Clinical geneticists are naturally most concerned with conditions that are common and serious, and all such conditions must have somehow escaped being wiped out by natural selection. Possible mechanisms include the following.

- A very high mutation rate. DMD is an example. Probably the remarkable structure of the dystrophin gene (*Chapter 3*) contributes to this.
- Heterozygote advantage for a recessive condition. Thalassemia (Case 12, Lawton family) is a clear example. As mentioned above, cystic fibrosis (Case 2, Brown family) must also have some heterozygote advantage, otherwise it could not be so common. In fact, unless there is evidence of a high mutation rate, as in CAH (Case 19, Stott family), it is reasonable to suppose that most of the more common severe recessive conditions in any large population, probably have some slight degree of heterozygote advantage.
- Symptoms mostly appear after reproductive age. Huntington disease (Case 1, Ashton family) is a classic example, as are the familial breast and colon cancers described in *Chapter 12*.
- Selection during spermatogenesis. As mentioned above, most cases of achondroplasia are new mutations, yet the condition is relatively common. The mutation rate is fairly high to account for this. This is only mildly surprising until we remember that only one very specific change, p.Gly380Arg in the FGFR3 protein will produce achondroplasia (see figure in *Box 6.3*). Most A→a mutation rates are the sum of the rates of mutation of hundreds of individual nucleotides, but for achondroplasia the whole mutation rate is the rate of this one specific change. The mutation rate at the nucleotide concerned is many orders of magnitude higher than the mutation rate at almost any other specific nucleotide in the entire genome. Inspection of the sequence does not suggest any reason for such an extraordinarily high mutability. The answer is believed to be that the mutation rate is not actually especially high, but cells in the male germ-line that carry the mutation are at a selective advantage, and so contribute disproportionately to the production of sperm.

What is the chance the offspring of a consanguineous marriage will have a recessive disease?

Consider Jack and Jill who are first cousins. Suppose the gene frequency of a disease gene is q. The chance that Jack is a carrier is $2pq$. For a rare disease p is virtually 1, so Jack's carrier risk is very nearly $2q$. Jill shares $1/8$ of her genes with Jack by virtue of their relationship. That is to say, for any gene in Jack, there is a 1 in 8 chance that Jill has the same gene. Therefore if Jack is a carrier, the chance that Jill is a carrier is $1/8$. If they are both carriers, the chance of a child being affected is 1 in 4. Overall the risk is $2q \times 1/8 \times 1/4 = q/16$. *Table 10.3* shows that the rarer a condition is, the greater is the relative risk for first cousins compared to unrelated people.

Table 10.3 – Inbreeding and the risk of a recessive disease

Disease gene frequency	Risk of affected child – unrelated parents	Risk of affected child – first cousin marriage	Relative risk for first cousins
q	q^2	$q/16$	$1/16q$
0.01	1 in 10 000	1 in 1600	6.25
0.005	1 in 40 000	1 in 3200	12.5
0.001	1 in 1 000 000	1 in 16 000	62.5

The calculation is only valid for rare diseases because it assumes the frequency of the normal allele is effectively 1, and it assumes that the only way first cousins would both carry a disease gene is if they both inherit it from a common ancestor.

Another way of looking at this, is that the rarer a recessive condition is, the greater the proportion of cases that are the offspring of consanguineous marriages. As mentioned before, this means that Hardy–Weinberg calculations of carrier frequencies are likely to be misleading when applied to rare recessives.

Can we abolish genetic disease?

Clinical geneticists are very clear that their goal is not to wipe out genetic disease, and their output must not be measured by the number of abnormal pregnancies terminated. Their goal is to enable people with genetic diseases, or at risk of them, to lead as normal lives as possible, including having families. Nevertheless, health planners might find it attractive if a by-product of genetic services were a reduction in the frequency of genetic disorders.

The discussion of mutations and selection above shows that abolishing genetic disease is not a generally realistic aim. Most serious dominant conditions have a high proportion of new mutations, while for recessives, the great majority of mutant genes are in healthy heterozygotes. If a country's dictator decided to sterilize all people with serious genetic diseases, this would not prevent fresh cases appearing in the next generation. Even continued over many generations this program could not succeed in its aim. A few dominant late-onset conditions such as Huntington disease could be largely prevented, but the only way to prevent recessive diseases would be to sterilize all carriers. This would rebound badly on the dictator and his family. Although carrier frequencies for individual recessive conditions are typically of the order of 1 in 100, OMIM lists thousands of different conditions, and every one of us is a carrier for several lethal recessive conditions. A sterilization program could prevent genetic disease only by sterilizing the dictator, along with the rest of the human race.

A slightly different question is whether medicine is storing up long-term problems by effectively combating natural selection (see *Box 10.4*).

Should treated people repay their debt to society by not having children?

Consider a treatable genetic condition such as phenylketonuria (PKU; see **Case 22, Vlasi family** in *Chapter 11*). Untreated phenylketonurics are severely mentally retarded and are likely to spend their lives in an institution. When the treatment works, an affected person is enabled to live a normal life, including having children. Genetically the person is still homozygous for the mutation, and any child will inevitably inherit a mutant allele. The treatment is expensive – should there be a bargain? Should we say that we agree to fund the treatment, but in return the treated person should agree not to pass on his or her mutant genes?

Most clinicians would find such a proposition deeply distasteful – but they may have at the back of their mind an uneasy feeling that as responsible physicians, perhaps they ought to face the question. The question should indeed be faced – because when it is examined, it goes away. We showed above that for a recessive condition the proportion of all mutant alleles that are present in affected people is q, where q is the gene frequency. In the UK, PKU affects about one person in 10 000. Thus q is 0.01. In other words, agonizing about whether or not a treated phenylketonuric has the right to pass on his genes is agonizing about 1% of the problem while ignoring the other 99%. Since we know we can have no influence on the 99%, it is pointless to worry about the 1%. Of course, each time a treated phenylketonuric passes on a mutant allele rather than failing to reproduce, that must marginally increase the frequency of mutant alleles in the next generation. Continued over 100 generations, a treatment program might double the gene frequency. Most people would feel that humanity has rather more serious problems to face over the next 2500 years than a doubling of the frequency of PKU mutant alleles.

Jewish diseases and Finnish diseases

Ashkenazi Jews and Finns are the two best-studied examples of populations with strong founder effects. Both have high levels of education and well developed medical services that provide good data on the range and frequency of genetic diseases. *Table 10.1* listed some Finnish diseases, and the table in this section shows some Ashkenazi Jewish diseases. Motulsky (1995) provides a good concise review of Jewish diseases.

Both populations have expanded greatly from a fairly small number of founders.

Some diseases that are unusually prevalent among Ashkenazi Jews

Disease	OMIM number	Mode of inheritance	Carrier frequency	Comments
Tay–Sachs disease	272800	AR	$1/30$	Three fairly common Ashkenazi mutations – see **Case 21 (Ulmer family)** and *Chapter 11*
Familial dysautonomia	223900	AR	$1/30$	Very few non-Jewish cases reported; 99.5% of Jewish cases have the same splicing mutation
Gaucher disease	230800	AR	$1/15$	Two common Ashkenazi mutations p.Asn380Ser (75%) and c.84insG (15%); p.Leu444Pro also frequent.
Canavan disease	271900	AR	$1/40$–$1/60$	Two common Ashkenazi mutations, p.Glu285Ala and p.Tyr231STOP
Fanconi anemia complementation group C	227645	AR	$1/90$	Most Ashkenazi cases have a splice site mutation in intron 4
Niemann–Pick disease Type A	257200	AR	$1/80$	Three mutations account for 65% of Ashkenazi cases
Bloom syndrome	210900	AR	$1/200$?	Most Ashkenazi cases affected have the same mutation, deletion of ATCTGA and insertion of TACATTC at nucleotide 2281
Familial breast cancer	113705 (*BRCA1*); 600185 (*BRCA2*)	AD	Total 2.5%	Three common Ashkenazi mutations: c.185delAG (1% of population), c.5382insC (0.15%) in *BRCA1*; c.6174delT (1.5%) in *BRCA2*
Torsion dystonia 1	128100	AD	$1/1000$–$1/300$ affected	Genetics heterogeneous; many Ashkenazi and non-Jewish patients have the same 3 bp deletion

- Of the 13–14 million Jews in the world, about 80% are Ashkenazi, descendants of a population that migrated to the Rhineland in Germany in the ninth century, and later moved into Poland, Lithuania, Belarus and surrounding regions. Ashkenazim have been distinct from Sephardic Jews, who are primarily from Spain, Portugal and North Africa, for over 1000 years. Until a few hundred years ago, Sephardim constituted the majority of all Jews, and their communities in Spain and Portugal may have existed since Roman times. The Ashkenazi population probably comprised a few thousand individuals in the early modern period. Motulsky

Disease box 10 – *continued*

Disease box 10 – continued

suggests that a small prosperous merchant class may have contributed disproportionately to succeeding generations, producing very strong founder effects.

- In Finland there were two phases of expansion, either of which could have produced strong founder effects: one in prehistoric times soon after the south of the country was first settled, and another in the seventeenth century when pioneer groups populated the largely empty north (De la Chapelle, 1993).

There has been controversy over whether the distribution of alleles in Ashkenazi diseases can be explained just in terms of population history. With a simple founder effect, one might expect one mutant allele, on one specific marker haplotype, to explain all the excess cases of a disease (excess over the levels found in other populations). That is what we see in familial dysautonomia, Fanconi anemia and Bloom syndrome. But in Tay–Sachs, Gaucher, Niemann–Pick and Canavan diseases, two or more alleles are relatively common. This has been taken as evidence of heterozygote advantage. It is noteworthy that three of the four diseases listed are lysosomal storage diseases (Tay–Sachs, Gaucher and Niemann–Pick disease), and in fact another lysosomal storage disease, mucolipidosis IV, is also relatively common in Ashkenazim. Is this just coincidence, or could there be something about being a carrier of a lysosomal storage disease that was advantageous at some time in the history of this population?

A natural observational bias could explain some of the data. For example, three different *BRCA1/2* mutations are fairly common in Ashkenazim and rare elsewhere (see *Chapter 12*). This seems remarkable – but it may be just an initial random fluctuation, amplified by the strong population expansion. Before demanding a special explanation, we should remember all the other genes where we don't find common Ashkenazi mutations. Maybe it is not so remarkable that one gene in a thousand should show a random fluctuation large enough to produce the present distribution.

10.5. References

De la Chapelle A (1993) Disease gene mapping in isolated human populations: the example of Finland. *J. Med. Genet.* **30**: 857–865.

Motulsky AG (1995) Jewish diseases and origins. *Nat. Genet.* **9**: 99–101.

Paw BH, Tieu PT, Kaback MM, Lim J and Neufeld EF (1990) Frequency of three Hex A mutant alleles among Jewish and non-Jewish carriers identified in a Tay-Sachs screening program. *Am. J. Hum. Genet.* **47**: 698–705.

10.6. Self-assessment questions

(1) 200 unrelated people were typed for a single nucleotide polymorphism that has two alleles, C and T. 87 people were CT, 93 TT and 20 CC. What are the gene frequencies of the C and T alleles? Is the population in Hardy–Weinberg equilibrium?

(2) Usher syndrome Type 1 is an autosomal recessive deaf–blindness syndrome that affects one person in 100 000 in a population. Although

all cases are clinically indistinguishable, genetic analysis has shown that mutations in several different genes can cause Usher syndrome (locus heterogeneity). What is the carrier frequency, (a) if all cases are due to mutations at a single locus, and (b) if homozygosity at any one of 10 different loci contributes equally to the overall incidence?

(3) Inability to taste low concentrations of bitter substances such as phenylthiourea and perhaps some types of cabbage is (usually) an autosomal recessive trait. People can be classified as tasters and non-tasters. 64% of people in a population dislike spring greens and won't eat them because they taste unpleasantly bitter. What is the frequency of the taster allele?

(4) As mentioned in *Disease box 8*, erythropoietic protoporphyria behaves as a dominant condition with reduced penetrance, but molecular analysis has shown that affected people are all compound heterozygotes, having a rare non-functioning allele and a common low-functioning allele ($q = 0.11$ in France). If the condition affects 1 person in 30000 in France, what is the frequency of the non-functioning allele? What is the risk that an affected person, married to an unaffected person, will have an affected child?

(5) A woman's only son has Duchenne muscular dystrophy. She has no brothers or sisters, and there is no history of the disease in the rest of the family. What is the chance her daughter is a carrier?

(6) The healthy sister of a boy with cystic fibrosis marries an unrelated man whose family has no history of the disease. Both are of Danish stock. She is pregnant. What is the risk the child will have cystic fibrosis? If she had consulted you beforehand, would you have advised her not to have children?

(7) An autosomal recessive disease affects one person in 40000. A woman's marriage breaks up under the stress of caring for her affected child. She finds solace with a sympathetic cousin; eventually they marry and now she is pregnant. What is the risk their child will be affected?

(8) Fred has an extremely rare autosomal recessive disease. What is the chance that both of his grandfathers are carriers?

(9) Waleed and Benazir (*Figure 10.4*) marry and have a deaf son, Aziz. Deaf people often prefer to marry a deaf partner, and Aziz marries Nasreen Choudhary. What is the chance their first child will be deaf? Calculate the coefficient of inbreeding of this child. Apart from deafness, is this child at high risk of other recessive conditions?

Chapter 11

When is screening useful?

Learning points for this chapter

After working through this chapter you should be able to:

- Distinguish between screening and diagnosis
- Describe the parameters commonly used to define the performance of a screening program
- Describe the technical, social and ethical requirements that a screening program should fulfil
- Give examples of prenatal, neonatal and postnatal screening programs, and discuss their advantages and disadvantages to individuals and to society

11.1. **Case studies**

| CASE 22 | Vlasi family | **271** | 276 | 376 |

- Valon, a 6-year-old boy
- Serious learning problems
- Small, microcephalic, blue eyes, fair skin and hair, eczema; hyperactive
- ? Phenylketonuria

Figure 11.1 – A patient with untreated PKU.

Valon, aged 6 years, was the only child of Adem and Flora Vlasi. They had had a very unsettled life and had travelled to Australia as refugees. Valon was born in Kosovo. The family lived in a remote rural area where only basic medical care was available. Soon after he was born the political situation became unstable and the family moved several times before entering Australia as refugees. Over the years, Adem had been worried about Valon's progress but Flora said the problems were likely to be due to all the moves he had experienced and the fact that he had not been to school. When they settled and Valon was enrolled in school, the teachers recognized at once that he had serious learning problems. They arranged for assessment by an educational psychologist and suggested that the family doctor refer him to a pediatrician. In the clinic the doctor was surprised to see that Valon had a condition he had only read about in textbooks. Valon was small and microcephalic and had blue eyes, very fair skin and hair, as well as eczema. He was hyperactive and when restrained he rocked his body. The pediatrician also thought that Valon had a musty smell about him in spite of him being well cared for by his parents. The doctor strongly suspected that Valon had phenylketonuria and arranged for measurement of phenylpyruvic acid in a urine sample and phenylalanine levels in a blood sample.

11.2. **Background**

Screening versus diagnostic tests

The word 'screening' is often used loosely as a synonym for testing, but the essentials of a true screening program are that it is applied to a whole population. In contrast to diagnostic tests, where a person has a problem and approaches the clinician for a test, screening is usually a top-down process, offered by some organization to a large cohort of people (probably defined by age, reproductive state, or ethnic origin). In any genetic screening program, ethical considerations are at least as important as technical questions. In this section we will consider some of the more straightforward technical matters, and return to some more general questions in the final section of this chapter.

Most screening tests do not result in a definite diagnosis, but serve to define a high risk group of people, who are then offered a definitive diagnostic test. Usually this involves setting an arbitrary cut-off point (*Figure 11.2*). This is always a compromise. Setting the cut-off too high means missing an unacceptably large proportion of the target group, while setting it too low means exposing too many people to further investigation, most of whom will turn out not to be affected. Population screening for mendelian disease mutations is unusual in that it provides a final diagnosis in a single step and in theory should not produce any false positives. However, as we shall see, even screening programs of this type rarely rely on mutation analysis as the first line of investigation, and the initial steps may bring the possibility of false positives; in any case, false negatives will occur, because no DNA screening test will identify every possible mutation in a gene. *Box 11.1* shows some of the measures used to define the validity of a screening test.

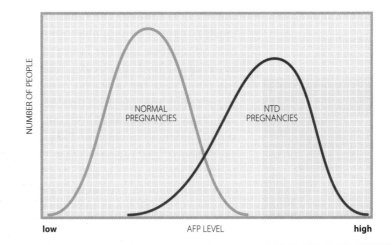

Figure 11.2 – A typical screening test.
In many hospitals maternal serum alpha-fetoprotein (MSAFP) screening is offered to pregnant women to assess the risk that their fetus has a neural tube defect (spina bifida or anencephaly). A raised level of AFP in the mother's blood indicates a higher risk, but the distributions in normal and affected pregnancies overlap. An arbitrary cut-off is used to select about 5% of women for further investigation. This involves detailed ultrasound examination and/or amniocentesis (see *Chapter 14*). Most women with raised AFP eventually deliver normal babies.

Parameters of a screening test

Considering, for example, the MSAFP test shown in *Figure 11.2*, women can be positive or negative on the test, and can have a fetus with or without a neural tube defect (NTD). In the table, a, b, c and d are actual numbers of women in each category.

	Fetus has NTD	**Fetus does not have NTD**
Positive on test	a	c
Negative on test	b	d

Sensitivity of test = proportion of affected picked up = a / (a+b)

Specificity of test = proportion of all unaffected that are true negatives = d / (c+d)

False positive rate = proportion of all tests that give a false positive result = c / (a+b+c+d);
Or = proportion of positive tests that are false = c / (a+c)

False negative rate = proportion of negative tests that are false = b / (b+d)

Positive predictive value = proportion of all positives that are affected = a / (a+c)

Relative risk = risk after a positive test compared to general population risk
= [a / (a+c)] / [(a+b) / (a+b+c+d)]

When might screening be done?

Genetic screening tests fall into three groups.

- **Prenatal screening** – pregnant women in the UK, for example, are usually offered screening for NTDs and for Down syndrome. Screening programs for thalassemia and sickle cell disease are currently being introduced. There may also be a more general fetal anomaly screen, consisting of a careful ultrasound examination of the fetus to look for structural anomalies. This should pick up most NTDs, in addition to other abnormalities, making a separate MSAFP test unnecessary. Screening for Down syndrome is discussed in relation to Case 8 (Howard family) in *Section 11.3*. Many individual mendelian and chromosomal conditions are also detectable prenatally, but these are not population screening tests; they are offered to individual couples who are known to be at high risk because of their family history.
- **Newborn screening** – as described in the next section, all newborn babies in many countries are screened for phenylketonuria. A variety of other tests may also be routinely offered (see *Section 11.4*). The list differs in different countries and often from institution to institution within a country. In the UK, newborn screening for hemoglobinopathies, congenital hypothyroidism and cystic fibrosis are in place or being introduced, and large-scale pilots are running for deficiency of medium chain acyl-CoA dehydrogenase (MCAD).
- **Adult screening** – this is most likely to be for carrier status for recessive, diseases – for example Tay–Sachs carrier screening in Ashkenazi Jews

(see *Section 11.3*, Case 21, Ulmer family). Particular groups of adults may be screened for other genetic risk factors, though this is usually conducted through family tracing rather than true population screening. For example, people with a strong family history of breast cancer are screened for *BRCA1/2* mutations (see *Chapter 12*), and people with high cholesterol levels may be screened for genetic hypercholesterolemia (see *Disease box 11*). As described in *Chapter 8*, screening for pharmacogenetic variants affecting drug metabolism is often discussed, and may perhaps become more common over the coming years.

For some conditions there are a variety of different ways in which screening might be offered. Carrier screening for a recessive condition might be performed on newborn infants, on school leavers, on couples of childbearing age selected by general practitioners, on pregnant women and their partners, or on anybody who cares to visit a drop-in centre. Each approach has its advantages and disadvantages. Points to consider include:

- can the subjects give properly informed consent?
- how easy is it to access the group to be screened?
- how relevant will the information be at that time to the person screened?
- what are the practical and ethical implications of a positive result?
- what will the program cost, and do the benefits justify the cost?

These considerations are discussed a little further below in relation to Tay–Sachs carrier screening.

Who should be screened?

Screening can be offered to the whole population or to specific groups. Singling out particular groups for screening may become politically fraught, no matter how sound the genetic case for doing so. When Down syndrome screening was restricted to older women because of their higher risk (see *Table 2.1*), some younger women who subsequently had a baby with Down syndrome complained that they had been unfairly discriminated against. Plans to screen specific ethnic groups have often caused trouble. In the UK, all babies are screened for sickle cell disease, and carrier screening is offered to all women early in pregnancy, even though the risk for white native British people is extremely low; however, the methodology used depends on the risk level in the local population.

In other cases screening is based on family history. This is done partly for economic reasons. Scanning the entire *BRCA1* and *BRCA2* genes for mutations is very expensive and, in the British NHS, testing is prioritized based on family history. These tests, and cascade screening (see *Disease box 11*) represent a halfway house between family-based clinical genetics and population screening.

How should screening be done?

A DNA test is seldom the best screening test. The cheap and rapid DNA tests that would be suitable for large-scale screening always check for specific mutations (see *Chapter 5*). However, what we usually want to know is whether *any* mutation is present, not just certain specific ones. For loss of function conditions with extensive allelic heterogeneity, it is usually more efficient to use a functional test for large-scale screening. PKU screening is based on measuring the level of phenylalanine in a blood spot; Tay–Sachs screening normally measures the ability of the affected enzyme to break down an artificial substrate; and cystic fibrosis screening relies on measuring the level of immunoreactive trypsin, although carrier screening would necessarily use a DNA test.

11.3. **Investigations of patients**

CASE 8	Howard family	26	38	68	100	**275**	376

- Helen – new-born daughter of Henry and Anne (33 years old)
- Down syndrome
- Risk of recurrence if they have more children?

Antenatal screening for Down syndrome (and other chromosomal anomalies) has been available for many years. Until the 1980s the screening test consisted of asking the mother's age. As *Table 2.1* shows, the risk of having a baby with Down syndrome rises sharply for older women. Over a certain cut-off (normally in the range 35–38 years, depending on resources available) women were offered a definitive prenatal diagnostic test. The test involved using amniocentesis or (more recently) chorion villus biopsy to obtain a sample of fetal cells for cytogenetic analysis. These procedures are invasive, unpleasant for the woman, and carry a 0.5–2% risk of causing a miscarriage. They are also expensive. They are only appropriate for women at the highest risk. The age cut-off puts around 5% of women in this group.

Screening by maternal age alone has low sensitivity. Although the individual risk is higher for a woman over 38 years, there are so many more pregnancies among younger women that the majority of babies with Down syndrome are in fact born to younger women. To improve sensitivity, several substances in the mother's blood are measured. For each, the distribution of levels in Down syndrome pregnancies (after adjustment for gestational age and maternal weight) is rather different from that in normal pregnancies. The level of AFP in Down syndrome pregnancies averages 70% of the level in unaffected pregnancies. The level of unconjugated estriols averages about 75%. On the other hand, levels of human chorionic gonadotrophin tend to be raised. All the Down syndrome and normal distributions overlap strongly, so that none of the levels is diagnostic by itself, but in combination, and including the mother's age, this 'triple test' gives a composite risk figure that is far more predictive than age alone. An additional test in some institutions uses ultrasound to measure the fluid under the skin of the neck of the fetus; those with Down syndrome tend to have more fluid, giving greater nuchal translucency.

Women whose composite risk is greater than a predetermined cut-off are offered the diagnostic test. Deciding what cut-off to use involves a trade-off between sensitivity and false positive rate. Any increase in sensitivity will be accompanied by a decrease in specificity. The performance of a test can be partly judged by how the trade-off varies. *Figure 11.3* shows theoretical calculations of how the trade-off for the triple test would be for various cut-off risks. Such curves are called, for historical reasons, receiver operating characteristic (ROC) curves. From April 2007, all pregnant women in the UK should be offered a

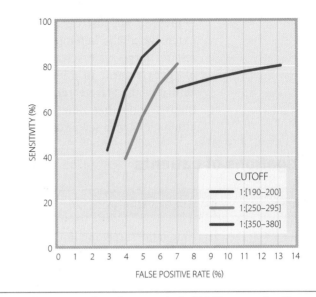

Figure 11.3 – Receiver operating characteristic (ROC) curves for the performance of the Down syndrome triple test as a screening test.
There is a trade-off between sensitivity (picking up the greatest number of affected pregnancies) and false positive rate (subjecting too many unaffected pregnancies to invasive diagnostic testing). Reproduced from Conde-Agudelo and Kafury-Goeta (1990) with permission from Lippincott Williams and Wilkins.

screening test with a detection rate above 75% and a false positive rate of less than 3%.

Women such as Helen's mother Anne, who had a previous child with Down syndrome, would normally be offered a diagnostic test regardless of their age or objective risk level. Although the recurrence risk for a younger woman is low, their anxiety level is naturally very high after having had an affected baby, and it would be cruel to refuse them the test.

There is considerable debate about the most appropriate test to use once fetal cells have been obtained (*Box 11.2*). As described in *Chapter 4*, Anne Howard opted for interphase FISH testing, and received a reassuring normal result within 2 days – but she had to understand that this did not mean that her fetus was chromosomally normal, only that it had the correct number of copies of chromosomes 13, 18 and 21.

CASE 22	Vlasi family	271	**276**	376

- Valon, a 6-year-old boy
- Serious learning problems
- Small, microcephalic, blue eyes, fair skin and hair, eczema; hyperactive
- ? Phenylketonuria
- Testing for subsequent baby?

When the family came to Sydney, Flora was already 6 weeks pregnant. Having learned that Valon had a serious genetic disease, she and Adem were extremely worried about the risk of the new baby being affected. With all their other problems, they felt they could not cope with a second affected child, and they discussed terminating the pregnancy despite their general reservations about abortion. When their family doctor explained that even if the baby was affected (a 1 in 4 risk), it could be treated, they immediately asked for the treatment for

What is the best prenatal diagnostic test for Down syndrome?

After antenatal screening by the triple test and/or nuchal translucency, women whose risk of a Down syndrome baby is above the cut-off are offered a diagnostic test. Fetal cells are obtained by amniocentesis or chorion villus biopsy, as described in *Chapter 14*. What is the best way of analyzing these cells?

- *Traditional karyotyping*, as described in *Chapter 2*, can detect every chromosome abnormality, but arguably this is not desirable. While autosomal trisomies are always pathological, detecting some other abnormalities would present the couple with very difficult decisions that they might rather not have to face. Some, such as Turner syndrome or XYY have well understood but relatively minor consequences, while the effects of others, such as *de novo* apparently balanced rearrangements or mosaicism for a small unidentified extra chromosome (a 'marker'), are unpredictable. Is it perhaps better not to know? The figure shows some data found by full karyotyping.

- *Molecular tests* check specifically for the common trisomies of chromosomes 13, 18 and 21. The technique used may be interphase FISH (see *Chapter 4*) or quantitative PCR. Both these methods can be applied to uncultured cells, avoiding the long wait required while the fetal cells are grown up for conventional cytogenetics.

In one UK survey, full karyotyping took 12 days and cost £253 per test; quantitative PCR took 24 hours and cost £30 per test. But around 10% of the abnormalities missed by the rapid test have a poor prognosis. Some of these will be picked up on routine ultrasound examination, and some will abort spontaneously, but some will result in live-born abnormal babies.

Chromosomal abnormalities found by full karyotyping of prenatal samples that would not have been detected by molecular trisomy testing. Data on 24 891 women tested because of increased risk of Down syndrome, from Ogilvie *et al.* (2005).

Valon – but the doctor explained that the treatment was only effective if started very soon after birth (see *Chapter 14*). So they asked if the new baby could be tested as soon as it was born, and were assured that it would be.

Flora delivered a healthy girl, and mother and baby were discharged from hospital. A few days later the midwife visited them at home. As well as checking on the health and progress of mother and baby, she pricked the baby's heel and collected a blood spot on to a special card (a Guthrie card). This is standard practice for every baby born in many countries, regardless of family history. The card was sent to a central laboratory and here the level of phenylalanine in

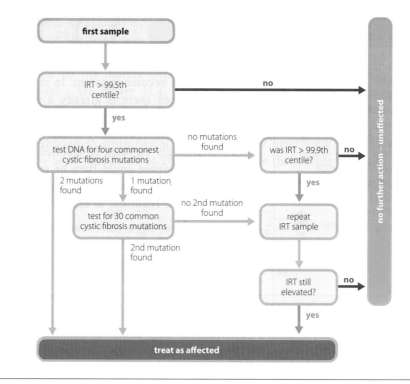

Figure 11.5 – Flowchart of scheme proposed in the UK for screening newborn babies to allow early identification and treatment of those with cystic fibrosis. IRT, immunoreactive trypsin.

mutation. The *CFTR* gene has 27 exons (see *Figure 3.8*) and there is currently no way of scanning the entire sequence of such a gene at a cost low enough to use in population screening. Because of founder effects (*Chapter 10*) a few specific mutations make up the bulk of all cystic fibrosis mutations in any particular community. Any carrier screening protocol therefore involves a trade-off between cost and sensitivity. Testing for the few commonest mutations is cheap but misses some proportion of carriers. Testing for many mutations is expensive, and however many individual mutations are checked, the sensitivity will never be 100%. *Table 11.1* shows the distribution of *CFTR* mutations detected by one large UK laboratory.

Inevitably, some couples who have tested negative will actually both be carriers, with a 1 in 4 chance of having an affected baby. Almost all of these will be couples where one partner was recognized to be a carrier, but the other carried a rare mutation and was a false negative on the test. If the carrier frequency is 1 in 23 (*Chapter 10*) and the sensitivity of the screening test is 0.9, then about 1 person in 25 will be found to be a carrier. Given the smaller number of such people compared to the number initially screened, it is possible to test the partner for a larger panel of mutations to try to minimize the number of false negatives. Ultimately, one criterion for a screening program could be that the risk for a positive–negative couple should be no greater than the initial risk for any couple before screening. It could then be argued that the program has left nobody in a worse position than they were in before screening. For a carrier frequency of 1 in 23, this requires a 99.8% sensitivity for testing the partner of a known carrier (so that the risk of a false negative is 1 in 500). The figures in *Table 11.1* suggest that reaching 99.8% sensitivity would be a challenge.

Table 11.1 – Distribution of *CFTR* mutations in 1754 cystic fibrosis chromosomes analyzed in Manchester, UK

Mutation	Exon	Number found	Percentage of cystic fibrosis	Cumulative %
p.F508del	10	1420	81.0	
p.Gly551Asp	11	62	3.5	84.5
p.Gly542X	11	20	1.1	85.6
c.621+1G>T	Intron 4	17	1.0	86.6
c.1898+1G>A	Intron 12	16	0.9	87.5
p.Arg553X	11	13	0.7	88.3
p.Arg117His	4	13	0.7	89.0
p.Arg560Thr	11	11	0.6	89.6
c.3272–26A>G	Intron 17a	10	0.6	90.2
c.3659delC	19	9	0.5	90.7
p.Asn1303Lys	21	8	0.5	91.2
c.1717–1G>A	Intron 10	7	0.4	91.6
c.2711delT	14a	7	0.4	92.0
Other detected		114	6.5	98.5
Unknown		27	1.5	
Total		**1754**		**100.0**

A sensitivity of 90% could be achieved by testing for the commonest nine mutations; 95% sensitivity would require testing for 26 mutations.
Data courtesy of Dr Martin Schwartz, St Mary's Hospital, Manchester.

CASE 21	Ulmer family	251	259	**281**	376

- Hannah, a 6-month-old baby girl
- Ashkenazi Jewish origin
- Tay–Sachs disease
- Test the sibs?
- Screening for Tay–Sachs disease?

Among Ashkenazi Jews the carrier frequency for Tay–Sachs disease is 1 in 30. Because of this, carrier screening programs have been established in the USA and many other countries, starting in the early 1970s. *Table 11.2* shows some statistics. In countries where the Ashkenazi community have embraced carrier screening enthusiastically, the majority of affected babies are now born to non-Jewish couples.

Screening uses a biochemical test, measuring the ability of hexosaminidase A in serum to hydrolyze an artificial substrate MUG (an *N*-acetyl glucosamine

Table 11.2 – Tay–Sachs carrier screening among Ashkenazi Jews, 1971–1998

Country	Number tested	Carriers	Carrier–carrier couples
United States	925 876	35 372	795
Israel	302 395	7277	380
Canada	65 813	3301	62
South Africa	15 138	1582	52
Europe	17 725	1127	37
Brazil	1027	72	20
Mexico	655	26	0
Argentina	84	5	0
Australia	3334	102	4
Total	**1 332 047**	**48 864**	**1350**

Data from Gravel RA *et al.* (2001) and reproduced here with permission from The McGraw-Hill Companies.

derivative of 4-methyl umbrelliferone). DNA testing is not used for population screening because not all carriers have one of the common Ashkenazi mutations (see *Table 10.2*). A more definitive diagnostic test is required after a positive screening result. About 2% of Jewish and 35% of non-Jewish people identified as carriers by the screening test in fact carry a so-called pseudodeficiency allele. Such alleles encode a variant form of the enzyme that is inactive against the artificial substrate used in the screening test, but retains enough activity against G_{M2} ganglioside to be non-pathogenic. Screening for Tay–Sachs disease is usually combined with screening for a variable selection of the other 'Jewish diseases' listed in *Disease box 10*.

There are various ways in which a screening program could be implemented, and various actions that might follow a positive test result. Which one is adopted is very much a matter for the community concerned. Whatever protocol is adopted, screening should be voluntary and requires fully informed consent.

- **Testing babies or children** is unethical and inefficient. The child cannot give proper consent and the result has no implications until many years later, by which time it may well have been forgotten.
- **Testing school leavers** raises issues of just how far consent is truly voluntary, and requires careful handling to avoid stigmatization of carriers. Some Orthodox communities try to solve the stigmatization problem by giving the results to a match-maker and not to the individual tested (see below).
- **Testing young single adult volunteers** minimizes problems of consent but will miss some fraction of the target group.

- **Testing couples** identifies the small number of at-risk couples without worrying the much larger number of carriers whose spouse is a non-carrier (compare the last two columns of *Table 11.2*). But it removes the possibility of choosing not to marry a carrier. In some Orthodox communities where marriages are semi-arranged, the match-maker has the results of testing young single people for a range of recessive conditions, and will indicate if a proposed marriage would be risky.

11.4. **Summary and extension**

What conditions should we screen for?

Technically, the possibilities for genetic screening seem almost unlimited – certainly they are already vast, and are increasing every year. In practice, however, what is on offer is very much more limited. Apart from the inevitable time-lag in bringing new developments into service, there are four main technical reasons why genetic screening is not more widespread (social and ethical factors are considered later).

- If you work through self-assessment questions 1–3, you will see that the positive predictive value of a test may be very low, even if the test performs well in the laboratory.
- A DNA variant may be indisputably associated with increased risk of a disease, but may be responsible for only a small fraction of the overall risk. The **Population Attributable Risk** (*Box 11.3*) is an important consideration in any screening program. If a variant explains only 5% of the total risk, what is the point of screening for it? If that 5% is concentrated in a few individuals who have a very high risk, it might be valuable for those individuals to know – but this is approaching the situation for mendelian diseases, where testing is mainly family-based. If the variant is common, so that the extra risk is spread across a large proportion of the population, there seems little value to anybody in knowing.
- It is important to consider not just the relative risk but also the absolute risk. Even a high relative risk may not be too worrisome if it translates into a low absolute risk. An example is Factor V Leiden (OMIM 227400). This is a well-authenticated risk factor for venous thromboembolism, for example, among long-haul airline passengers and oral contraceptive users. The *relative* risk among oral contraceptive users is high (around 15) but the *absolute* risk still quite low, because oral contraceptive users are generally young and the risk of embolism is very age-dependent.
- In general, there is no point in screening unless a positive result leads to some useful action. This might mean lifestyle changes, prophylactic drugs to reduce the risk, or maybe increased surveillance, for example, where the risk is of cancer and early diagnosis improves the prognosis. Sometimes genetic testing is done simply to provide people with information for planning their future as, for example, in predictive testing for Huntington disease, but normally a screening test should lead to some practical outcome.

Box 11.3

The Population Attributable Risk

This is the proportion of the total disease risk in the population that is attributable to the factor in question. It is sometimes called the Population Attributable Fraction. If the PAR is low, it calls into question the value of screening for the factor.

If the overall risk in the population is r, but a proportion p of the population have a variant that gives them an additional risk of R, on top of the general risk, then the PAR for that variant is pR/r.

The Office of Genomics and Disease Prevention at the Centers for Disease Control and Prevention in the USA has provided a framework that can be used for assessing any genetic (or other) test, not just a screening test. The ACCE framework suggests a test should be assessed against four sets of criteria.

- **Analytical validity:** how accurately does the test measure what it is supposed to measure? For a DNA test this might translate into asking what proportion of all mutations in a gene are picked up by the test protocol.
- **Clinical validity:** how accurately does the test detect or predict the presence or absence of disease? For example, most people with hereditary hemochromatosis (OMIM 235200) have mutations in both copies of their *HFE* gene, usually p.Cys282Tyr and/or p.His63Asp. But testing for these mutations has low clinical validity because the great majority of homozygotes or compound heterozygotes for the mutations do not have clinical hemochromatosis.
- **Clinical utility:** how useful are the test results in providing clinical benefits? Everybody with Type 1 Waardenburg syndrome (OMIM 193500) has a mutation in the *PAX3* gene. The test has high analytical and clinical validity – but detecting the mutations does not provide much obvious clinical benefit to most patients, beyond satisfying their curiosity.
- **Ethical, legal and social implications**

Population-based screening programs, where individuals opt out rather than opt in, need to be funded by the state or insurance companies. Funders will evaluate any proposed scheme critically against technical, financial and ethical criteria. The criteria used are usually based on a set formulated by Wilson and Jungner in a 1968 report for the World Health Organization (see *References*). *Box 11.4* shows a selection of the criteria used by UK National Screening Committee. In the directly marketed sector the arguments may look very different. Companies will offer a genetic test if they see a likely profitable market for it, regardless whether or not it might result in useful actions or long-term benefits. This has resulted in various companies offering 'lifestyle' genetic screening – testing for variants associated with increased risk of some common disease, coupled with advice on how to mitigate any increased risk (see *Box 11.5*). Profitability may, however, depend on being able to pass part of the cost on to somebody else. Somebody in the UK who gets a disturbing test result from an internet-based company, will probably expect their family doctor and NHS genetics service to deal with their worries.

Box 11.4

Criteria used by the UK National Screening Committee

For a complete list of the 22 criteria see www.nsc.nhs.uk/pdfs/criteria.pdf.

The condition:

(1) The condition should be an important health problem.

(2) The epidemiology and natural history of the condition ... should be adequately understood...

(3) All the cost-effective primary prevention interventions should have been implemented as far as practicable.

(4) If carriers of a mutation are identified as a result of screening, the natural history of people with this status should be understood, including the psychological implications.

The test:

(5) There should be a simple, safe, precise and validated screening test.

(7) The test should be acceptable to the population.

(9) If the test is for mutations, the criteria used to select the subset of mutations to be covered by screening, if all possible mutations are not being tested, should be clearly set out.

The treatment:

(10) There should be an effective treatment or intervention for patients identified through early detection, with evidence of early treatment leading to better outcomes than late treatment.

The screening programme:

(13) There should be evidence from high quality randomised controlled trials that the screening programme is effective in reducing mortality or morbidity. Where screening is aimed solely at providing information to allow the person being screened to make an 'informed choice' (e.g. Down syndrome, cystic fibrosis carrier screening) there must be evidence from high quality trials that the test accurately measures risk. The information that is provided about the test and its outcome must be of value and readily understood by the individual being screened.

(14) There should be evidence that the complete screening programme (test, diagnostic procedures, treatment / intervention) is clinically, socially and ethically acceptable to health professionals and the public.

(15) The benefit from the screening programme should outweigh the physical and psychological harm (caused by the test, diagnostic procedures and treatments).

(16) The opportunity cost of the screening programme (including testing, diagnosis and treatment, administration, training and quality assurance) should be economically balanced in relation to expenditure on medical care as a whole (i.e. value for money).

(19) All other options for managing the condition should have been considered (e.g. improving treatment, providing other services), to ensure that no more cost-effective intervention could be introduced...

(20) Evidence-based information, explaining the consequences of testing, investigation and treatment, should be made available to potential participants to assist them in making an informed choice.

(22) If screening is for a mutation, the programme should be acceptable to people identified as carriers and to other family members.

Box 11.5

'Lifestyle' genetic testing

Searching the internet, you can easily find companies offering to genotype you for certain common DNA variants in order to help you decide your most healthy lifestyle. All these offers are based on reports of associations between common DNA polymorphisms and risk of specific diseases. The reports are likely to be by reputable scientists in peer-reviewed journals. Impressive though the list of references may look, there are several questions you need to ask.

(a) Has the association been validated? The proportion of reported associations that are replicated in independent studies is depressingly low – see *Chapter 13* for further discussion of this problem.

(b) Has it been validated in all ethnic groups? Many identified risk factors are specific to certain ethnic groups.

(c) What is the risk ratio? That is, does the variant increase your risk by a factor of 20, 5, 2 or 1.1? Do you care about a 10% increase in your risk? It is important to distinguish between the statistical significance and the size of an effect. A large survey can identify a highly significant association (that is, there is no doubt that it is real) with a quite trivial risk ratio. Note incidentally that it is well known that initial risk ratios almost always come down in subsequent studies, even when the risk is confirmed.

(d) What is the population attributable risk?

Assuming a test is satisfactory by all these criteria, the question remains, so what? From a public health point of view, 'lifestyle' genetic testing risks simply diluting universally valid messages about the need to eat sensibly, get some exercise and stop smoking. Companies looking at market opportunities may be less bothered by such thoughts – but no company could risk saying to people who come out as low risk on their test that they can therefore cheerfully indulge in an unhealthy lifestyle. The lawyers would have a field day when, as will inevitably happen, some people succumb to diseases for which their reported risk was low. The risk never was zero, it was simply rather lower than for some other people. Therefore, quite regardless of the test result, the advice from the company must be the same routine healthy living advice, just delivered a bit more emphatically for high-risk people. It might therefore be argued that such testing has no ethical implications. The same advice may be available to everybody free of charge, but some people will only take notice of it if they have paid $250 and got a scientific-looking piece of paper. The public health question is, what is the balance between those who would be motivated to act appropriately by receiving advice of a high risk and those who would act inappropriately on receiving advice of a lower risk?

A separate scientific question, normally ignored by proponents of lifestyle testing, is the relation of the test result to overall health, rather than risk of a specific disease. All these tests are based on research that compares the frequency of a certain DNA variant in a cohort of people with a particular disease, to the frequency in controls who don't have that disease. A variant may increase the risk of that disease – but maybe there is a compensating decrease in the risk of some other disease. This is not as far-fetched as it may sound. All our metabolic settings are a balance, optimized over thousands of generations to cope with a variety of circumstances. Such balances involve compromises. A variant that shifts the balance may just change the compromises. Variants that are common in the population cannot be wholly bad, or natural selection would have eliminated them. It is possible of course that a variant might only have had benefits in the environment of cavemen, and is wholly bad in people living in affluent Western societies, as suggested by the 'thrifty genotype' theory of diabetes susceptibility (Hales and Barker, 2001). But at present we have almost no information on the effects of any variants on overall health. This is particularly relevant to concerns that insurance companies might want to use data on common DNA variants in their underwriting, but it also sounds a cautionary note about the value of genetic testing as a guide to healthy living.

Newborn screening is the least ethically contentious area of population screening, because the targets are treatable conditions and the aim is to ensure early treatment to avoid irreversible damage. The American College of Medical Genetics has recommended that all newborns should be screened for 29 conditions (*Table 11.3*). These recommendations have been widely accepted. Although implementation inevitably varies from state to state, in 2006 nearly two-thirds of newborns across the USA will be screened for at least 20 conditions – a near-doubling of activity compared to the previous year. *Figure 11.6* shows the distribution of activity by state. In most other countries newborn screening is limited to a shorter list, mainly for reasons of cost.

Attitudes towards prenatal screening, or screening children or adults for carrier status or risk of developing a late-onset condition, are more engrained in local cultures. Criteria 7, 14, 15, 20 and 22 of the UK NSC set cover ethical and social issues. Screening is an expression of the desires and values of the society in which it takes place. Antenatal screening will have little place in a society where abortion is unacceptable under any circumstances, even though the two are not necessarily linked. Some societies are more accepting of abnormal people, or more fatalistic about abnormalities, while in others the desire for a normal child

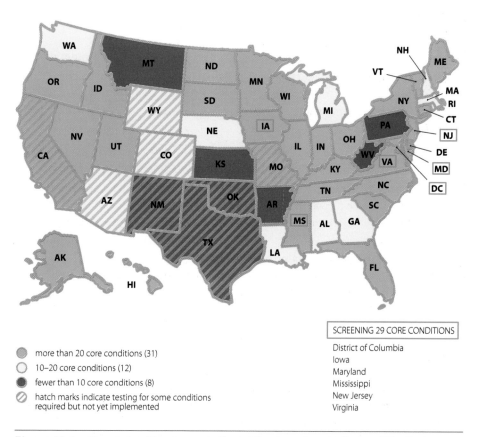

more than 20 core conditions (31)

10–20 core conditions (12)

fewer than 10 core conditions (8)

hatch marks indicate testing for some conditions required but not yet implemented

SCREENING 29 CORE CONDITIONS

District of Columbia
Iowa
Maryland
Mississippi
New Jersey
Virginia

Figure 11.6 – The state of implementation of the American College of Medical Genetics recommendations on newborn screening as of June 2006.
Data from the March of Dimes Birth Defects Foundation, and reproduced here with permission.

Table 11.3 – The 29 conditions for which the American College of Medical Genetics (2005) recommends that every newborn baby should be screened

Condition	OMIM number	Treatment
Medium chain acyl-CoA dehydrogenase deficiency	201450	Nutritional supplements; avoid fasting
Congenital hypothyroidism	**	Oral thyroid hormone
Phenylketonuria	261600	Low-phenylalanine diet
Biotinidase deficiency	253260	Daily oral biotin
Sickle cell anemia	603903	Vigilant medical care, avoid infections
Congenital adrenal hyperplasia	201910	Genital surgery; hormone replacement
Isovaleric acidemia	243500	Low protein diet, nutritional supplements
Very long chain acyl-CoA dehydrogenase deficiency	201475	High carbohydrate, low fat diet; supplements; avoid fasting
Maple syrup urine disease	248600	Low protein diet
Galactosemia	230400	Avoid milk and dairy products
HbS/β thalassemia	141900	As for sickle cell anemia
HbS/C disease	141900	As for sickle cell anemia
Long chain 3-hydroxyacyl-CoA dehydrogenase deficiency	609016	High carbohydrate, low fat diet; supplements; avoid fasting
Glutaric acidemia Type I	231670	Low protein diet with oral carnitine
Hydroxymethylglutaric aciduria	246450	High carbohydrate, low fat, low protein diet; avoid fasting
Trifunctional protein deficiency	609015	Low fat diet, supplements, avoid fasting
Multiple carboxylase deficiency	253270	Oral biotin
Methylmalonic acidemia (mutase deficiency)	251000	Vitamin B_{12} and other supplements; low protein diet
Homocystinuria	236200	Diet, supplements including vitamins B_6 and B_{12}
3-methyl crotonyl-CoA carboxylase 1 deficiency	210200	Low protein diet
Hearing loss	**	Communication strategy; hearing aids, maybe cochlear implant
Methylmalonic acidemia (cblA or cblB deficiency)	251100	Vitamin B_{12}, low-protein diet
Propionic acidemia	606054	Low-protein diet, supplememts
Carnitine – acylcarnitine translocase deficiency	212138	Carnitine
β-keto thiolase deficiency	203750	Vigilant medical care, low-protein diet
Citrullinemia	215700	Low-protein diet, supplements
Argininosuccinic aciduria	207900	Low-protein diet, supplements
Tyrosinemia Type I	276700	NTBC (see *Section 14.4*)
Cystic fibrosis	219700	Vigilant medical care

They are listed in order of priority, based on frequency, severity, effectiveness of treatment and practicality of screening. Some rare conditions rank high because they can be added in to a multiplex tandem mass spectrometry, or high performance liquid chromatography screen, for very little extra cost. ** Congenital hypothyroidism and hearing loss have many causes, not all genetic.

is very strong. Views on individual responsibility, and on the relative values of individual freedom and public health will affect the acceptability of specific programs. Attitudes to children are important – how far do parents own their children, and have the right to know about their genetic make-up, or how far must children's autonomy be respected, and no tests performed until the child is old enough to give properly informed consent? It is a general principle that screening should be voluntary and needs informed consent, but even here the issues are not clear-cut. A baby cannot consent to being screened for PKU. If the parents object, do they have the right to risk condemning their child to life in an institution, while expecting the general public to meet the costs? Nevertheless, people must in general be free to opt out of screening if they wish. This does not simply mean that they can decline testing; it also means that if, say, after declining prenatal testing they have an affected child, they should not be in any way blamed or penalized.

In Britain, the Greek Cypriot community have taken up screening for β-thalassemia with enthusiasm, whereas the Pakistani community, also at high risk, have by and large not wanted it. In Israel there is said to be a strong popular demand for every possible screening test, whereas in the UK the approach is much more cautious. For example, a chain of British high-street stores stopped offering a set of 'lifestyle' tests after public disquiet about the implications – even though many would argue that such tests are no more harmful than a horoscope, and at worst, only a waste of money. According to the stores, the reason for discontinuing the offer was lack of public interest which, if true, reflects better on the good sense of the British public.

Concerning the economics of screening, it is interesting to see how Criterion 16 in the UK NSC list is rather cautiously worded. Assessing the financial benefits of a screening program usually involves balancing the immediate costs of screening against claimed savings in the longer term. This is a difficult area, though of course a vital one in many areas of policy. It is handled using *discounted cash flow*. To compare a present cost with a saving in 10 years' time, the present cost is treated as an investment, whose value in 10 years is calculated using compound interest. The interest rate used (the discount rate) obviously affects the outcome, but different types of institution may have different views about the relevance of potential savings in the distant future. Moreover, these calculations have their limitations as guides to action. Applied to normal childbearing, the discounted cash flow method suggests that reproduction is financially disastrous for society: it is very unlikely that an individual's contribution to society in taxes as a working adult can ever repay the discounted cost of his delivery, upbringing and education.

If the cost calculations look reasonable, the decision on whether to implement a screening program revolves round public demand and social acceptability. Since public opinion is never unanimous about such issues, decisions are in the end political.

Familial hypercholesterolemia

We are all familiar with a high cholesterol level as a sign of unhealthy eating – but about 1 person in 500 has an extremely high cholesterol level as a result of a genetic condition and regardless of diet. Familial hypercholesterolemia (FH; OMIM 143890) is an autosomal dominant condition. In most populations it is the commonest of all clinically significant mendelian conditions. Heterozygotes typically have serum cholesterol and LDL-cholesterol levels of 250–450 and 200–400 mg/dl (normal range 150–250 and 75–175 mg/dl, respectively). They develop tendon xanthomata (subcutaneous cholesterol deposits) and suffer coronary artery disease in mid-life, with many premature deaths from myocardial infarction. Rare homozygous affected people have these features to a more extreme degree.

(a)　　　　　　　　　　(b)　　　　　　　　　　(c)

Cholesterol deposition in patients heterozygous for familial hypercholesterolemia. (a, b) Tendon xanthomata, and (c) corneal arcus. Photos courtesy of Dr Paul Durrington, Manchester Royal Infirmary.

Michael Brown and Joseph Goldstein won the 1985 Nobel Prize for Medicine for their work on FH that has led to a detailed understanding of cholesterol homeostasis (see *References* for further information). They demonstrated that FH was usually caused by mutations in the low density lipoprotein receptor (*LDLR*) gene. This cell surface receptor imports cholesterol-containing LDL into liver cells (an example of receptor-mediated endocytosis), where it represses endogenous cholesterol synthesis as part of a homeostatic mechanism. The mutant receptor is either absent or fails to bind LDL, depending on the particular mutation, leading to uncontrolled endogenous production of cholesterol. Sometimes FH can be caused by mutations in either of two other genes:

- some people produce LDL that is not recognized by the LDL receptor because a mutant *APOB* gene encodes an abnormal form of the lipoprotein
- occasional patients have gain of function mis-sense mutations in *PCSK9*, a gene encoding a protein-processing enzyme that is part of the homeostatic mechanism.

The normal action of internalized LDL is to repress 3-hydroxy-3-methylglutaryl coenzyme A (HMG CoA) reductase, which catalyzes the rate-limiting step in cholesterol synthesis. In FH patients, statin drugs are used to inhibit the enzyme. This is a very effective clinical management, which can normalize cholesterol levels and health risks. Because the condition is common, has serious health implications and can be effectively treated, there is a good case for screening the whole population for FH. However, the resource implications are considerable. Screening based on cholesterol levels and tendon xanthomata has poor sensitivity, especially in younger people. DNA-based screening is expensive because the *LDLR* gene on chromosome 19p13.2 has 18 exons and several hundred different mutations have been described.

Since this dominant condition affects large extended pedigrees, a very cost-effective method of ascertaining large numbers of affected people is to test relatives of known affected cases, a procedure known as **cascade screening** or cascade testing. The principle was mentioned earlier in connection with testing relatives of **Joanne Brown (Case 2)** for cystic fibrosis mutations. The best developed cascade screening program for FH, in the Netherlands, has run since 1994. Relatives are contacted directly by a genetic field-worker. Family tracing is exceptionally thorough, leading to an average of 25.7 relatives per proband being tested. Of those who turned out to be affected, only 39% were already on statins. Details of this and other programs are reviewed by Hadfield and Humphries (2005).

Studies of the Dutch program have demonstrated very clear clinical benefits: 93% of affected people ascertained through the program subsequently took statins, thus greatly reducing their risk of premature death. Various ethical issues can be raised. The direct contacting of relatives is considered ethically problematic in some countries and instead probands are left to suggest to their relatives that they might benefit from talking to a geneticist. This avoids some problems, but greatly decreases the number of relatives tested per proband. There are questions about identifying affected children – does the benefit of early treatment outweigh the risk of stigmatization or impaired self-image? It is also necessary to think about insurance implications for people contacted out of the blue. Some companies at least have accepted the argument that underwriting should be based on the phenotype – the actual cholesterol level in the treated patient – and not on the genotype. Since statin treatment is effective, this largely disposes of the insurance issues. Careful studies of the Dutch program have shown none of the predicted ill effects, though it is possible that this partly reflects the admirable qualities of Dutch society, and might not be so easily replicated elsewhere.

11.5. **References**

Conde-Agudelo A and Kafury-Goeta AC (1990) Triple marker test as screening for Down syndrome: a meta-analysis. *Obstet. Gynecol. Survey* **53**: 369–376.

Hadfield SG and Humphries SE (2005) Implementation of cascade testing for the detection of familial hypercholesterolaemia. *Curr. Opin. Lipidol.* **16**: 428–433.

Hales CN and Barker DJP (2001) The thrifty phenotype hypothesis. Type 2 diabetes. *Br. Med. Bull.* **60**: 5–20.

Ogilvie CM, Lashwood A, Chitty L, Waters J, Scriven PN and Flinter F (2005) The future of prenatal diagnosis: rapid testing or full karyotype? An audit of chromosome abnormalities and pregnancy outcomes for women referred for Down syndrome testing. *Br. J. Obstet. Gynae.* **112**: 1369–1375.

Wilson JMG and Jungner G (1968) *Principles and Practice of Screening for Disease.* World Health Organization, Geneva.

Useful websites

The UK National Electronic Library website has a good section on screening: http://www.library.nhs.uk/screening/.

See also the UK Newborn Screening Programme Centre: http://www.newbornscreening-bloodspot.org.uk/.

An example of an antenatal screening service (one among many, but with good documentation on Down syndrome and cystic fibrosis) is the UK Leeds Antenatal Screening Service: http://www.leeds.ac.uk/lass/Index.htm.

The Brown-Goldstein lab website at UT Southwestern Medical Center tells a fascinating story of their Nobel Prize-winning work on cholesterol regulation: http://www4.utsouthwestern.edu/moleculargenetics/pages/brown/past.html

11.6. Self-assessment questions

(1) A hypothetical disease is caused by mutations in the *IGNO* gene. 1 person in 100 carries a mutation. You have a genetic testing protocol that detects 80% of all mutations. You receive 10000 blood samples from newborn babies – but 1% of the samples were taken into contaminated tubes that give a false positive result on your test. What is the positive predictive value of your test?

(2) A scientist has been studying people who suffer severe adverse effects of a certain drug. In the general population one person in 10 000 suffers these effects. He has identified a DNA polymorphism that is strongly associated with the risk. In blind testing in the laboratory, $^{99}/_{100}$ people who had shown the adverse drug reaction tested positive for the variant, while only $^{1}/_{100}$ people who had taken the drug without ill-effects tested positive. He proposes to screen the entire 1 million population of his city for the variant. Calculate the positive predictive value of his test.

(3) Repeat the calculation of the previous question, assuming the adverse reaction occurred in 1 person in 10 rather than 1 in 10000. What does this tell us about the potential of screening in general?

(4) Assuming an incidence of neural tube defect of 1:100 pregnancies tested, use the curves in *Figure 11.2* to estimate the sensitivity and positive predictive value of the MSAFP test, using cut-offs of:

(a) everybody above the normal mean value
(b) everybody above the minimum abnormal value
(c) everybody above the maximum normal value

(5) In cystic fibrosis carrier screening, some couples will have one partner test positive and the other negative. Calculate the sensitivity required of a screening test so as to ensure that such couples are at no greater risk of really both being carriers that they were before any screening was done. Assume the carrier frequency in this population is 1 in 40.

(6) You are a health administrator charged with establishing a population screening program for carriers of cystic fibrosis (who make up 1 person in 25 in your population).

(a) Decide at what stage in their life and under what circumstances people should be tested; write a brief justification of your choice.
(b) You have proposals from two companies for performing the high-throughput genotyping. One offers to test a limited panel of mutations, covering 70% of all mutations; the other tests a larger panel covering 90% of all mutations. Naturally the costs are different, but before you can make decisions you need to know the likely results. For each option, calculate the expected outcomes from screening 1 million people, in terms of cystic fibrosis births avoided and cystic fibrosis births to couples who were not both carriers on the screening test.

Chapter 12

Is cancer genetic?

Learning points for this chapter

After working through this chapter you should be able to:

- Describe carcinogenesis as an evolutionary process within an individual
- Define oncogenes and tumor suppressor genes, giving examples
- Describe the types of genomic instability found in cancer cells and the roles of cell cycle checkpoints in avoiding these
- List the essential capabilities of malignant tumors and describe the types of somatic genetic change that lead to their development, including activation of oncogenes or inactivation of tumor suppressor genes by somatic mutation, epigenetic changes, deletions leading to loss of heterozygosity, and chromosomal rearrangements leading to fusion genes
- Describe at least three inherited cancer syndromes and discuss their relationship to common sporadic cancers
- Describe the roles of genetics in diagnosis, treatment and prevention of cancer

12.1. Case studies

- ? Familial breast cancer

Wendy Wilson saw a television program about breast cancer running in families that raised her concerns about her own family history. She had mentioned her worries some years before to her family doctor but had been reassured. Her mother Wanda had developed the disease at the age of 42 years and sadly died when she was 44 years old. Her mother's sister Amy who lived in New Zealand also developed breast cancer in her 40s but after surgery and chemotherapy was well 7 years later. The previous Christmas Wendy had received a card from an elderly great aunt in which she mentioned that one of her grandsons was undergoing treatment for breast cancer as well, and expressed her shock that a man could be affected. Wendy got in touch with her brother William and sister Veronica and they decided they should look into things in more detail. Veronica was the family genealogist and before long had contacted several relatives they had lost touch with. They found one of Wanda's cousins had died at a young age of breast cancer. The television program had mentioned that tests for familial breast cancer were available through genetic clinics so Wendy made an appointment with her family doctor to ask for a referral. At the surgery Wendy gave as many details as possible to the doctor and he consulted the online guidelines provided by the genetics center. Wendy's family fulfilled the criteria for a high risk and so a referral was made. Before the appointment the genetic counselor from the center contacted Wendy to draw up a family tree. She also asked Wendy for details of her mother and where she was treated so that her medical records could be obtained to confirm the details of her illness.

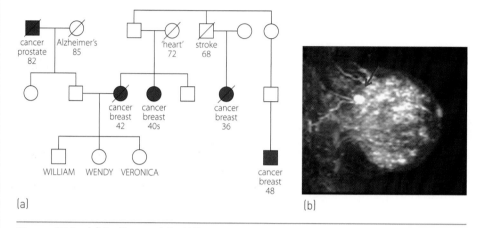

(a)

(b)

Figure 12.1 – (a) Pedigree of the Wilson family, showing types of cancer and age at diagnosis. (b) Carcinoma of the breast detected in a 40-year-old woman by magnetic resonance imaging. This lady had a *BRCA1* mutation. Photo. courtesy of Dr Gareth Evans, St Mary's Hospital, Manchester.

| CASE 24 | Xenakis family | **294** | 315 | 376 |

- Family history of bowel problems
- ? FAP

Christos was one of three children born in Cyprus in the 1960s to Xavier and Demi Xenakis. Xavier started having bowel symptoms at the age of 41 but didn't go and see his doctor until he became really unwell. At the hospital, bowel cancer with liver metastases was diagnosed and only palliative treatment was possible. He died later that year, and soon afterwards Christos moved to Seattle to open his own restaurant with his wife and young son and daughter. Demi came to live with them. Life was very busy but the restaurant did well. At an insurance medical examination some years later, Christos mentioned that he had recently noticed some rectal bleeding which he thought might be due to hemorrhoids. Because of the family history the doctor recommended that Christos had a sigmoidoscopy and to everyone's concern this revealed multiple polyps.

The surgeon explained that this indicated Christos had Familial Adenomatous Polyposis (FAP) and that the only sensible treatment was to remove the colon, since it was inevitable that cancer would develop in one or more of the polyps. While Christos was still in hospital, the surgeon recommended he be referred to the genetic clinic when he was recovered to find out about risks for his children, and also about screening tests that they could have in due course. After a few months the family attended the genetic clinic. The counselor explained dominant inheritance, and they worked out that each child was at 50% risk of having inherited the mutated gene. They learned that genetic testing would be possible if a mutation was found in Christos and that, in children who were at risk or who were found to be mutation carriers, regular sigmoidoscopies were offered from 10 years of age.

(a)   (b)

Figure 12.2 – Familial adenomatous polyposis coli.
(a) Pedigree of the Xenakis family. (b) Part of a surgically resected colon with polyps. Photo. courtesy of Medical Illustration Department, Manchester Royal Infirmary.

12.2. **Background**

Natural selection and the evolution of cancer

Imagine an isolated wood in which a population of voles lives. One vole acquires a heritable mutation that makes it able to reproduce faster than the other voles. When you visit the wood 100 vole generations later you would expect to find that most of the voles were descendants of that one faster breeding mutant. Exactly the same simple Darwinian argument applies to the cells of your body. Cell division is under genetic control. If one cell acquires a mutation that makes it divide faster than others then, all things being equal, its descendants will take over your body. Thus cancer is not a specific disease with one cause, and one cure waiting to be discovered. All things being equal, it is simply the natural end-point of evolution within the body of any multicellular organism.

Fortunately, all things are not equal. Multicellular organisms could not survive if they did not have mechanisms to control and repress the evolution of their somatic cells, at least until their reproductive life is over. Over the billion years through which they have been evolving, multicellular organisms have developed sophisticated and many-layered defenses against rogue cells. Cell growth is tightly controlled. Most somatic cells do not have the capability of dividing indefinitely. Any cell that behaves inappropriately and whose antisocial behavior cannot be remedied is made to kill itself (**apoptosis**). In an important paper, Hanahan and Weinberg (2000) listed six functional capabilities that a malignant tumor needs to acquire in order to develop and survive (*Box 12.1*). Acquiring each capability means overcoming a separate regulatory mechanism or line of defense in the organism. Consistent with this, classic studies of the age-specific incidence of the common epithelial cancers, suggested that four to seven independent events were needed to generate a malignant tumor.

Box 12.1

The six essential capabilities of a malignant tumor

According to Hanahan and Weinberg (2000), a malignant tumor needs to acquire the following six capabilities during its development:

- ability of cells to divide independently of external growth signals
- ability of cells to ignore external anti-growth signals
- ability of cells to avoid apoptosis
- ability of cells to divide indefinitely without senescence
- ability to stimulate sustained angiogenesis
- ability to invade tissue and establish distant secondary tumors

Tumors contain a diversity of cells and these capabilities probably belong to only a small population of cancer stem cells. Acquiring each capability is likely to require a specific genetic or epigenetic change in order to circumvent a regulatory mechanism. Possible exceptions are the ability to divide indefinitely, if the founding cell is already a stem cell, and the ability to metastasize – it is controversial how often this is a specifically acquired capability and how often it is just a frequent result of acquiring the other five capabilities.

Overcoming the defenses

Given typical mutation rates, the chance of any cell in a person's body sequentially acquiring six specific mutations would appear to be negligibly low. Assuming a mutation rate of 10^{-6} per gene per cell, the chance of a cell picking up six successive specific mutations is 10^{-36}. There are only of the order of 10^{14} cells in a human body, so it would appear that the defenses against cancer are impregnable. Since we know that one person in three will nevertheless develop cancer, there has to be some way round the defenses.

The trick is that the mutations early in the process must somehow greatly increase the probability of later mutations. They can do this in either of two ways.

- They can give the cell a growth advantage. If the mutant cell can generate 1000 mutant daughter cells, the chance that one mutant cell will acquire the next mutation has increased 1000-fold. Pathologists have long known that tumors develop through stages that are marked by increasing growth potential, and that rapidly dividing tissues are the ones most likely to develop tumors. It is believed that the founding cells of many tumors have stem cell-like properties, so that they already have unusual growth potential (Pardal *et al.*, 2003).
- They can increase the general mutation rate by destabilizing the genome. All cancer cells show one of two types of genomic instability:
  (i) **chromosomal instability** – most tumor cells have bizarre karyotypes with grossly abnormal numbers of chromosomes and many structural rearrangements (*Box 12.2*);
  (ii) **microsatellite instability** – a few tumors are chromosomally normal, but DNA testing shows that normal checks on the accuracy of DNA replication have been lost (see below).

As a result of these changes, the early stages of tumorigenesis are likely to produce a growing population of cells with a great variety of random mutations, making fertile ground for subsequent developments. The genes that become mutated in these early stages are classified as **oncogenes** or **tumor suppressor genes**. The classification is primarily dependent on the type of mutation required – gain of function or loss of function – but this in turn depends on the normal function of the gene. Broadly speaking, oncogenes are genes whose normal role is to stimulate cell division, while the normal role of tumor suppressor (TS) genes is to restrain cell division.

Chromosomal instability in cancer cells

Cancer cells usually have grossly abnormal karyotypes with many gains, losses and rearrangements. Solid tumor cells normally give very poor chromosome preparations that are difficult or impossible to analyze using conventional cytogenetic techniques. M-FISH or SKY are multicolor versions of chromosome painting (see *Section 4.4*) that make each original chromosome appear in a different color. These methods allow detailed analysis of the cytogenetic changes in cancer cells. As an example, here is the karyotype recorded for the human HT29 colon carcinoma cell line by Dr T Reid:

> 67–71,XX,del(X)(p11.2)[19], del(3)(p21)[11], der(3)ins(3;12)(p12;?)[16], der(3)del(3)(p25)
> ins(3;12)(p12;?)[5], der(3)t(X;3)(?;qter)[11], i(3)(q10)[21], del(4)(q31.3) [21],
> +der(5)t(5;6)(q11;?)[10], del(6)(q12)[9], t(6;14)(q21;q13)[15], der(6)t(6;14)(q21;q13)[5],
> +del(7)(p15)[17], –8[20], der(8)i(8)(qter->q10::q10->q24::hsr::q24->qter)[21], +11[20],
> –13[9], der(13)i(13)(q10)del(q14)[11], der(13)t(5;13)(p13;p11.1)[12], i(13)(q10)[18], –14[21],
> –14[4],+15[20], der(17)t(17;19)(p11;p11)[21], i(18)(p10)[19], –19[13],
> i(19)(q10)dup(19)(q13.1q13.4)[19], +i(20)(q10)[21], –21[21], der(?22)t(17;?22;17)[20]

21 cells were analyzed. The chromosome number varied between 67 and 71. The numbers in square brackets are the number of cells having each specified abnormality. This and many other cases can be viewed as 'Skygram' karyotype diagrams on the National Cancer Institute website at http://www.ncbi.nlm.nih.gov/sky/

Box 12.2

Living for ever: the importance of telomeres

Cancer cells are immortal: they have acquired capability number 4 in *Box 12.1*. HeLa cells, a standard laboratory cell culture workhorse, have been growing in culture for half a century. Ordinary human cells won't do this. They grow in culture for a few dozen divisions, but then they stop growing, a condition called senescence. Cells with certain cancer-related mutations (in *TP53* and *RB1*, see below) avoid senescence. After some further divisions they reach a stage called crisis. Crisis is marked by death of the great majority of the cells. The few survivors have acquired extensive chromosomal rearrangements and the immortality of cancer cells.

These events are related to a problem with replicating chromosome ends. Recall that the two strands of the double helix are anti-parallel, and that DNA strands can only grow in the 5′→3′ direction (*Box 3.2*). One strand of the double helix has a free 5′ end. When this strand is used as a template for synthesis of a complementary strand, the polymerase moves towards the end of the strand and there is no problem extending the new strand up to the end of the template (*Figure 12.3a*). The other, with a free 3′ end, has problems. When this strand is used as a template, the polymerase moves in the direction from the end towards the interior of the template, against the direction of movement of the replication fork. The new strand is made discontinuously in 100–200 nt segments (**Okazaki fragments**). Each fragment starts with a short (10 nt) RNA primer. The last primer does not necessarily start on the very last nucleotide of the chromosome, and even if it did, the 10 nt corresponding to the primer would be lost as the primer is removed when the Okazaki fragments are ligated together. Thus a linear DNA double helix inevitably loses some sequence at the end each time it is replicated.

Bacteria solve this problem by having circular chromosomes; eukaryotic cells use **telomeres**. Human chromosomes end with about 10 kb of repetitive sequence, $(TTAGGG)_n$. With each round of cell division the telomere shortens by 50–100 nt. Within limits, this doesn't matter because the telomeric repeats contain no genetic information. Repeated division will lead to complete loss of telomeres. One function of the telomeres is to protect chromosome ends against DNA repair mechanisms that recognize broken DNA ends and try to join them together (*Figure 12.3b*). This is what happens to cells in the post-senescence crisis.

Every cell of our body is descended by a chain of cell divisions from the original fertilized egg, which in turn is descended through a chain of cell

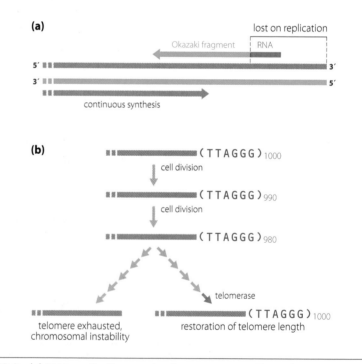

Figure 12.3 – (a) DNA replication mechanisms cannot replicate the extreme 3′ end of a molecule. (b) Telomeres of human chromosomes contain tandemly repeated TTAGGG units. Some repeats are lost each time a cell replicates its DNA. Continued loss in cultured cells leads to chromosomal instability. In the germ-line and in cancer cells, telomerase can restore telomeres to full length.

divisions from the zygotes that created our parents, and so through an unbroken chain of cell divisions through the generations and back through time right to the very dawn of life. So how do we still have telomeres? The answer is that certain cells possess an enzyme, **telomerase**, that can restore telomeres to full length. Telomerase adds TTAGGG units using its own inbuilt RNA template, and is therefore not dependent on an external template. Telomerase restores telomere length in the germ-line of each generation. Normal somatic cells lack telomerase (the gene is there but not expressed) – but most cancer cells possess it. Reactivation of telomerase is an important step in acquiring the capability to divide indefinitely. Equally, of course, telomerase looks like an excellent target for an anticancer drug – though the results of trials have been disappointing.

Oncogenes

The oncogene story begins with investigations of cancer viruses in the 1970s. Viruses never cause cancer in the way they cause flu – cancer is never infectious and no virus causes cancer in every infected person. Nevertheless, a few cancers in humans and animals are causally associated with the presence of certain viruses – for example, cervical cancer is associated with human papilloma virus. In the laboratory, **acute transforming retroviruses** could be recovered from certain animal tumors. These viruses were non-infectious but were able efficiently to transform cells in culture into cells that, when transplanted into recipient animals, formed tumors. Retroviruses have a very simple RNA genome consisting of just three transcription units (*Figure 12.4*). When the genomes of acute transforming retroviruses were analyzed they were seen to contain an extra gene, the oncogene. Several dozen oncogenes were identified through studies of such viruses, and named after the animal tumors from which the viruses were isolated (see *Table 12.1*). Other oncogenes were discovered by identifying DNA fragments from tumor cells that could transform mouse cells in tissue culture, causing them to grow in a manner similar to tumor cells.

These discoveries led to a brief flurry of speculation that all cancer might be the result of infection by oncogene-carrying viruses, and so might be preventable

Figure 12.4 – (a) A retrovirus. The RNA genome comprises three transcription units, *gag*, *pol* and *env*. There are short terminal repeats (TR). (b) An acute transforming retrovirus. In a random processing error, part of the viral genome has been replaced by a cellular proto-oncogene. Over-expression or random mutations may render the cellular gene oncogenic when the virus enters a host cell. The viral genes are partially deleted and the virus is unable to replicate.

Table 12.1 – Viral oncogenes and their cellular counterparts

Gene	Animal source	Cellular proto-oncogene	
		Location	Function
ABL	Abelson murine leukemia	9q34	Signal transduction (tyrosine kinase)
ERBB2	Avian erythroblastic leukemia	17q21	Signal transduction (receptor tyrosine kinase)
FES	Feline sarcoma virus	15q26	Signal transduction (tyrosine kinase)
FMS	Friend murine leukemia	5q33	M-CSF receptor tyrosine kinase
HRAS	Harvey rat sarcoma	11p15.5	Signal transduction (small GTPase)
KRAS	Kirsten mouse sarcoma	12p12	Signal transduction (small GTPase)
MYB	Avian myeloblastosis	6q22	Transcription control (nuclear protein)
MYC	Avian myelomacytosis	8q24	Transcription control (nuclear protein)
SIS	Simian sarcoma virus	22q12	Platelet-derived growth factor B chain
SRC	Rous chicken sarcoma	20q12	Signal transduction (tyrosine kinase)

by vaccination. This beguiling idea lost its luster when it was discovered that normal cells contained homologs of viral oncogenes. Some complex viruses do indeed contain virus-specific oncogenes, but the acute transforming retroviruses are in fact transduction vectors: they pick up genes at random from an infected cell and deliver them into the next cell they infect. The transduced gene replaces part of the normal viral genome, so the viruses are replication-defective.

Clearly there must be some difference between the oncogene in the virus, which transforms cells, and the normal cellular version, which does not. Viral oncogenes are activated versions of the cellular genes (**proto-oncogenes**). The proto-oncogene terminology is often ignored in current research literature and the genes are usually simply called oncogenes – but the distinction between activated and non-activated forms is crucial.

Function and activation of oncogenes

A great breakthrough in molecular understanding of carcinogenesis was achieved when the normal functions of cellular oncogenes were identified, starting in the early 1980s. As *Table 12.1* shows, the normal, non-activated versions of these genes have roles in the control of cell proliferation. Given their normal function, it is entirely understandable that pathogenically activated versions of these genes should be oncogenic. Activation involves a gain of function. This can be achieved in a variety of ways.

- *Point mutations* – as always, a gain of function requires a specific mutation. For example, bladder cancers may have the mutation p.Gly12Val in the *HRAS* (proto)oncogene. The three human *RAS* genes (*KRAS, HRAS, NRAS*) encode small GTPases which activate an intracellular signaling cascade (RAS →RAF → MEK →MAPK) that leads to changes in gene expression. Gain of function mutations produce a hyperactive version of the GTPase that triggers excessive expression of the target genes.

- *Amplification* – some tumors contain many tandemly repeated copies of oncogenes, sometimes in the form of small extra chromosomes, sometimes as duplications within a chromosome. The *MYC* oncogene, for example, is frequently amplified in tumors.

- *Chromosomal rearrangements* can bring together exons of two distant genes to make a novel chimeric gene. As mentioned above, cancer cells usually have many chromosomal abnormalities. Much painstaking research has been dedicated to identifying changes that are specific to particular tumor types, and distinguishing them from the large numbers of random changes. Most of the changes have been identified in leukemia, which is easier to study than solid tumors. *Table 12.2* gives examples and *Box 12.3* illustrates one well-known case. These rearrangements are exceptionally interesting because cloning the breakpoints reveals the chimeric genes and has been a route to discovery of many oncogenes. Some genes are involved in many different rearrangements – the *MLL* gene at 11q23 has been noted with over 30 different fusion partners in leukemia patients. Tests for specific rearranged genes are an important part of molecular diagnosis of cancer. Often, as in the case of the Tierney family (Case 20), defining the chimeric oncogene provides a guide to prognosis and treatment. Research into the function of the chimeric gene also provides an important entry into understanding the biology of the tumor.

- *A chromosomal rearrangement can up-regulate expression of an oncogene* by moving it into a transcriptionally highly active region of chromatin. The classic case is Burkitt's lymphoma, a childhood tumor particularly affecting the jaw and found mainly in Africa. Incidence is associated with infection by malaria and Epstein–Barr virus. Tumor cells have a characteristic somatically acquired balanced reciprocal translocation, t(8;14)(q24;q32), *Figure 12.5*. The effect of the translocation is to move the *MYC* oncogene from chromosome 8 to the neighborhood of the *IGH* immunoglobulin heavy chain gene on chromosome 14. Unlike most tumor-specific rearrangements, the move does not create a chimeric gene. However, in lymphocytes, but not in other cells, *IGH* is expressed at a very high level. Thus lymphocytes, but not other cells with the translocation, greatly over-express *MYC*. The result is a lymphoma. Sometimes an alternative translocation moves *MYC* to the immunoglobulin light chain gene regions on chromosomes 2 or 22.

(a)   (b)

Figure 12.5 – Burkitt's lymphoma.
(a) Histology, and (b) a karyotype showing the characteristic 8;14 translocation. Additional chromosome abnormalities are also present, as is usually the case in neoplasia. Reproduced from *Molecular Cancer*, **2**: 30; © 2003 Duensing *et al.*; licensee BioMed Central Ltd.

Table 12.2 – Tumor-specific balanced chromosomal rearrangements that create chimeric genes

Rearrangement	Genes	Disease
t(1;22)(p13;q13)	*RBM15/MKL1*	Acute megakaryoblastic leukemia (FAB–M7)
t(2;13)(q35;q14)	*PAX3/FKHR*	Alveolar rhabdomyosarcoma
t(3;8)(p21;q12)	*PLAG1/CTNNB1*	Pleomorphic salivary gland adenoma
inv(3)(q21q26)	*RPN1/EVI1*	AML without maturation (FAB–M1)
t(4;11)(q21;q23)	*MLL/AFF*	ALL/lymphoblastic lymphoma
t(6;11)(q27;q23)	*MLL/MLLT4*	AMML (FAB–M4)
t(9;11)(p22;q23)	*MLL/AF9*	ALL/lymphoblastic lymphoma
t(11;19)(q23;p13)	*MLL/MLLT1*	ALL/lymphoblastic lymphoma
t(7;11)(p15;p15)	*NUP98/HOXA11, HOXA13, HOXA9*	AML with maturation (FAB–M2)
t(9;22)(q34;q11)	*BCR/ABL1*	Chronic myeloid leukemia
t(11;14)(q13;q32)	*IGH/CCND1*	Chronic lymphocytic leukemia, Mantle cell lymphoma
t(15;17)(q22;q12)	*PML/RARA*	Acute promyelocytic leukemia (FAB–M3)
t(12;16)(q13;p11)	*FUS/DDIT3*	Liposarcoma
inv(16)(p13q22)	*CBFB/MYH11*	AMML (FAB–M4)
t(X;18)(p11;q11)	*SS18/SSX1, SSX2, SSX4*	Synovial sarcoma
t(14;18)(q32;q21)	*IGH/BCL2*	Follicular lymphoma
t(12;21)(p13;q22)	*ETV6 (TEL)/RUNX1 (AML1)*	ALL/lymphoblastic lymphoma
t(8;21)(q22;q22)	*RUNX1/ETO*	AML with maturation (FAB–M2)

See http://cgap.nci.nih.gov/Chromosomes/RecurrentAberrations for a large database of rearrangements established by Dr Felix Mitelman. Rearrangements have been particularly defined in leukemias and lymphomas because in these conditions the cells are usually a single clone and are more amenable to cytogenetic analysis than those in solid tumors. ALL, acute lymphoblastic leukemia; AML, acute myeloblastic leukemia; AMML, acute myelomonocytic leukemia.

Box 12.3

The Philadelphia chromosome and the chimeric *BCR–ABL* gene

Lymphocytes from 90% of patients with chronic myeloid leukemia (CML) contain an abnormal small chromosome, the Philadelphia (Ph[1]) chromosome (*Figure 1*). It is a sufficiently constant feature of the disease to make the diagnosis of CML questionable in its absence. The Ph[1] chromosome was shown to be one product of a balanced reciprocal 9;22 translocation, t(9;22)(q34.1;q11.2). The translocation junction creates a novel chimeric gene on the Ph[1] chromosome by joining the 5′ part of the *BCR* gene from chromosome 22 on to the 3′ part of the *ABL* gene from chromosome 9. The resulting *BCR–ABL* gene always contains exon 1 of *BCR* and usually the next 10 or so exons, joined to exons 2–11 of *ABL* (*Figure 2*).

ABL is a known oncogene, having been first identified in an acute transforming retrovirus isolated from the Abelson rat sarcoma (*Table 12.1*). Its product is a tyrosine kinase that is part of a signaling system controlling cell growth. Activity of the kinase is tightly controlled, probably in part by the domain encoded by

Figure 1 – Karyotype of metaphase with t(9,22).
The abnormal chromosomes 9 and 22 (Philadelphia chromosome) are on the lefthand side of each pair. Photo. courtesy of Dr Christine Harrison, University of Southampton.

exon 1. The chimeric gene is transcribed and translated; its product is a tyrosine kinase that is constitutively active. Such a gain of function in an important growth control could clearly tip a cell towards uncontrolled growth.

Figure 2 – Joining the *BCR* and *ABL* genes to make the chimeric *BCR–ABL* gene. The breakpoint in *BCR* can be in any of several different introns.

As mentioned in *Chapter 8*, because this abnormal tyrosine kinase is so characteristic of CML, a drug that specifically targets it has proved extremely effective at inducing remission in CML patients.

Tumor suppressor genes

The rare forms of cancer that are heritable have been hugely important in furthering our understanding of carcinogenesis. Back in 1971 Alfred Knudson formed a hypothesis about the relationship between the inherited and sporadic versions of a cancer. He hypothesized that the early rate-determining steps of carcinogenesis required the founder cell of a tumor to suffer two 'hits' – these might be simple mutations or some other genetic change. In sporadic cancers both hits were chance events, each with a low probability. In the familial version one hit was inherited. Every cell of a susceptible person carried one hit, so it only required one cell in the target tissue to suffer one further hit for the tumor to develop. The familial susceptibility was inherited from one parent as a dominant trait. The cellular phenotype that allows a cell to found a tumor is recessive, requiring two hits (this is a useful reminder that dominance and recessiveness are properties of phenotypes and not of genes or mutations, see *Figure 1.13*).

Knudson formulated his hypothesis in relation to retinoblastoma (RB), a rare childhood tumor of the retina. RB can be unilateral or bilateral, and an additional persuasive observation was that while the familial form is often bilateral, sporadic RB is always unilateral. A similar observation can be made about breast cancer. In familial RB there are sometimes multiple independent tumors in one eye. Clearly retinoblasts in people with familial RB have a strong tendency to become tumorigenic – though considering the size of the target cell population, the probability of such a transformation is compatible with typical mutation rates (*Figure 12.6*).

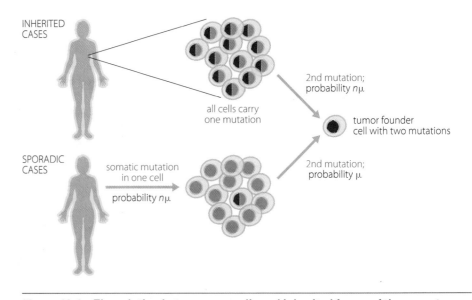

Figure 12.6 – The relation between sporadic and inherited forms of the same tumor. The target tissue contains *n* cells and the chance of one cell suffering a loss of function mutation in the tumor suppressor gene is μ.

Proving the two-hit hypothesis

A seminal paper in 1983 by Cavenee *et al.* showed how Knudson's hypothesis for RB could be confirmed, and set the agenda for the next 20 years of research into familial cancers. There was a suspicion that the 'hits' in RB might be on chromosome 13, because of a family in which familial RB co-segregated with an abnormality of that chromosome. Cavenee and colleagues collected cells and DNA from tumors in patients with sporadic RB. Using a combination of cytogenetic analysis and Southern blotting with probes from chromosome 13, they looked for differences between the tumors and the normal cells of the same patients. The cytogenetic analysis showed that some tumors had missing or extra copies of chromosome 13. The Southern blots showed that in some cases, where the normal (blood) DNA of a patient was heterozygous for a polymorphism, the tumor was homozygous. Correlating the cytogenetic observations and the occurrence of **loss of heterozygosity** in individual tumors, the researchers were able to put together a convincing description of chromosomal mechanisms for producing one of Knudson's 'hits' (*Figure 12.7*).

Later work added to the picture by showing that in inherited cases, the second hit always worked so as to eliminate the normal sequence. Tumor cells retained just the sequence that the patient had inherited from the affected side of his family. Some years later, when the *RB1* gene had been cloned and PCR made it possible to scan it for mutations, a variety of loss of function mutations were identified in the inherited RB-susceptibility allele. Acquired somatic mutations could also be demonstrated in the wild-type gene in tumors that had no relevant chromosome abnormality.

Figure 12.7 – Mechanisms in retinoblastoma.
The initial mutation may be inherited or somatic. Mechanisms A, B and D result in loss of heterozygosity (in B, only for markers close to the *RB* locus; in D only for markers distal to the crossover). In Cavenee's original study, some tumors duplicated the remaining copy of chromosome 13 after loss of the wild-type chromosome by mechanism A.

The RB work confirmed the existence of TS genes and showed that the two-hit hypothesis explained the basis of familial cancer syndromes. It suggested two ways of identifying TS genes:

- identifying chromosomal regions of loss of heterozygosity in sporadic tumors by comparing tumor and constitutional (blood) DNA from the same patient
- mapping and positional cloning of the genes mutated in familial cancers

Loss of heterozygosity analysis has yielded disappointing results from a huge amount of work. The problem is that fully developed tumors contain a heterogeneous collection of cells with so many chromosomal changes that it is difficult to extract clean patterns of loss specific to one small chromosome region. The introduction of array-CGH (see *Figure 4.7*) promises to make this line of enquiry more productive, because for the first time it will provide a genome-wide picture of the changes in a tumor. Meanwhile the family linkage approach has allowed the identification of the inherited susceptibility in many familial cancer syndromes. Once the gene responsible has been identified, sporadic tumors can be checked for mutations in the same gene. In this way a significant number of TS genes have been identified (*Table 12.3*).

Table 12.3 – Familial cancer syndromes with inherited mutations in tumor suppressor genes

Syndrome	OMIM number	Gene	Location
Retinoblastoma	180200	*RB1*	13q14
Familial adenomatous polyposis	175100	*APC*	5q21
Hereditary non-polyposis colon cancer	120435 120436	*MSH2* *MLH1*	2p22 3p21
Familial breast cancer	113705 600185	*BRCA1* *BRCA2*	17q21 13q12
Li–Fraumeni syndrome	151623	*TP53*	17p13
Gorlin syndrome	109400	*PTC*	9q22
Ataxia-telangiectasia	208900	*ATM*	11q23
Neurofibromatosis 1	162200	*NF1*	17q11
Neurofibromatosis 2	101000	*NF2*	22q12
Von Hippel–Lindau disease	193300	*VHL*	3p25
Multiple endocrine neoplasia 1	131100	*MEN1*	11q13
Multiple endocrine neoplasia 2	171400	*RET*	10q11
Familial melanoma	155601	*CDKN2A*	9p21

The normal functions of tumor suppressor genes

TS genes act to restrain cell growth, and are involved in a variety of checkpoints and controls. Two of the main areas are cell cycle checkpoints and the control of apoptosis.

In a set of continuously growing cells the cell cycle can be divided into four stages (*Figure 12.8*). Progression through the cycle is controlled by a series of checks. These include:

- *the G1–S checkpoint* – cells should not be able to start replicating their DNA until all DNA damage has been repaired; cells with unrepairable damage are triggered to commit suicide by apoptosis
- *the S-phase checkpoints* operate while DNA replication is underway; different replication origins become active at different times during S-phase, and the checkpoints prevent initiation at new origins while there is DNA damage
- *the G2/M checkpoint* prevents cells from initiating mitosis when there is unrepaired DNA damage
- *the spindle checkpoint* prevents the separation of chromatids in anaphase until every chromosomal centromere is attached to spindle fibers

The first three checkpoints represent different downstream responses to the machinery that detects DNA damage, especially double-strand breaks. This machinery involves several TS genes. Checkpoint mechanisms are strongly conserved through evolution. Much of our understanding of human cell cycle controls comes from studies of model organisms, especially yeast. The 2001 Nobel Prize for Medicine was awarded to Leland Hartwell, Tim Hunt and Paul Nurse for their work unraveling these controls (you can read their accounts of how they did it at http://nobelprize.org/medicine/laureates/2001/). Progress through the cycle is particularly controlled by cyclins, a family of proteins whose level in the cell fluctuates according to the phase of the cycle. Cyclins

Figure 12.8 – The cell cycle and its checkpoints.

operate by activating a series of protein kinases, the cyclin-dependent kinases. Specific CDK inhibitors counteract the cyclins.

The G1–S checkpoint in particular involves an impressive cast of TS genes (*Box 12.4*).

- *The RB protein (pRB)* binds and inhibits E2F, a transcription factor that activates expression of many genes required for moving through G1 phase into S phase. Phosphorylation of pRB by CDKs inactivates it and releases active E2F.

- *p53*, the product of the *TP53* gene, is normally bound by MDM2 and degraded. p53 stimulates transcription of *MDM2*, thereby regulating its own activity to a very low level. Various signals inactivate *MDM2*, allowing the p53 level to rise. Depending on the circumstances, this can either cause cell cycle arrest through the action of p21 or target the cell for apoptosis. p53 is inactivated by somatic mutations in a high proportion of all cancer cells; inherited mutations cause the Li–Fraumeni familial cancer syndrome.

The G1–S checkpoint

Box 12.4

Progression through the cell cycle is primarily governed by the availability of specific cyclin proteins. These activate CDKs. The kinases act as effectors by phosphorylating a range of downstream targets; they are regulated by the availability of their cognate cyclins and by various inhibitors. Progression through G1 phase and into S phase is governed by cyclins D and E with their kinases. A complex network of upstream controls modulates their activity. The figure shows only part of the network and more detail can be found in any cell biology textbook.

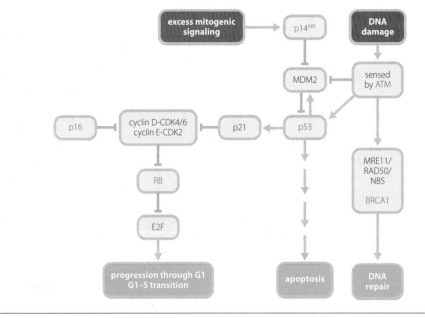

Some of the controls and interactions governing G1–S progress. TS genes identified through familial cancers are shown in red. ━▪ shows an inhibitory action, ━▶ shows a stimulatory action.

EXON 2 OF p16/INK4A

GT	CAT	GAT	GAT	GGG	CAG	CGC	CCG	AGT	GGC	GGA	GCT	GCT	GCT	GCT
Gly	His	Asp	Asp	Gly	Gln	Arg	Pro	Ser	Gly	Gly	Ala	Ala	Ala	Ala

EXON 2 OF p14ARF

GTC	ATG	ATG	ATG	GGC	AGC	GCC	CGA	GTG	GCG	GAG	CTG	CTG	CTG	CTC
Val	Met	Met	Met	Gly	Ser	Ala	Arg	Val	Ala	Glu	Leu	Leu	Leu	Leu

Figure 12.9 – The *CDKN2A* gene encodes two completely different proteins, p16 and p14ARF, both of which function in cell cycle control.
CDKN2A is very often deleted in tumor cells. ARF, alternative reading frame.

- *p16 and p14ARF* are both products of the same gene, *CDKN2A* (*Figure 12.9*). The use of alternative promoters and first exons causes the coding sequence in exon 2 to be read in different reading frames for the two products, which end up sharing no amino acid homology. Remarkably, both function in cell cycle control. Deletion of this gene is a very efficient way of disrupting cell cycle controls, and is a common occurrence in tumor cells. p16 is a cyclin-dependent kinase inhibitor. Inherited p16 mutations are found in some familial melanomas; these affect only the p16 product of the gene. Inherited mutations affecting only p14ARF are very uncommon but the p14 promoter is often epigenetically silenced in tumors.

- *ATM protein* may be the primary sensor of DNA double-strand breaks. Activated ATM phosphorylates several proteins including MDM2 (inactivating it), and p53, CHK2, BRCA1 and the MRE11/RAD50/NBS DNA repair complex (all of which are activated by phosphorylation).

It is noteworthy that several TS genes encode extremely large proteins. Examples include the proteins encoded by *APC* (2843 amino acid residues), *ATM* (3056 residues), *BRCA1* (1863 residues), *BRCA2* (3418 residues) and *NF1* (2839 residues). Not all TS genes encode large proteins (the two products of the *CDKN2A* gene are just 156 and 173 residues long), and not all large proteins have any role in cancer (some of the largest known proteins are muscle structural proteins like dystrophin, 3685 residues, and titin, 19946 residues). Nevertheless, the list in *Table 12.3* suggests that loss of function of genes encoding very large non-structural proteins is a frequent initiating event in tumorigenesis. Such proteins do in fact often have a structural role at the molecular, though not the microscopic, level. They interact with many other proteins and serve as scaffolds for assembling the large multi-protein machines that carry out many cellular tasks. Loss of function at such nodal points in the networks of interactions within cells may be a powerful way of disrupting normal cellular functions.

A desperate solution: apoptosis

Apoptosis is a specific active process that is triggered by various abnormal cellular states as well as being an important part of normal development (for separating the fingers of the hand in a developing embryo, for example). The mechanism involves activation of a cascade of proteolytic enzymes called caspases. Caspases can be activated through perturbations of mitochondria, with release of cytochrome C, or through the actions of FAS protein in conjunction with so-called death receptors. Such potent suicide machines naturally need to be kept under tight control, and the regulatory circuitry for apoptosis is extremely involved.

Among the conditions that can trigger apoptosis, are irreparable DNA damage and excessive growth signaling. The p53 protein is a central link in these processes. It is activated by phosphorylation of specific residues and/or inactivation of its inhibitor MDM2. As shown in *Box 12.4*, p53 stimulates expression of the p21 protein which acts to promote cell cycle arrest. p53 also stimulates transcription of several proteins that are involved in both the mitochondrial and the FAS-mediated pathways of apoptosis. Because of its key role in all these processes, p53 has acquired the label 'guardian of the genome'. *TP53* is one of the most frequently mutated genes in all cancers.

12.3. **Investigations of patients**

CASE 20	Tierney family	200	213	**310**	376

- 4-year-old boy, Jason
- Pale with extensive bruising and tachycardia
- ? Acute lymphocytic leukemia
- Bone marrow test and check diagnosis
- TPMT enzyme analysis prior to 6-mercaptopurine treatment

Childhood acute lymphoblastic leukemia (cALL) is a neoplasm of B cell precursors or stem cells. About 25% of cases have a balanced reciprocal 12;21 translocation, with breakpoints at 12p13 and 21q22.3. At the translocation junction, the 5′ portion of the *TEL* (*ETV-6*) gene and almost the entire coding sequence of the *AML1* (*RUNX1* or *CBFA2*) gene, are brought together to create a fusion gene. Loss of function experiments in mice show that both *TEL* and *AML1* are critical genes for hemopoiesis. Each gene encodes a transcription factor. *AML1* encodes the alpha subunit of core binding factor, a master regulator of the formation of hemopoietic stem cells. The fusion inhibits normal AML1-mediated transcriptional activity, resulting in alteration of the capacity of hemopoietic stem cells to self-renew and to differentiate. Both genes are found as fusion partners with a variety of other genes encoding kinases or transcription factors in both lymphoid and myeloid leukemias. The *TEL–AML1* fusion appears to be unique to B cell progenitor ALL.

The positions of the *TEL/AML1* breakpoints in the pale-staining subtelomeric chromosome regions make the translocation hard to spot by conventional karyotyping. Diagnosis is based on FISH. Interphase cells from Jason were hybridized to differently colored FISH probes for the *TEL* and *AML1* genes. One of the colored spots marking the *TEL* genes always lay adjacent to one of the *AML1* spots, confirming the presence of the *TEL/AML1* fusion gene (*Figure 12.10*). This was good news because individuals with *TEL* rearrangements usually show an excellent response to chemotherapy. As described in *Chapter*

8, the induction and consolidation treatments were successful, but there were initial problems with his long-term maintenance treatment because Jason had thiopurine methyl-transferase deficiency which made him hypersensitive to one of the drugs used, 6-mercaptopurine. With a suitably low dose of the drug he remained healthy and disease-free.

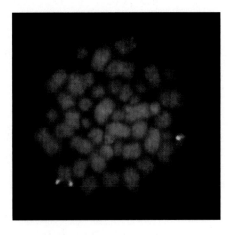

Figure 12.10 – Metaphase with *TEL–AML1* fusion.
The green signal is on the normal chromosome 12, one red signal is in the normal chromosome 21 and one is on the derived chromosome 12. The yellow *TEL–AML1* fusion signal is on the derived chromosome 21. Photo. courtesy of Dr Christine Harrison, University of Southampton.

| CASE 23 | Wilson family | 293 | **311** | 376 |

- ? Familial breast cancer
- DNA analysis for mutation

Since one woman in eight in the USA or UK is likely to develop breast cancer at some time in her life, it is not surprising that many families have more than one case. In affected women, 5–10% have a mother or sister with breast cancer, and about twice as many have either an affected first- or second-degree relative. Many of these represent chance coincidences, but statistical analysis suggests that in 5–10% of families the condition is truly familial. In 1990, linkage analysis in a large collection of multicase families pinpointed a possible susceptibility locus for early-onset breast cancer on chromosome 17. After 4 years of intensive work the *BRCA1* gene was identified by positional cloning. A further round of analysis in *BRCA1*-negative families led to identification of the *BRCA2* gene on chromosome 13.

BRCA1 and *BRCA2* are both large genes (*Figure 12.11*). *BRCA1* has 24 exons encoding a 1863 amino acid protein, and *BRCA2* has 28 exons encoding a 3418 amino acid protein. As mentioned above, such large proteins are likely to have multiple functions and many interacting partners. Our understanding of the roles of these proteins in the cell is still very incomplete. One main role is in detecting DNA damage and signaling its presence to cell-cycle checkpoints. There is also evidence for roles of these proteins in transcription control. *BRCA1* and *BRCA2* behave as TS genes, in that familial cases often involve inherited loss of function mutations, and tumors in familial cases show loss or inactivation of the remaining wild-type allele. Curiously, however, sporadic breast tumors very seldom have *BRCA1/2* mutations, although 10–15% of sporadic tumors silence *BRCA1* epigenetically. It may be that although cells with two *BRCA1/2* mutations have a significant tumorigenic potential, those with a single mutation have no enhanced potential over normal cells. In that case, there may be alternative routes that have a higher probability of leading to a sporadic tumor. Supporting this, expression array studies show different patterns of gene expression in sporadic breast tumors without *BRCA1* involvement, compared to those with either mutation or silencing of *BRCA1*.

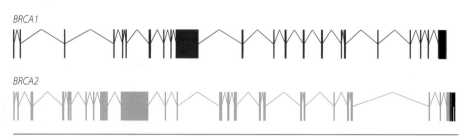

Figure 12.11 – Exon structure of *BRCA1* and *BRCA2* genes.
The two genes and proteins share no homology, and the expression array study shown in *Figure 12.16* suggests that they are involved in different pathways within cells. Both genes have one very large central exon (3426 and 4932 bp, respectively).

The Breast Cancer Information Core of the National Human Genome Research Institute (http://research.nhgri.nih.gov/bic/) lists about 1500 *BRCA1* and 1800 *BRCA2* sequence changes. An unknown number of these are coincidentally discovered non-pathogenic variants. Most definitely pathogenic changes are small frameshifting deletions or insertions, splice site mutations, or deletions of one or more whole exons. They can be identified through sequencing or any of the standard methods for scanning a gene (*Chapter 5*). The whole exon deletions are best detected by MLPA (*Figure 5.8*). Like most premature termination mutations, these are expected to trigger nonsense-mediated decay of the mRNA, so that the mutations act as null alleles, producing no (or maybe very little) truncated protein.

Ashkenazi Jews are a special case. Three specific frameshifting mutations (c.185delAG and c.5382insC in *BRCA1*, and c.6174delT in *BRCA2*) are common in this population, presumably because of founder effects (*Chapter 10*). A survey of 5318 healthy Ashkenazi women found 120 (2.2%) were carriers of one or other of the three mutations. This frequency contrasts with the 0.2% frequency of all *BRCA1/2* mutations in non-Ashkenazi white women in the USA or UK. The high frequency of these specific mutations makes genetic testing among Ashkenazim important and relatively straightforward. Of course, excluding those three mutations does not remove the risk that some other *BRCA1/2* mutation, or a mutation in another gene, may be putting the person at high risk. Other populations, for example French–Canadians, Icelanders and Pakistanis, also have their own particular founder mutations.

The lifetime risk for a mutation carrier has been variously estimated at between 30% and 85%. This illustrates an interesting feature of susceptibility testing. The initial estimates were made in the large multi-case families in which the mutations were first found. But these families were selected for having many affected cases, and so the initial estimates of risk are from a biased set of families. Population-based surveys show a lower risk. Nevertheless, the risk is still substantial compared to the risk for people who do not carry the mutations, and possibly particularly so in women with a strong family history. Thus there is considerable demand for mutation screening. Because these are large genes, and loss of function mutations may be found anywhere within the gene, screening for mutations is laborious and expensive. Clinicians need to prioritize families for screening, and this is done largely on the basis of the family history.

Markers of *BRCA1/2* mutations include:

- cases with unusually early onset
- bilateral cases (compare with the RB example)
- cases with male breast cancer (particularly a feature with *BRCA2* mutations)
- families with both breast and ovarian cancer (particularly a feature with *BRCA1* mutations)

None of these features is completely specific to *BRCA1/2* breast cancer, but risk indices have been developed based on these factors. *Table 12.4* shows one such index (Evans *et al.*, 2004). The indices allow physicians to assess the probability that any given case is likely to have a *BRCA1/2* mutation.

Table 12.4 – A scoring system to assess the likelihood of finding a *BRCA1* or *BRCA2* mutation in a family

Cancer, age at diagnosis (yr)	Points for *BRCA1*	Points for *BRCA2*
Female breast cancer, <30	6	5
Female breast cancer, 30–39	4	4
Female breast cancer, 40–49	3	3
Female breast cancer, 50–59	2	2
Female breast cancer, >59	1	1
Male breast cancer, <60	5 if *BRCA2* excluded	8
Male breast cancer, >59	5 if *BRCA2* excluded	5
Ovarian cancer, <60	8	5 if *BRCA1* excluded
Ovarian cancer, >59	5	5 if *BRCA1* excluded
Pancreatic cancer	0	1
Prostate cancer, <60	0	2
Prostate cancer, >59	0	1

Scores are summed for all cases in the family that are compatible with a dominantly inherited susceptibility. The total score is intended to represent the % chance of finding a mutation. Data from Evans *et al.* (2004) and reproduced here with permission from the BMJ Publishing Group.

β-catenin regulatory sequence
β-catenin-binding module
axin-binding module

Figure 12.12 – The APC protein and its role in regulating β-catenin levels.
The protein has 2843 amino acid residues. Three 15-amino acid modules bind
β-catenin and seven 20-amino acid modules down-regulate the level. APC
functions in a complex with axin and GSK3β. Somatic mutations are clustered in
the mutation cluster region (MCR). Because of the unusual exon–intron structure
of the *APC* gene only truncations in the green shaded part of the protein would be
eliminated by nonsense-mediated decay. Most mutations produce truncated APC
proteins that are unable to bind axin but can still bind β-catenin and have some
limited ability to down-regulate it.

This complexity depends on the unusual structure of the *APC* gene (*Table 12.5*).
The extremely large 3′ exon includes 6580 bp of the 8538 bp coding sequence.
Normally, nonsense and frameshifting mutations would produce none of the
predicted truncated protein because of nonsense-mediated decay (*Chapter 6*).
However, premature stop codons in the last exon of a gene, or within 50 nt of
the last splice site, are generally exempt from decay (*Figure 6.3*). The mutation
cluster region and all the β-catenin binding and regulatory modules are encoded
by the large last exon. Only stop codons before codon 640 of the *APC* gene
would be expected to trigger nonsense-mediated decay. Mutations in the 5′ end
of the gene are associated with an attenuated phenotype, with relatively few
polyps. Presumably these are true null mutations. Elsewhere it seems likely that
at least some of the truncated protein is produced, and its properties determine
the selective advantage of the second hit.

Christos Xenakis gave a blood sample, from which DNA was extracted for *APC*
mutation testing. This showed that he was heterozygous for a nonsense mutation
at codon 1309 of the *APC* gene (p.Glu1309X). This is a frequent mutation in
FAP. It is highly penetrant, so that mutation carriers have a near-100% risk
of developing colon cancer if untreated. Identifying it allowed at-risk family
members to be tested. Christos's mother Demi contacted several relatives of her
late husband in Cyprus to let them know about the newly discovered high risk in
the family, and gave them a contact number of the Seattle geneticist for use by
their local genetics service if any of them opted for testing. Meanwhile there were
Christos's two young children to consider. Each was at 50% risk, and they would
need annual sigmoidoscopy examinations from age 10 to check for development
of polyps. All this could be avoided if a DNA test showed that the child had not
inherited the mutation. The question arose whether to test them now or leave
it until later. Testing now would mean that an at-risk child could grow up with
the knowledge that he would need annual bowel screening and not have this
suddenly sprung on him; postponing testing would mean that the child, by age
10, would be more able to understand and consent to the procedure.

This family illustrates some of the ethical arguments about DNA testing in
children. Normally it is felt improper to test children for genetic susceptibility

Table 12.5 – The unusual structure of the *APC* gene

Exon	Size (bp)	Intron	Size (bp)
1	39	1–2	16 947
2	153	2–3	11 300
3	85	3–4	778
4	202	4–5	8238
5	109	5–6	5052
6	114	6–7	11 542
7	84	7–8	8749
8	105	8–9	14 111
9	99	9–10	3372
10	379	10–11	2551
11	96	11–12	5116
12	140	12–13	681
13	78	13–14	849
14	117	14–15	5978
15	215	15–16	2387
16	8686		
Total	**10 701**		

The open reading frame is 8538 nt, encoding a 2843 amino acid protein. Most mutations in polyposis coli are frameshifting or nonsense, but only those in exons 1–15 would be expected to trigger nonsense-mediated decay. Data from ENSEMBL (June 2006).

– for example in Case 21, Hannah Ulmer's parents were dissuaded from having their other children tested for Tay–Sachs carrier status. In the present case there are benefits for a child in being tested by age 10. For children at 50% risk of FAP, annual sigmoidoscopy surveillance needs to start around this time. It is clearly beneficial to a child to avoid this unpleasant procedure if he can be shown not to carry the family mutation. Only parental consent would be formally required for testing, but good practice would include discussing the issue with the child and obtaining consent as far as possible.

12.4. **Summary and extension**

Hereditary non-polyposis colon cancer

FAP, the condition in the Xenakis family (Case 24) is not the only form of inherited susceptibility to colorectal cancer. Some families show a clear history of dominantly inherited early-onset colon cancer but do not have polyps. The susceptibility maps to chromosome 2p22 in some families and to 3p21.3 in others. A study of loss of heterozygosity in the tumors gave the first clue to the molecular events. Genotyping with microsatellite markers showed a quite unexpected effect: instead of loss of heterozygosity at specific chromosomal locations, the investigators found the tumors often showed additional novel alleles of the marker. Moreover, the effect was not specific to one particular chromosomal location but was seen with microsatellites from all over the genome.

Microsatellites are short stretches of repetitive DNA sequence, often $(CA)_n$ (see *Chapter 9*). When DNA polymerase replicates such sequences it quite often makes mistakes, putting in an extra repeat unit or leaving one out. Such replication slippage occurs during PCR amplification, and is the cause of the extra bands ('stutter bands') seen when microsatellites are scored on gels (see *Figure 7.15b*). The same thing can happen during cellular DNA replication, but *in vivo* proof-reading mechanisms detect mismatches between the template and the newly synthesized strand, and correct the errors. The microsatellite instability seen in hereditary non-polyposis colon cancer (HNPCC) is a result of failure of this **mis-match repair** (MMR) machinery.

The MMR machinery is quite highly conserved from *E. coli* through to man, and one route by which the human MMR genes were cloned was by searching for the human homologs of so-called mutator genes in yeast. Six genes are involved in the process in man (*Table 12.6*). Of these, mutations in *MSH2* and *MLH1* are the usual causes of HNPCC. They act as TS genes: one loss of function mutation can be inherited, and the remaining functional allele is inactivated in the tumor by somatic mutation or epigenetically (see below). Sporadic cases have both gene copies silenced somatically, by mutation or promoter methylation.

Why should a defect in a general mechanism like MMR specifically cause colon cancer? Partly the answer is that it can in fact cause other cancers. Microsatellite instability is sometimes seen in other tumors, especially gastric and endometrial tumors. Partly the answer can be found by looking for the likely consequences of a failure of MMR. Transforming Growth Factor B (TGFβ) is a strong inhibitor

Table 12.6 – Genes involved in mismatch repair

Gene	OMIM number	Location	Percentage of HNPCC
MSH2	609309	2p22p21	60%
MLH1	609310	3p21.3	30%
MSH6	600678	2p16	5% (atypical)
MLH3	604395	14q24.3	Rare or absent
PMS1	600258	2q31q33	Rare or absent
PMS2	600259	7p22	Rare or absent

Mutations in *MSH6* (*GTBP*) have been mainly described in women with endometrial cancer rather than colon cancer.

of cell proliferation in the colorectum. It acts through a cell-surface receptor of which the TGFBR2 (TGFβ receptor 2) protein is part. The *TGFBR2* gene contains a run of 10 consecutive A nucleotides in exon 3 of the coding sequence (*Figure 12.13*). MMR-deficient cells are liable to insert or skip one or more As. This creates a frameshift and renders the new copy non-functional. One survey found somatic *TGFBR2* mutations in the tumors of 100/111 cases of colon cancer with microsatellite instability. Several other relevant targets have been noted, that is, genes with relevant functions that contain microsatellite-like sequences.

```
743  TGC  ATT  ATG  AAG  GAA  AAA  AAA  AAG  CCT  GGT  GAG  ACT  TTC
120  Cys  Ile  Met  Lys  Glu  Lys  Lys  Lys  Pro  Gly  Glu  Thr  Phe
```

Figure 12.13 – Part of the sequence of exon 3 of the *TGFRB2* gene.
A run of 10 consecutive As makes replication of the gene vulnerable to defects in mismatch repair.

A rather similar effect has been suggested in the *APC* gene. A mis-sense variant, p.Ile1307Lys, is carried by about 6% of Ashkenazi Jews, and a much smaller proportion of other people. The variant appears to be a low-penetrance susceptibility allele for colon cancer, roughly doubling the normal risk. The DNA sequence change creates an unbroken run of As (*Figure 12.14*), suggesting a vulnerability to MMR defects. However, unlike with *TGFBR2*, there is no evidence that this run is preferentially mutated in HNPCC, so the susceptibility effect may operate at the protein level.

```
GCA  GAA  ATA  AAA  GAA  AAG     →     GCA  GAA  AAA  AAA  GAA  AAG
Ala  Glu  Ile  Lys  Glu  Lys           Ala  Glu  Lys  Lys  Glu  Lys
```

Figure 12.14 – The p.Ile1307Lys colon cancer susceptibility allele of the *APC* gene.
Note the run of 8 As created by the mutation.

The multistage development of cancer

Pathologists have long known that malignant tumors develop through stages marked by increasing growth and de-differentiation. FAP offers exceptional opportunities for studying the process. When the colon is surgically removed from an FAP patient, it often contains lesions showing every stage of tumor development. Vogelstein and colleagues (summarized in Kinzler and Vogelstein, 1996) analyzed such series, together with sporadic colon tumors, for mutations in candidate genes and loss of heterozygosity. They found some alterations that were often present in the early stages, and others that only appeared in later stages. Putting their observations together, they proposed the developmental scheme shown in *Figure 12.15*.

The earliest stages are the most critical, because these mutations must cause instability or a growth advantage in a relatively normal cell that still has most of its defenses intact. Probably there are only a small number of ways of achieving this, but a larger number of ways of developing once the initial stages are negotiated. Cells with HNPCC mutations may have a wider range of possible evolutionary paths towards cancer, but many of the same players are involved. Tumors lacking *APC* mutations often have mutations in other

Figure 12.15 – A possible common pathway for the development of colon cancer.
The scheme (see Kinzler and Vogelstein, 1996) summarizes the way that some
genes are often inactivated in early lesions, while others are inactivated only
in late-stage lesions. There has been some controversy about the general
applicability of this scheme, and there is no suggestion that every colon cancer has
developed exactly in this way.

components of the same pathway, for example, β-catenin or axin. Tumors
lacking *RAS* mutations commonly have mutations in the *BRAF* gene, which has
similar functions. As mentioned above, TGFβ signaling is an important negative
regulator of cell growth in the colon. Within the cell, the TGFβ receptor signals
by phosphorylating serine or threonine residues in SMAD proteins. This pathway
is commonly subverted in colorectal cancer, by *TGFBR2* mutations in cancers
with MMR defects, or in non-HNPCC cancers by loss of chromosome 18 where
the *SMAD4* gene is located.

Broadening this approach, Vogelstein considered the balance between cell birth
and cell death. Since adult tissues and organs remain a constant size, there must
be some mechanism to regulate this balance. Vogelstein suggested that in each
tissue there is one critical gene that governs the balance. He called such genes
'gatekeepers'. Mutations in tissue-specific gatekeepers would be initiating events
in tissue-specific cancers. Once the tumor has initiated, progression will depend
on the ability of the cell to maintain its defenses against disordered growth. He
named the genes responsible for this as 'caretakers'. Thus tumors initiate with
mutations in gatekeepers and progress with mutations in caretakers. This picture
clearly fits colorectal cancer; how far it is generally applicable is debatable. At
the very least, it is a nice tool for thinking about carcinogenesis.

Epigenetics in cancer

As we noted in *Chapter 7*, it is not clear how extensive is the role of epigenetic
mechanisms in inherited disease. However, there is no dispute about their
importance in cancer. Studies of DNA methylation in tumor cells show a
somewhat paradoxical picture. On the one hand, the general level of methylation
is reduced in many tumor cells compared to their normal counterparts. On the
other, many CpG islands are hypermethylated. About half of all genes have
a CpG island associated with their promoter (see *Chapter 7*). In normal cells
these islands are not methylated, regardless of whether the related gene is
active or silent. Promoter methylation (of isolated CpG dinucleotides) controls
expression of genes that lack CpG islands, but not of those with islands. In
cancer cells, however, genes that have CpG island promoters are often silenced

by methylation. There is some evidence that tumors can be divided into those where many islands are methylated and those where this does not occur, implying the existence of some general mechanism favoring aberrant island methylation. It is claimed that tumors with extensive methylation of islands are clinically and etiologically distinct from those lacking this feature.

TS genes are silenced by promoter methylation at least as frequently as by mutation. The relative importance of these two routes varies from gene to gene. Several genes are known that are always silenced epigenetically and never by mutation, while for others the reverse is true, and for yet others both processes are common. For example *MLH1* is often silenced epigenetically, but *MSH2* never is. Jones and Baylin (2003) provide a review of this topic, with many examples and some speculation about mechanisms. One such speculation is that the hypomethylation of centromeres might predispose cancer cells to chromosomal instability. This is based in part on the observation that in ICF syndrome (OMIM 242860), deficiency of the *DNMT3B* DNA methyltransferase results in aberrant packing of centromeric heterochromatin.

Are familial breast and colon cancer really multifactorial conditions?

In the case of the Wilson family (Case 24), the result of mutation screening explained the strong family history. However, many multicase breast cancer families do not have mutations in either of the *BRCA1/2* genes. Mutations in *BRCA1* or *BRCA2* explain only around 25% of the overall familial tendency of breast cancer. Sustained searches have failed to reveal any *BRCA3* gene that could account for any significant proportion of the remaining cases. It seems likely that the remaining familial tendency is polygenic, made up of the combined effects of several low-penetrance loci (Antoniou *et al.*, 2002). A consortium has been set up to test candidate genes for such low penetrance effects on susceptibility (National Cancer Institute Breast and Prostate Cancer Cohort Consortium, 2005).

One such locus has been definitively identified. *CHEK2* (OMIM 604373) is a gene involved in the detection and signaling of DNA damage. A frameshifting deletion, c.1100delC, was found in the *CHEK2* gene in 201/10860 (1.9%) unselected breast cancer patients but only 64/9065 (0.7%) controls. This gave a relative risk of 2.34. The data suggested that the variant doubled whatever risk a woman had due to other factors. Overall, a female carrier of the 1100delC mutation had a lifetime risk of breast cancer of 13.7%, compared to 6.1% for a non-carrier. However, by itself the variant accounted for only 0.7% of the total population incidence of breast cancer, a figure lower than many lifestyle factors such as parity, weight and physical activity. Thus it is not clear under what circumstances it would be worth screening for the variant. Other possible low penetrance factors are variants in the *STK15* and *PTPRJ* genes (Lesueur *et al.*, 2005). Looking for these low penetrance susceptibility factors, and deciding what to do when they are found, takes us into the area of susceptibility to common multifactorial disease, which is the subject of the following chapter.

A somewhat similar but less striking situation is seen in colon cancer. The lifetime risk in the USA is 5–6%. About 20% of all colorectal cancer patients have two or more first or second degree relatives with colon cancer; 5–10% of cases show more or less mendelian inheritance. FAP and HNPCC account for about 4% of all colon cancers; the rest of the familial tendency is probably the effect of several low-penetrance susceptibility alleles.

Expression profiling of tumors

Every tumor is genetically unique. As Hanahan and Weinberg (2000) show, there are many different ways of achieving the six capabilities listed in *Box 12.1*. Different genes in a pathway can be activated or inactivated by point mutations, epigenetic changes or chromosomal events. Many of the gene products are multifunctional, and so in addition to the effect that is the target of natural selection, there may be all sorts of other incidental effects. Tumors evolve in a sea of genetically unstable cells harboring a diversity of relevant and incidental mutations. The real targets for therapy must be the small minority of the cancer cells in a tumor that have stem cell-like properties. For a physician trying to decide the optimal management and prognosis for a patient, there is a great need to define a shortlist of relevant changes. For Jason Tierney (Case 20) identifying the *TEL–AML1* fusion gave this information. For breast cancer patients, looking for amplification of the *HER* receptor is a start, as it defines the responsiveness to Herceptin. But this is still a long way from using all the genetic information in a tumor.

Tumor expression profiling holds out the hope of doing this. Bulk mRNA or cDNA from the tumor is dye-labeled and hybridized to a microarray, probably in a competitive assay to compare it with the repertoire of mRNA in the relevant normal tissue. The microarray carries oligonucleotides corresponding to unique regions of cDNA from every gene in the genome, and hopefully all the major splice variants. The University of Utah Genetic Science Learning Center (see *References*) has a very nice animated website explaining from ground level the principles of expression array analysis in cancer. These experiments generate huge amounts of data. The investigator has to try to extract a 'signature' or pattern of expression of a limited number of genes that defines the prognosis or the response of the tumor to anticancer drugs. *Figure 12.16* shows an example of expression signatures. An editorial placing this work in a broader context is available (Hedenfalk, 2002).

Statistical analysis by hierarchical clustering, as in *Figure 12.16*, allows signatures to be extracted that in several cases have been shown to be predictive of drug response or prognosis (see, for example, Glinsky *et al.*, 2005). It remains to be seen whether these signatures can be translated into useful clinical tools. There are two problems to be overcome. The first is that a single microarray experiment produces a vast volume of data that can be analyzed in many ways. This makes it hard to know the significance of any reported signature. The second problem is a very common one in translating research into clinical practice. A test may discriminate efficiently between two groups, but that does not necessarily mean that it can assign an individual accurately to the

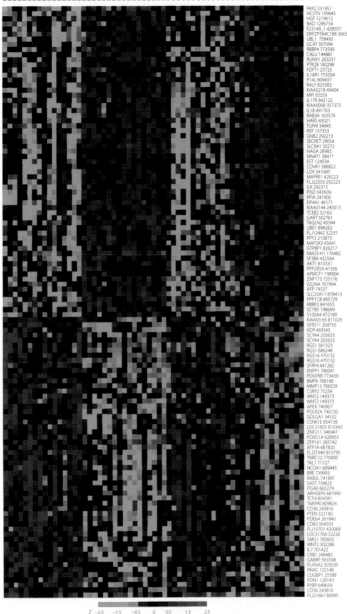

Figure 12.16 – Expression profiling of ovarian tumors.
This is not a picture of a microarray; it is a large table showing the expression pattern of 110 genes, selected from 7651 on the microarray, in 61 individual ovarian tumors. Each column is the data from one tumor, each row is the data for one gene. Expression levels are color coded (green = significantly reduced expression, red = significantly raised expression). Results are clustered by statistical analysis in a way that reveals common patterns: 18 of the tumors carried a *BRCA1* mutation, 16 had a *BRCA2* mutation and 27 had neither ('sporadic'). The expression profiles distinguish the *BRCA1* and *BRCA2* patterns, and show that different sporadic tumors fit one or other of these two patterns. Evidently *BRCA1* and *BRCA2* mutations cause ovarian cancer by different routes, and sporadic tumors follow one or other of these pathways. Reproduced from Jazaeri *et al.* (2002) with permission from Oxford University Press.

appropriate group. Some expression signatures do allow a statistical prediction, and can distinguish between groups of tumors with good and poor prognosis – the question is whether they are sufficiently specific to give a useful prediction for an individual patient. Some researchers feel it will be more profitable to study the total protein repertoire in a tumor using proteomic technology (2-dimensional gel electrophoresis, mass spectrometry, etc.).

von Hippel–Lindau disease

Patients with von Hippel–Lindau disease (OMIM 193300) are at risk of developing a variety of tumors (*Table 1*). The most frequent causes of death are renal cell carcinoma or hemangioblastomas in the central nervous system. The disease is autosomal dominant, with an incidence of 1 in 35 000–45 000. 95% of gene carriers have developed one or more of the characteristic tumors by age 65. Because the different manifestations of the disease may be treated by different clinicians, the connection between them is not always made promptly, leading to delays in establishing the diagnosis. One role of clinical geneticists can be to act as a central point of reference for the family, and to co-ordinate the different surveillance programs that need to be put in place for family members.

Table 1 – Patients with von Hippel–Lindau disease may develop a variety of tumors and require careful surveillance

Tumor	Frequency	Mean age at presentation	Screening	Age to start screening
Hemangioblastoma of CNS	60–80%	33 years	Annual craniospinal MRI	11 years
Hemangioblastomas of retina	60%	25 years	Annual ophthalmoscopy	Infancy
Endolymphatic sac tumors	11%	22 years	CT or MRI	When symptoms occur
Renal carcinoma	24–45%	39 years	Annual CT scan of abdomen	18 years
Pheochromocytoma	10–20%	30 years	Annual plasma or 24 hr urinary catecholamine	2 years

Data from Lonser *et al.* (2003).

The *VHL* locus was mapped to 3p25–26, and the gene was identified by positional cloning. It behaves as a classic TS gene. Patients inherit one loss of function mutation, and in their tumors the second copy is inactivated by mutation, deletion or methylation. 70–80% of sporadic renal clear cell carcinomas show inactivation of both copies of the gene. The gene is small (3 exons encoding a 213 amino acid protein) and mutation detection is relatively straightforward.

The expression of the disease varies between families (*Table 2*). In some families affected people never seem to develop pheochromocytomas, while in other families these are frequent. This has led to the disease being divided into Types 1 and 2. Type 2 has been further subdivided into 2A, 2B and 2C. All forms are caused by mutations in the *VHL* gene. Loose genotype–phenotype correlations have been established: deletions and truncating mutations usually cause Type 1, while Type 2 families usually have mis-sense mutations. Particular mis-sense mutations are associated with the different sub-types of Type 2. Renal cell carcinoma is more frequent in Type 1 than in Type 2 families.

Table 2 – Clinical subtypes of von Hippel–Lindau disease tend to breed true within families

Type	Pheo.	RCC	Hem.
1	–	+	+
2A	+	–	+
2B	+	+	+
2C	+	–	–

Pheo, pheochromocytoma; RCC, renal cell carcinoma; Hem, hemangioblastoma.

Investigation of the pathogenic mechanism has focussed on the relation of the VHL protein to the HIF-1α (hypoxia-inducible factor 1α) protein. The VHL protein is part of an E3 ubiquitin ligase complex (VCB-Cul2) that controls the level of HIF-1α by degrading it when oxygen levels are normal (*Figure*). HIF-1α is flagged for degradation by hydroxylation of specific proline residues in an oxygen-dependent reaction. VHL protein acts as the recognition component of the ubiquitin ligase: it directly binds hydroxylated HIF-1α. Pathogenic mis-sense mutations in VHL cluster in the HIF-1α-binding region of the protein. Under conditions of hypoxia HIF-1α is stabilized. It then acts as a multifunctional transcriptional activator. Among its many targets are VEGF (vascular endothelial growth factor), a powerful promoter of angiogenesis. It is noteworthy that the tumors in von Hippel–Lindau disease are all particularly highly vascularized. Other targets of HIF-1α include the growth factor TGFα and enzymes promoting glycolysis and glucose transport.

Hypoxia-inducible factor 1α causes major adjustments to cell metabolism in response to hypoxia. Cul2, cullin-2; EloB, elongin B; EloC, elongin C; Rbx1, cullin regulatory protein. In VHL cells, HIF is constitutionally active.

VHL protein appears to have other functions independent of HIF-1α (Barry and Krek, 2004). Although this protein is much smaller than the giant scaffold proteins encoded by some other tumor suppressor genes (see above), a surprising number of possible binding partners have been identified. VHL protein binds cyclin D1, leading to possible effects on the cell cycle. Effects on the extracellular matrix, via binding to fibronectin, and on the cytoskeleton via association with microtubules, may be significant in invasiveness and metastasis. In addition, VHL protein has recently been shown to bind directly to p53 and stabilize it against MDM2-mediated degradation.

12.5. References

Albuquerque C, Breukel C, van der Luijt R, *et al.* (2002) The 'just right' signaling model: *APC* somatic mutations are selected based on a specific level of activation of the β-catenin signaling cascade. *Hum. Molec. Genet.* 11: 1549–1560.

Antoniou AC, Pharoah PDP, McMullen G, *et al.* (2002) A comprehensive model for familial breast cancer incorporating BRCA1, BRCA2 and other genes. *Br. J. Cancer,* **86:** 76–83.

Barry RE and Krek W (2004) The von Hippel–Lindau tumor suppressor: a multi-faceted inhibitor of tumorigenesis. *Trends Mol. Med.* **10:** 466–472.

Cavenee WK, Dryja TP, Phillips RA, *et al.* (1983) Expression of recessive alleles by chromosomal mechanisms in retinoblastoma. *Nature,* **305:** 779–784.

Evans DGR, Eccles DM, Rahman N, *et al.* (2004) A new scoring system for identifying a *BRCA1/2* mutation outperforms existing models including BRCAPRO. *J. Med. Genet.* 41: 474–480.

Glinsky GV, Berezovska O and Glinskii AB (2005) Microarray analysis identified a death-from-cancer signature predicting therapy failure in patients with multiple types of cancer. *J. Clin. Invest.* **115:** 1503–1521.

Hanahan D and Weinberg RA (2000) The hallmarks of cancer. *Cell,* 100: 57–70. *Readers who are not strong on cell biology may need to skip the detail, but this is an excellent introduction to a modern view of cancer.*

Hedenfalk IA (2002) Gene expression profiling of hereditary and sporadic ovarian cancers reveals unique *BRCA1* and *BRCA2* signatures. *J. Natl. Cancer Inst.* **94:** 960–961. *Free full text at* http://jncicancerspectrum.oxfordjournals.org/cgi/content/full/jnci;94/13/960

Jazaeri AA, Yee CJ, Sotiriou C, *et al.* (2002) Gene expression profiles of *BRCA1*-linked, *BRCA2*-linked, and sporadic ovarian cancers. *J. Natl. Cancer Inst.* **94:** 990–1000.

Jones PA and Baylin SB (2003) The fundamental role of epigenetic events in cancer. *Nature Rev. Cancer,* 3: 415–428.

Kinzler KW and Vogelstein B (1996) Lessons from hereditary colorectal cancer. *Cell,* **87:** 159–170.

Lesueur F, Pharoah PD, Laing S, *et al.* (2005) Allelic association of the human homologue of the mouse modifier *Ptprj* with breast cancer. *Hum. Molec. Genet.* **14:** 2349–2356.

Lonser RR, Glenn GM, McClellan W, *et al.* (2003) Von Hippel–Lindau disease. *Lancet,* 361: 2059–2067.

National Cancer Institute Breast and Prostate Cancer Cohort Consortium (2005) A candidate gene approach to searching for low-penetrance breast and prostate cancer genes. *Nature Rev. Cancer,* **5:** 977–985.

Pardal R, Clarke MF and Morrison SJ (2003) Applying the principles of stem-cell biology to cancer. *Nature Rev. Cancer*, 3: 895–902.

Useful websites

Cancer Genome Anatomy Project Education resources: http://cgap.nci.nih.gov/info/EducationResources

University of Utah Genetic Science Learning Center section on expression analysis in cancer: http://gslc.genetics.utah.edu/units/biotech/microarray/

12.6. Self-assessment questions

(1) In relation to tumorigenesis, for each of the following statements decide if it is:
  (a) true of both oncogenes and tumor suppressor genes
  (b) true of oncogenes but not tumor suppressor genes
  (c) true of tumor suppressor genes but not oncogenes
  (d) true of neither tumor suppressor genes nor oncogenes.

  (1) May show nonsense mutations in sporadic cancers
  (2) May encode proteins involved in cell cycle regulation
  (3) Frequently mutated in familial and sporadic cancers
  (4) Often involved in loss of heterozygosity in sporadic cancers
  (5) Frequently mutated in familial but not sporadic cancers
  (6) May indirectly act to inactivate telomerase
  (7) Often involved in chromosomal rearrangements in sporadic cancers
  (8) May show inherited mis-sense mutations in familial cancers
  (9) Frequently mutated in sporadic but not familial cancers
  (10) May show gene amplification in familial and sporadic cancers

(2) Blood and tumor DNA was extracted from two unrelated children with retinoblastoma and typed for a 2-allele DNA marker that maps close to the *RB1* gene. One child has a family history of retinoblastoma while the other has a sporadic unilateral tumor. The genotypes were:

	Child A	Child B
Blood	Heterozygous 2–1	Homozygous for allele 1
Tumor	Homozygous for allele 2	Homozygous for allele 1

Mark each of the following statements as true or false:
(a) the result indicates that Child B has the sporadic form of the disease
(b) the result indicates that Child A has the familial form of the disease
(c) the result indicates that the tumor in Child B could be either homozygous or hemizygous for the marker.
(d) the result indicates that if Child A has the inherited form of the disease, he inherited it on the chromosome that carries allele 2 of the marker.

(3) Neurofibromatosis 2 (OMIM 101000) is the result of inherited and/or somatic mutations in the *NF2* tumor suppressor gene. Inherited NF2 shows 90% penetrance. Assuming a mutation rate of 2×10^{-4} per gene per cell, what is the size of the target cell population? What is the expected incidence of sporadic NF2?

(4) The *Figure* shows two families in which there are several cases of cancer (B, breast; O, ovarian; P, prostate; numbers are the age at diagnosis). Which of the two women marked with a question mark would you prioritize for *BRCA1/2* mutation screening?

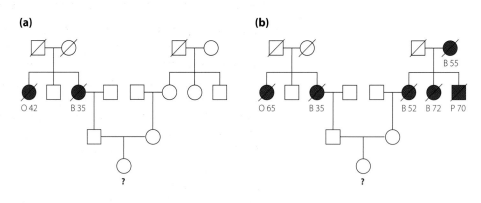

Chapter 13

Should we be testing for genetic susceptibility to common diseases?

Learning points for this chapter

After working through this chapter you should be able to:

- Describe how modifier genes, and stochastic and pleiotropic effects, result in variable expressivity and incomplete penetrance, even for mendelian conditions
- Describe in principle how genes interact with other genes and with various environmental factors to produce phenotypes including disease
- Describe the multifactorial nature of most human traits, both normal and abnormal, and the principles of multifactorial inheritance
- Explain quantitative trait loci
- Describe Falconer's threshold theory and use it to make qualitative predictions of risk
- Describe the principle of affected sib pair analysis
- Define and compare linkage and association between a marker and a disease
- Describe and explain the haplotype block structure of the human genome
- Describe the problems and prospects for identifying susceptibility factors through association studies

13.1. Case studies

CASE 25	Yamamoto family	**329**	341	376

- Family history of dementia
- ? Alzheimer disease
- Test for ApoE4?

Bill Yamomoto's mother had been getting increasingly forgetful. After a series of incidents including one when she left a pan on the cooker and set the kitchen on fire, it became clear that she was not coping with life on her own. She moved into sheltered accommodation in the same Californian town as Bill and his wife. She never adjusted to her new surroundings and soon required residential care.

Over the next 3 years her dementia progressed until she seldom recognized Bill and was unable to do anything for herself. It was almost a relief when she died at the age of 71 – as Bill said, 'my real mother died several years ago'.

When a friend of his wife said that Alzheimer disease was hereditary, Bill started to worry. He knew that his aunt Yumiko – his mother's sister who had always lived in the old family home in Hawaii – had been diagnosed with Alzheimer

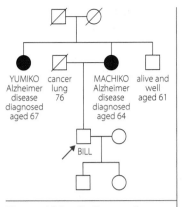

Figure 13.1 – Pedigree of Yamomoto family.

disease at the age of 67. His wife suggested he should to talk to his physician. The doctor told him that only the rare forms of the disease with onset before age 60 were inherited. Bill was still not entirely reassured.

Searching on the internet, he discovered that a genetic factor, ApoE4, was associated with susceptibility to the common late-onset form of the disease, and he came across companies offering to test for ApoE4. He wondered whether he should take the test, and decided to consult a geneticist. He wanted to know whether the test was reliable for somebody of Japanese ancestry like himself, and what he should do if the result was positive.

CASE 26	Zuabi family	**330**	345	376

- Woman aged 52 years, Zafira
- Overweight; sedentary lifestyle; insatiable thirst
- Type 2 diabetes
- Test son

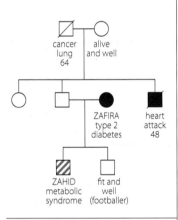

Figure 13.2 – Pedigree of the Zuabi family.

Zafira was 52 when she consulted her physician about a 3-month history of dizziness, headaches and blurry vision. She also mentioned that she had developed a terrible thirst, leading her to drink large amounts of water every day and produce correspondingly large amounts of urine. Her urine was found to contain sugar, and a fasting glucose test showed a level of 9 mmol/l. This confirmed the diagnosis of Type 2 diabetes (T2D). She was given a thiazolidenedione drug as the first line of treatment. Enquiry showed that she had an entirely sedentary lifestyle, and her body mass index (BMI) was 30; she was enrolled on a program of graded moderate exercise. Both exercise itself and weight loss help minimize morbidity in T2D.

The shock of diagnosis made Zafira think about her family. Her brother had died of a heart attack aged 48. He had been badly overweight and completely inactive, though she did not remember him drinking especially large amounts of water. When she learned that first-degree relatives of T2D patients were at high risk of developing the condition (her physician quoted a risk of 38% for a child of an affected parent), her thoughts turned to her elder son Zahid. He did not have overt disease, but he shared several risk factors. He went to work by car, took the lift to his office, spent all day sitting at his desk, enjoyed a good meal then spent the evening watching television. Not surprisingly he was overweight. He agreed to come for some tests. These showed that his BMI was 30 with a waist measurement of 99 cm. His fasting plasma glucose was 6.4 mmol/l, below the 7.0 threshold for T2D, but above normal. He was hypertensive (blood pressure 142/90 mmHg) and had dyslipidemia (triglycerides 1.9 mmol/l). His combination of obesity, impaired glucose tolerance, dyslipidemia and hypertension defined him as having the 'metabolic syndrome' (*Table 13.1*). This is a rather loosely defined but well-known precursor of T2D and a major risk factor for cardiovascular disease (reviewed by Eckel *et al.*, 2005). He was prescribed exercise and antihypertensive drugs.

Table 13.1 – World Health Organization definition of the metabolic syndrome (1999)

Feature	Measure
Diabetes	Fasting glucose > 7.0 mmol/l
Or impaired fasting glycemia	Fasting glucose 6.1–7.0 mmol/l
Or impaired glucose tolerance	
Or insulin resistance	Hyperinsulinemic
PLUS 2 or more of:	
Obesity	BMI > 30 or waist-to-hip ratio >0.9 (male) or 0.85 (female) (different figures may be appropriate for non-white people)
	Triglycerides ≥1.7 mmol/l or
Dyslipidemia	HDL cholesterol (male) <0.9 or (female) 1.0 mmol/l
Hypertension	>140/90 mm Hg
Microalbuminuria	Albumin excretion >20 µg/min

Other bodies have produced somewhat different but overlapping definitions. The list shows the complex of interacting characters that indicate susceptibility to Type 2 diabetes and cardiovascular disease. The prevalence of the syndrome rises with age, among US adults from 7% at age 20–29 to 44% at age 60–69. Prevalence is 50% in severely obese US youngsters, and is increasing at all ages and in most countries of the world.

13.2. **Background**

Two models of genetic determination

Traditionally, genetic characters have been divided into mendelian and **polygenic**. Polygenic conditions depend on the combined action of a very large number of genetic factors, each of which makes only a very small contribution to the final phenotype. Both categories, mendelian and polygenic, are conceptual models, useful tools for thinking about inheritance – but in reality, all conditions fall somewhere between the two. For any particular character, you need to decide what mix of the two conceptual models gives the best description, and then you need to add in environmental effects. *Figure 1.15* showed a linear spectrum of genetic phenotypes. Adding in environmental effects, the overall etiology of any disease might be represented by a point somewhere inside the triangle of *Figure 13.3*. 'Multifactorial' or 'complex' are useful non-committal terms for conditions that fall in the interior of the triangle.

Genes are always mendelian, but *characters* are never wholly dependent on the genotype at a single locus. Closer acquaintance with any mendelian disease reveals that these 'simple' conditions are actually not so simple. As described in *Chapters 6* and *8*, the quest for genotype–phenotype correlations seldom yields the desired neat result. The long road between a DNA sequence variant and an observable phenotype allows many additional players, environmental, genetic and simply chance ('stochastic'), to join the action. The concept of *penetrance* allows you to lump all these other factors together and not try to analyze them. Identified genes that influence the expression of a basically mendelian character are called **modifier genes**.

Figure 13.3 – Etiology of diseases.
For any condition the overall balance of genetic and environmental determinants can be represented by a point somewhere within the triangle.

Dichotomous versus quantitative characters

You can divide all human characters into two sorts:

- dichotomous or discontinuous characters, like diseases and malformations, that you either have or do not have
- continuous or quantitative characters, that everybody has, but to differing degrees; examples would be height, weight or blood pressure.

Characters of either sort can be genetically determined, though continuous characters cannot be mendelian. Gene loci involved in determining continuous characters are called **quantitative trait loci (QTL)**. The whole QTL field has been mainly developed by animal and plant geneticists concerned with improving continuous characters like milk yields or corn production. Some QTL may be the result of the same simple loss of function or gain of function mutations that underlie most mendelian characters. However, in many cases QTL variants are likely to have more subtle effects on gene function. Variants in promoters or other control elements could result in small changes in the level of expression. Sequence changes might slightly alter the stability of the mRNA or the balance of splice isoforms. The lactase gene variant responsible for persistence of intestinal lactase (see *Box 8.4*) might be a typical example. The same gene could cause a mendelian condition if it has a mutation of major effect, and act as a QTL with more subtle changes. Equally, a genetic change may have a major effect on one character and be a QTL for another.

Polygenic theory

Models of polygenic inheritance consider characters that depend on the combined action of a large number of genetic factors, each of which makes only a small contribution to the final phenotype. The main use of these models in human genetics is not to make predictions, but to provide a framework for thinking about complex genetic conditions. For any actual condition the framework needs to be populated by empiric epidemiological data. The two elements of the framework that are most relevant to clinical genetics are the concepts of **heritability** and of **thresholds**, as described below.

Heritability is estimated by comparing the incidence of a character in relatives of affected people with the incidence in the general population. For continuous characters it is calculated from the correlation between relatives. It is a number between 0 (no genetic involvement) and 1 or 100% (no non-genetic factors). Heritability is symbolized as h^2, reflecting its origin in polygenic theory as a correlation coefficient. The concept of heritability is often misunderstood, leading at times to its misuse in political arguments about whether or not to try to prevent a condition by social action. As long as its limitations are understood, heritability is a useful measure for researchers investigating a complex condition because it gives a guide to the relevance of genetic factors under the circumstances prevailing at the time.

The heritability of a condition is not a measure of how the condition is caused physiologically or biochemically in a person. In fact, it is not a statement about individuals at all, but about a population. Mathematically, it is the proportion of the phenotypic variance that is attributable to genetic variance. The question that heritability answers is, how much of the differences between people, in this particular society and at this particular time, are the result of the genetic differences between them, and how much are they the result of differences in people's environments?

Heritability is not a fixed property of a condition. If occurrence of a condition is affected by both genetic and environmental factors, its heritability will be high if most members of the population share a relatively uniform exposure to the relevant environmental factors, and low if exposure differs greatly between people. For example, a part-genetic condition that is also associated with poverty and social deprivation will have a higher heritability in an egalitarian society than in one with great inequalities. New environmental factors can change the heritability. For example, 100 years ago phenylketonuric mental retardation was wholly genetically determined. Nowadays, in societies where neonatal screening and dietary treatment are available, its causes are almost entirely environmental – lost samples, a family that couldn't be traced or that are unable to make sure a homozygous child sticks rigidly to the diet. This example underlines the fact that heritability is a property of a character at a particular place and time, and not an intrinsic property of a gene.

Thresholds are concepts used to explain how dichotomous characters can be polygenic. In its simplest form, polygenic theory applies only to continuously variable quantitative characters that show a Gaussian distribution in a population. The geneticist DS Falconer, used the concept of thresholds to show how the polygenic theory could be extended to dichotomous characters (*Box 13.1*). In clinical genetics, thinking about thresholds helps make sense of the way risks for complex conditions, unlike risks for mendelian conditions, depend on family history.

Investigating the genetics of complex diseases

Claims for genetic factors in complex disease need to be backed by evidence. This normally comes from three types of study.

- *Family studies* look at relatives of affected probands and ask how much more likely they are to be affected, compared to an unrelated person. The risk ratio is symbolized as, λ, with a subscript denoting the relationship. For example, λ_s is the relative risk for a sib of a proband (*Table 13.2*). High values of λ suggest genetic factors – but it is important to remember that the same effect could be produced by shared family environment. Because we give our children their environment as well as their genes, it is not safe simply to rely on family studies, especially for behavioral traits.
- *Adoption studies* separate the effects of genes and family environment. For example, children of schizophrenic parents who were adopted at birth into unaffected families have a significantly increased risk of developing schizophrenia, compared to their adoptive sibs. This suggests that the familial tendency of schizophrenia is due to genetic factors rather than parental behavior.

Box 13.1

Polygenic susceptibility to a disease

Although diseases are dichotomous characters (some people have the disease and others do not), threshold theory postulates that susceptibility to the disease is a continuous character. The susceptibility is a quantitative character that depends on the combined small effects of many genes. It shows a bell-shaped distribution in the population. Most people have a middling susceptibility; a few have very high or very low susceptibility. Only people whose susceptibility exceeds a certain threshold develop the disease (see top part of figure).

Distribution of susceptibility in the general population (top), with threshold. Distribution in relatives (bottom).

If you have an affected relative, that person must have had a high genetic susceptibility. They have a 'bad hand' of high-susceptibility genes. You share genes with your relatives (see *Box 10.3*). You may be lucky and share only a few of your relative's high susceptibility genes, or you may be unlucky and share many. Overall, there will be a wide distribution of susceptibility among relatives of affected people, but the curve will be displaced towards the high-susceptibility end compared to the distribution in the general population (see bottom part of figure). Relatives of affected people are more likely than unrelated people to end up above the threshold. The closer the relationship, the more likely this is. Therefore complex diseases tend to run in families, but the tendency is much weaker than with mendelian diseases (*Table 13.2*).

The idea can be extended in several ways.

- To allow for environmental factors, we could suppose that, rather than a single fixed threshold, there will be an increasing risk of developing the disease across some range of high susceptibilities.

- Thresholds can be sex-specific. The classic example is pyloric stenosis. This is much more common in boys than girls (5M : 1F). The threshold must be lower in boys than girls, for some physiological reason. To be affected, a girl must have a particularly high susceptibility. On average, affected girls have higher susceptibility genes than affected boys. Therefore relatives of affected girls are at higher risk of pyloric stenosis than relatives of affected boys.

Although these models can be developed mathematically, they are mainly useful as qualitative tools for thinking about recurrence risks. They lead to the general rule:

Box 13.1 – continued

In complex disease, the worse luck (many affected people; the less common sex affected) a family have had in the past, the greater is the risk of a recurrence.

Note the complete contrast between complex and mendelian diseases in this respect. If by bad luck all your three children have cystic fibrosis, the risk your next child will be affected is still 1 in 4. But if you had two babies rather than one baby with a neural tube defect, the risk to the next baby changes from 1 in 25 to 1 in 12. Having a second affected child didn't change your risk, but it changed our understanding of the risk you always had.

Table 13.2 – **Examples of recurrence risks for mendelian and multifactorial diseases**

Disease	λ_s	Lifetime risk (to age 80)
Cystic fibrosis	500	0.05%
Huntington disease	5000	0.01%
Celiac disease	60	3%
Multiple sclerosis	25	1%
Type 1 diabetes	15	6%
Type 2 diabetes	4–6	7–35%
Testicular cancer	8	2%
Alzheimer disease	4	35%
Breast cancer	2	14%

λ_s is the relative risk for a sib of a proband, compared to an unrelated person. Compare the risks for the mendelian conditions (shaded rows) with the complex conditions. These are **empiric risks**, derived from surveys of families, not from theoretical calculations. They can vary between populations and also over time (the latter presumably because of environmental changes). When using such risks for counseling it is important to use risks derived from studies appropriate to the consultand's background. Data from Dr Alison Stewart, Cambridge.

- *Twin studies* look at affected people who have a twin. They compare monozygotic (MZ) and dizygotic (DZ) twins to see how often the co-twin is also affected. MZ twins share all their genes while DZ twins share on average half their genes; twins should share their environment to the same degree regardless of zygosity. Thus a higher concordance among MZ twins is evidence for genetic factors. MZ twins separated at birth and brought up in different environments form the perfect study, but their numbers are too small to provide anything more than fascinating anecdotes.

The end result of family, twin or adoption studies is an estimate (see *Figure 13.4*) of the heritability of the condition.

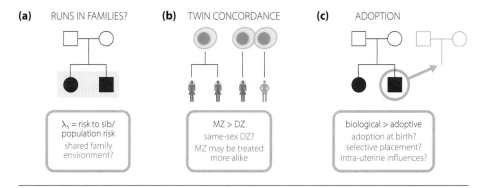

Figure 13.4 – Methods of demonstrating genetic effects in complex diseases, and reasons for caution in interpreting the results.

Linkage studies to identify susceptibility factors

Having decided that genetic factors do play a role in susceptibility to your chosen disease, the next step is to identify the factors. This is a great deal easier said than done. As with mendelian diseases the usual first approach is through linkage analysis (*Chapter 9*). The laboratory method is the same: appropriate family members are typed for a large panel of genetic markers, and the data analyzed to find markers that co-segregate with the disease. However, the analysis is different. Standard lod score analysis requires the researcher to tell the computer the penetrance for each genotype, the gene frequencies, and the mutation rate. For mendelian diseases it is usually possible to make a plausible guess about these parameters, but there is no way this can be done for complex conditions. It is therefore necessary to use **non-parametric linkage analysis.**

Non-parametric analysis uses families with more than one affected person and considers the extent to which the affected family members share genes. Genes, unlike characters, are always mendelian, and it is easy to calculate the expected sharing among any set of relatives. Affected relatives should show excessive sharing of any gene or marker that is involved in causing the disease, quite regardless of the mode of inheritance. The commonest approach uses affected sib pairs.

Affected sib pair analysis

The principle of affected sib pair (ASP) analysis is to form a collection of affected sib pairs (100–500 pairs would be typical) and to type them for a genome-wide panel of markers. Consider a pair of sibs with a mendelian recessive condition. *Figure 13.5* shows how they would share alleles at a marker locus that either was or was not closely linked to their disease locus. *Table 13.3* generalizes this. Regardless of the mode of inheritance, markers that are linked to a susceptibility locus should be shared by the affected sibs more often than by chance.

ASP analysis is an extremely robust method of non-parametric linkage analysis. There are no built-in assumptions that might be proved wrong. However, the chromosomal regions it defines are very large. With a mendelian disease, as we saw in *Chapter 9*, you can pursue linkage analysis in big families down to

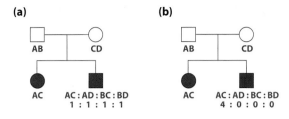

Figure 13.5 – Sharing of marker alleles by a pair of sibs who are both affected by a mendelian recessive disease.
(a) A marker that is on a different chromosome from the disease locus. (b) A marker that is closely linked to the disease locus. A, B, C, D represent different alleles at the marker locus.

Table 13.3 – Expected sharing of marker alleles by a pair of affected sibs

Marker	Sibs share no alleles	Sibs share 1 allele	Sibs share 2 alleles
Not linked to disease locus	¼	½	¼
Tightly linked to rare mendelian dominant	0	½	½
Tightly linked to rare mendelian recessive	0	0	1
Linked to common disease susceptibility locus	< ¼	> ½	> ¼

The figures for mendelian diseases assume that both sibs have the same alleles at the disease locus, which will normally be true as long as disease alleles are rare in the population. For a common disease susceptibility locus, one cannot predict the exact proportions, only the direction in which the proportions will deviate from the random expectation.

the last recombinant, and can hope to define a candidate region that contains only a handful of genes. But the complex disease susceptibility factors are neither necessary nor sufficient for disease to develop. As a result, even when a significant result is found, the candidate region is likely to be 20–50 Mb. Such a large region has somehow to be narrowed down before mutation testing becomes possible. Association studies are ideal for this.

Detecting susceptibility factors by association

Ancestral chromosome segments

During prophase I of meiosis there are an average of 60 crossovers per cell in males and 90 in females. An average chromosome might be split into two or three segments. Thus when sibs share chromosome segments, these tend to be large. As we move from sibs to more and more distant relatives, the likely size of any shared ancestral segment gets smaller. Consider a chromosomal segment that two distant relatives, Bob and Carol, have inherited from a shared ancestor

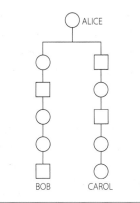

Figure 13.6 – Bob and Carol both inherit a chromosomal segment from their great-great-great grandmother Alice. Recombination events in ten meioses have reduced the size of the segment that is shared by Bob and Carol.

(*Figure 13.6*). A segment 10 cM long will have only a 1% chance of not being broken up by recombination in one or more of the ten meioses that separate Bob and Carol.

Bob and Carol probably did not know they were related. They each have 32 great-great-great grandparents, and even if they were both enthusiastic family historians, it is highly unlikely they would know about all 32 of them and would have identified all their many descendants. The same argument applies to every segment of every chromosome in every person. People who thought themselves unrelated, share small chromosome segments that are inherited from a distant common ancestor. The more distant the ancestor, the smaller the shared segment will be, but the larger will be the number of people who share it. N generations ago you had 2^N ancestors (*Figure 13.7*). Each ancestor in turn would have on average 2^N descendants if the population size remained constant. Going back even 20 generations (say 500 years, to 1500), 2^{20} is over 1 million. Ultimately we are all related. The word 'unrelated' will be used here, as elsewhere in genetics, to mean people who do not share any great grandparent.

The relevant shared ancestor is the most recent common ancestor. This ancestor is likely to be more recent in a small isolated population than in a large outbred population, and the shared segments will be correspondingly larger (for a recent ancestor) or smaller (for a distant ancestor). For different chromosomal segments the common ancestor will be different, and the people with whom we share the

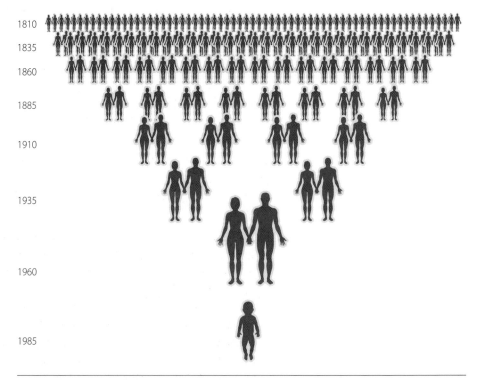

Figure 13.7 – N generations ago a person has 2^N ancestors. This number quickly exceeds the population of most countries a few hundred years ago. Even allowing for inbreeding and the isolation of communities, we are all related through distant common ancestors. (From an idea by Dr Bryan Sykes.)

segment will be different. Each chromosome segment will include polymorphic markers that have particular allelic variants on that chromosome. Whatever set of marker alleles an ancestral segment carried, those same alleles will be shared by all the present-day people who inherited it, barring occasional mutations.

Shared ancestral segments and disease associations

Suppose one such ancestral segment contained a gene conferring susceptibility to diabetes. A collection of present-day unrelated diabetics would tend to share that chromosome segment. The gene is neither necessary nor sufficient to cause diabetes, so not every diabetic will share this segment, and some non-diabetic people will have it – but insofar as having the gene increases susceptibility, affected people are more likely than unaffected people to have that ancestral segment.

Looking for such shared segments is the basis of association studies in complex disease. A few hundred or a few thousand unrelated affected people are collected, and typed for a large number of genetic polymorphisms. SNPs are the polymorphisms of choice, partly because of their abundance and the availability of high-throughput SNP genotyping methods, but also because they are less likely than microsatellites to mutate. Microsatellites are liable to mutate by replication slippage (see *Section 12.4*); the rate of mutation is low enough to make them stable markers for the linkage studies in nuclear families that are used for mendelian diseases, but when you are looking for ancestral chromosome segments that have been transmitted through a hundred generations, it is safer to use SNPs.

As we have seen, the shared segments are expected to be small. The HapMap project (see below) suggests a few kb would be typical. Thus it is necessary to test the samples for markers located every few kilobases in order not to miss a shared segment. If an ancestral segment carries a disease susceptibility factor, a marker allele that is found on that segment will be present at higher frequency in the affected people than in controls.

Using association to find susceptibility factors

There are three ways in which association studies can contribute to identifying susceptibility factors for complex diseases. In increasing order of difficulty, these are as follows.

- *Checking candidate genes.* Knowledge of the pathology of a disease or of animal models will usually suggest some plausible candidate genes. SNPs in and around a candidate gene are often tested for disease associations. The choice of SNPs can be informed by knowledge of the haplotype block structure around the candidate gene (see below).
- *Combined linkage and association strategy.* Linkage defines large segments shared by closely related people, which can be detected with a few hundred markers spaced across the genome. Association defines very short segments shared by 'unrelated' people. The dbSNP database lists around 10 million SNPs, one per 300 bp on average. Therefore, for the most part there are sufficient SNPs available to be able to detect shared segments that are only a few kb long. A natural strategy is therefore to

use linkage (affected sib pairs) to define large candidate regions, and then to try to narrow down the candidate region by high-density SNP genotyping to seek associations.

- *Whole genome association studies*. Continuing development of high-throughput genotyping technology has made it feasible to conduct association studies across the whole genome. One SNP every 5 kb, or even every 1 kb would be needed to sample every possible ancestral chromosome segment. That translates to 600 000 to 3 000 000 SNPs. As described below, an exceedingly stringent threshold for statistical significance of an association must be used, because of the large number of potential associations studied. This in turn means that very large sample sizes are needed. The resulting scale of work is beyond the means of all but the most lavishly funded institutions or collaborations. One approach to reducing the scale is to work in small isolated populations. Because most people share relatively recent common ancestors, the shared segments are on average larger, and can be detected with fewer markers. That is the basis of, for example, the DeCode project (see www.DeCode.com) that studies the population of Iceland.

The results of these approaches in Alzheimer disease and Type 2 diabetes are described in the next section. In the final section we will take a more general look at the promise and limitations of linkage and association studies in complex disease.

Interpreting associations

A successful association study might show that allele X of marker Y is 20% more frequent in people with disease Z than in controls. This does not necessarily mean that X confers susceptibility to Z. Alternative explanations include:

- the association is a statistical fluke (a Type 1 error) and would not be found in a second independent sample
- the cases and controls were badly matched; X is irrelevant to the disease, but cases were drawn from a population subgroup that happened to have a higher frequency of X than the controls
- X does not itself confer any susceptibility to disease Z, but it is present on the same ancestral chromosome segment as the true susceptibility factor; this is an example of **linkage disequilibrium** – see *Box 13.2*.

In *Section 13.4* we discuss how to distinguish between these possibilities and identify the true cause of an association.

13.3. **Investigations of patients**

For multifactorial diseases there is seldom any benefit from genetic investigations of *individual* patients – whether in the future there might be more benefits is discussed in the final section. However, investigations of *groups* of patients have been the mainstay of research into genetic susceptibility for all complex diseases. Such studies are now the mainstream of clinical genetic research. Therefore for the two diseases described in Cases 25 and 26 for this chapter, we

Box 13.2

Linkage and association

Linkage is a relation between **loci**, not between alleles. In the example shown in *Table 9.1* the *D1S252* locus is linked to the dyschromatosis locus. That is the case regardless which allele a particular chromosome carries at the disease and marker loci.

Association (in a genetic example) is a relationship between **alleles** or phenotypes. A particular marker allele, not the marker locus, is associated with a disease. The association is with the actual disease (the phenotype), not with a disease susceptibility locus that might have high-risk and low-risk alleles. An allele at one marker locus may also be associated with an allele at another marker locus.

Linkage does not imply a population-based association. For example, in *Figure 9.7*, a variety of different alleles are seen for each marker, both on disease-carrying and on normal chromosomes. Within a family, there is an association – for example, within Family 1 all but one of the 10 affected individuals have *D1S2777* allele 1 on their disease-carrying chromosome. But the association is only within that family. Affected people in the other families have allele 3 or 5 of this marker.

Linkage and association overlap when the family and the general population overlap. Where many members of the present day population share ancestral chromosome segments, to that extent they are all members of one huge extended family, and loci that are linked within those segments will produce population associations between the relevant alleles. This is usually called **linkage disequilibrium**. Strictly speaking, linkage disequilibrium is a phenomenon that can have other evolutionary causes. However, when human geneticists talk about linkage disequilibrium they always mean allelic association due to shared ancestral chromosome segments.

will first describe the advice that a geneticist might give to an anxious relative, and then describe the research on groups of affected individuals. The final section will set these examples into a more general framework.

| **CASE 25** | Yamamoto family | 329 | **341** | 376 |

- Family history of dementia
- ? Alzheimer disease
- Test for ApoE4?

When Bill Yamomoto talked with the geneticist, she confirmed his physician's statement that only early onset Alzheimer disease was strongly inherited. The condition in Bill's mother and aunt was the common late-onset form. Both forms are defined by the same post-mortem brain pathology, with abundant extracellular senile plaques and intracellular neurofibrillary tangles (*Figure 13.8*), but the late-onset form is not simply inherited. Bill pressed the geneticist about ApoE4. She confirmed that there is a statistical association with late-onset Alzheimer disease, and that this was valid in Japanese as well as in people of European origin. A number of studies had shown an E4 allele frequency of 0.25–0.3 in Japanese Alzheimer disease patients, compared to 0.10 in controls. However, she advised against testing. She showed him a statement on ApoE testing issued by a working group of the American College of Medical Genetics and the American Society of Human Genetics (1995) which concluded '... at the present time it is not recommended for use in routine clinical diagnosis nor should it be used for predictive testing'.

When Bill suggested this attitude was patronizing, she asked what he would do if the result was positive. 'Ask you what I must do to avoid developing the disease' he replied. 'But there's nothing I could tell you. There is no proven way of preventing Alzheimer disease, though there are drugs that may slow the progression. The best you can do is keep your mind active – but I would say that to anybody, regardless of their circumstances. And what would you do if the result was negative?' 'Celebrate!'. 'But you would be wrong – plenty of ApoE4-negative people go on to develop Alzheimer disease. The association is only statistical. It is not predictive for an individual.' She gave him a copy of an article by Holzman on genetic testing to take away and read, as a caution against some of the persuasive sounding offers on the internet (Holzman, 1999). The consultation did not reassure Bill about his risk, but it did persuade him that spending money on testing would not provide the reassurance he wanted.

(a) (b)

Figure 13.8 – The characteristic brain pathology of Alzheimer disease
(a) Amyloid plaques and (b) neurofibrillary tangles. Photos courtesy of Dr Simon Lovestone, Institute of Psychiatry, London.

About 1% of Alzheimer disease cases have onset before age 60. These early onset cases are often familial and often behave as mendelian dominant conditions. Those that do are amenable to standard linkage analysis and positional cloning. These approaches have identified three causative genes (*Table 13.4*).

Table 13.4 – Known causes of early onset Alzheimer disease

Gene	OMIM no.	Location	Number of recorded families	Product
APP	104760	21q21	39	Amyloid precursor protein
PSEN1	104311	14q24	258	γ-secretase subunit
PSEN2	600759	1q31	15	γ-secretase subunit

The total number of recorded families is from Bertram and Tanzi (2004). In total these causes explain only a tiny fraction of all Alzheimer disease; the great majority of cases are late-onset and non-familial.

The senile plaques in Alzheimer disease consist largely of β-amyloid protein, while the neurofibrillary tangles consist of tau protein. β-amyloid is derived from the amyloid precursor protein (APP) by proteolytic cleavage. APP is a 695 amino acid brain protein that is cleaved by the γ-secretase enzyme, producing $A\beta_{40}$ and $A\beta_{42}$ peptides. $A\beta_{42}$ is thought to be the pathogenic variant. γ-secretase is a complex of five polypeptides including the PSEN1 and PSEN2 gene products. The rare mendelian forms of Alzheimer disease have clearly implicated amyloid as a cause of the pathology, and not just a side effect of some other cause.

Geneticists have much to offer members of families affected by early onset Alzheimer disease. Linkage and mutation detection can be used to try to identify a causative mutation. If one is discovered, predictive testing can be offered, similarly to Huntington disease. A suitable protocol is described in the following chapter (*Box 14.2*). However, as Bill Yamomoto discovered, with the late onset form we are still in the research phase and, at present, genetic services have nothing useful to offer. Many linkage and association studies have been performed to try to identify susceptibility factors, but with the exception of *APOE*4*, discussed below, the results have not yet identified either useful predictors of disease or valuable new drug targets.

For linkage analysis, affected sib pairs are the most obvious material. People classed as unaffected may develop Alzheimer disease later, so studies are best limited to affected people. Multi-generation families are seldom available, and seeking out such families biases the research sample towards earlier onset cases, that may not be typical. Many genome-wide linkage studies have been reported, but all have shown low lod scores. *Box 13.3* shows a widely accepted set of significance thresholds for whole-genome screens. Using these criteria, no investigation has found a *highly significant* result. Among *significant* or *suggestive* results, chromosomal regions implicated in one genome-wide trawl have seldom been replicated in others. These rather disappointing results are

---

Box 13.3

Thresholds of significance in genome-wide linkage studies

In *Chapter 9* we saw that the threshold for significance of a lod score is 3.0. The probability of getting so high a lod score if there is really no linkage to that marker is 0.05. If we use hundreds of markers to scan the whole genome, the chance that one or another of them will give a false positive result is clearly higher than if we use just a single marker. The question of how much higher is quite difficult statistically. Following Lander and Kruglyak (1995), the results of a whole genome linkage trawl can be categorized as:

- highly significant evidence for linkage (lod score > 5.4)
- significant evidence for linkage (lod score > 3.6)
- suggestive evidence for linkage (lod score > 2.2)

These thresholds are chosen to give chances of 0.001, 0.05 and 1, respectively, of finding such a high lod score once in a whole-genome linkage scan on the null hypothesis of no true linkage. Scores in the lower categories carry little weight until independent studies have replicated them.

typical of linkage studies of complex diseases; possible reasons are discussed in *Section 13.4*. However, there is some support for several possible locations. The review by Bertram and Tanzi (2004) lists 12 chromosomal regions with evidence for linkage from more than one study, and discusses the evidence supporting each. In total, this work has suggested several chromosomal regions that are worthy of further investigation, but has not mapped any definite susceptibility factors other than 19q13, the location of the *APOE* gene.

About 100 genes in all have been examined for Alzheimer disease-associated variants. These include positional candidates suggested by the linkage studies, and candidate genes suggested from the pathology of Alzheimer disease. Many associations have been reported but none apart from *APOE*4* has been convincingly confirmed. Again, Bertram and Tanzi (2004) review the evidence. Apart from *APOE*4*, the findings of the many studies provide intriguing pointers to further research, but they do not identify any definite Alzheimer disease susceptibility factors. The relevance of *APOE*4*, however, has been confirmed in many studies and is undisputed.

The *APOE* gene on chromosome 19q13 encodes apolipoprotein E. Many variants of ApoE have been described (see OMIM 107741) but only three are common polymorphisms. E2, E3 and E4 are coding sequence variants producing ApoE proteins with either cysteine or arginine at positions 112 and 158 (*Table 13.5*). These differences produce functional differences in lipid handling. The E4 variant is associated with higher levels of plasma total cholesterol and LDL cholesterol than in E3 homozygotes. The gene frequencies have been studied in many populations. E4 is the ancestral allele, found in non-human primates, and it remains frequent in populations where foraging is still important. In settled agricultural populations the frequency of E4 is low.

Table 13.5 – The common apolipoprotein E variants and their gene frequencies in various populations

	Residue 112	Residue 158	Spanish	UK	Chinese	Japanese	Native American	Khoi San
E2	Cysteine	Cysteine	0.052	0.089	0.105	0.048	0.0	0.077
E3	Cysteine	Arginine	0.856	0.767	0.824	0.851	0.816	0.553
E4	Arginine	Arginine	0.091	0.144	0.071	0.101	0.184	0.370

Data from Corbo and Scacchi (1999) *Ann. Hum. Genet.* **63**: 301–310.

E4 is a risk factor for both coronary artery disease and late-onset Alzheimer disease among people living in Westernized environments. Among Europeans and North Americans of European origin, heterozygosity or homozygosity for *APOE*4* result in a 3-fold and 15-fold increase, respectively, in risk of Alzheimer disease; *APOE*4* accounts for 20–30% of the total risk. It is associated with both higher risk and earlier age of onset. However, the mechanism producing this increased risk is unclear.

Bertram and Tanzi (2004) conclude their review by asking 'What should we tell the patients?'. Their answer is, not much, yet. They echo the views of several expert panels that have advised against using ApoE or any other alleged risk factor for clinical purposes. ApoE4 is neither necessary nor sufficient for Alzheimer disease. ApoE genotyping would not assist the diagnosis in a person with possible Alzheimer disease, and it would not usefully predict the likelihood of somebody developing Alzheimer disease. A British study concluded that the predictive power was too low to affect insurance underwriting, even for long-term care insurance (Warren, 1999). ApoE is quite properly tested as part of the investigation of dyslipidemias, and this raises the tricky question of whether patients should be told results that are irrelevant to their lipid problem and may be disturbing. Inevitably ApoE testing is also available over the internet – but the result can only be false optimism or false pessimism for anybody who takes it seriously.

| CASE 26 | Zuabi family | 330 | **345** | 376 |

- Woman aged 52 years, Zafira
- Overweight; sedentary lifestyle; insatiable thirst
- Type 2 diabetes
- Test son

Diabetes mellitus, defined by hyperglycemia > 7 mmol/l fasting, > 11 mmol/l non-fasting, or a glucose tolerance test, is a heterogeneous condition. In addition to many minor types, the two major types are:

- Type 1 (T1D) – a sudden onset disease in young people, the result of an autoimmune attack on the pancreatic β-cells, and not associated with obesity
- Type 2 (T2D) – normally with adult onset, associated with obesity and physical inactivity, without autoimmune features, and resulting from a combination of inadequate secretion of insulin and resistance to its effects

These two separate diseases both involve genetic susceptibility and environmental factors. For T2D, evidence for environmental factors comes from the alarming recent increases in prevalence (in the USA a 40% increase among adults during the period 1990–1999, with further increases since 1999), and from intervention studies showing the efficacy of weight control and exercise. Evidence for genetic factors comes from family and twin studies, and from the ethnic variations in prevalence. λ_s is 4–6 and many studies have reported higher concordance in monozygotic compared to dizygotic twins. A positive family history confers a 2.4-fold increased risk; 15–25% of first-degree relatives of T2D patients develop impaired glucose tolerance or overt diabetes. The prevalence varies greatly between different ethnic groups, even when members of the groups live intermingled in multiethnic communities. Some variants of T2D (MODY and mitochondrial T2D, see below) are inherited as single-gene conditions, but these make up less than 10% of the total.

As regards genetic advice, the Zuabi family is fairly typical. An overlapping set of problems – T2D, cardiovascular disease, coronary heart disease – cluster loosely in families. The metabolic syndrome is a clear predictor of risk, as are its individual components. While a strong family history predicts increased risk, there is little scope for specifically genetic advice: the general advice for every overweight and inactive person, regardless of family history, is to get some exercise and lose some weight. The many possible drugs are prescribed according to the physiology and not the genetics.

The recent epidemic increases in T2D in many countries have stimulated intensive efforts to understand its causes. As regards genetic causes, more than 50 family or sib pair linkage studies and numerous association studies have been reported. The results for T2D have been typical of many complex diseases.

Linkage studies: using the Lander–Kruglyak criteria (*Box 13.3*), no investigation found a highly significant result. Only a few regions gave significant evidence in a single scan, or have been consistently replicated in other studies. Most studies found lod scores that were suggestive at best, and that did not coincide with suggestive locations from other studies. Almost every chromosome region has shown suggestive evidence of linkage in one or another study, and almost none of the suggestive linkages has been replicated. *Table 13.6* summarizes the most positive results from this huge amount of work.

Association studies: only one putative susceptibility factor has been identified by following through the two-stage strategy outlined in the previous section. Positional cloning under the linkage peak at 2q37 eventually pointed to the

Table 13.6 – **Possible locations for T2D susceptibility loci suggested by linkage analysis**

Initial study			Supportive study	
Population	**Location**	**Lod**	**Population**	**Lod**
Pima Indians	1q25.3	4.1	American Caucasians	4.3
			French Caucasians	3.0
			UK Caucasians	1.5
Mexican–Americans	2q37.3	4.1	American Caucasians	2.2
			Chinese	2.1
Mexican–Americans	3p24.1	3.9	Mexican–Americans	1.3
			Mexican–Americans	2.7
			Finnish Caucasians	1.1
French Caucasians	3q28	4.7	Japanese	1.4
			Australian Aborigines	1.8
Mexican–Americans	10q26.13	3.8	UK Caucasians	2.0
Finnish Caucasians	12q24.31	3.6	American Caucasians	1.5
			Pacific Islanders	3.7
			Finnish Caucasians	1.9
Finnish Caucasians	18p11.22	4.2	American Caucasians	2.4

These have been selected from the much larger number of studies that showed insignificant lod scores at these locations. Reproduced from Florez *et al.* (2003) with permission. © 2003 Annual Reviews www.annualreviews.org.

calpain-10 (*CAPN10*) gene. Calpain-10 had not been on anybody's list of likely susceptibility factors, showing the power of positional cloning to produce novel insights into pathogenesis. In the original study, susceptibility was ascribed to a combination of three non-coding SNPs whose functional significance was completely unclear. However, many subsequent studies have failed to clarify the nature of the susceptibility determinant, and not all have confirmed its existence. In a possible second example, SNPs in the calsequestrin (*CASQ1*) gene under the 1q25 linkage peak, have been tentatively associated with increased risk of T2D.

Most association studies have picked genes thought likely to be involved in the pathogenesis, rather than chromosomal regions suggested by linkage studies. *Figure 13.9a* shows the self-reinforcing pathogenic cascade that produces the hyperglycemia and increased free fatty acids of T2D, while *Figure 13.9b* shows the complicated events controlling insulin signaling. Clearly the list of possible candidate genes is very long.

These studies have reported more than 30 other genes as harboring susceptibility variants, but as with the linkage studies, very few of the claimed associations have been replicated. A huge **meta-analysis** including over 25 000 cases has confirmed the role of a mis-sense variant (p.Pro12Ala) in the *PPARG* gene which encodes a nuclear hormone receptor. The common Pro allele (frequency 85% in Europeans) confers a modestly increased risk (risk ratio 1.27), but because it is so common, this polymorphism accounts for about 25% of the population attributable risk (see *Chapter 11*) for T2D. Variants in two of the targets of drugs commonly used to treat T2D have also been fairly convincingly implicated in disease susceptibility (*ABCC8* and *KCNJ11*).

The relationship between single-gene and complex forms: a common view of complex disease susceptibility is that genes in the relevant pathways will have major mutations causing mendelian disease and minor variants acting as susceptibility factors in complex disease. Mendelian forms of T2D are well-known. MODY (maturity-onset diabetes in the young) is an autosomal dominant condition with early onset. There is no association with obesity or lifestyle, but otherwise it closely resembles the adult onset form. Linkage, positional cloning and candidate gene approaches, have identified seven different genes in which mutations can cause MODY (see OMIM 606391). Identification of these genes has shed light on the mechanisms controlling glucose homeostasis and the insulin response. Has it also helped us understand T2D susceptibility? The present answer has to be 'very little'. Only one of the MODY genes (*HNF4A, MODY1*) falls under a replicated T2D linkage peak (at 20q13, too weak to include in *Table 13.3* but supported by lods of 2.2 and 2.9 in Finns and Chinese). Initial studies found no association in adult onset disease, but some recent studies lend cautious support to a role of *HNF4A* SNPs in T2D susceptibility.

Several different mutations in mitochondrial DNA have been linked to diabetes, often complicated by other features such as deafness. There is some evidence of mitochondrial malfunction in typical T2D (see Stumvoll *et al.*, 2005), but no mitochondrial DNA variant has been significantly associated with the common type of T2D.

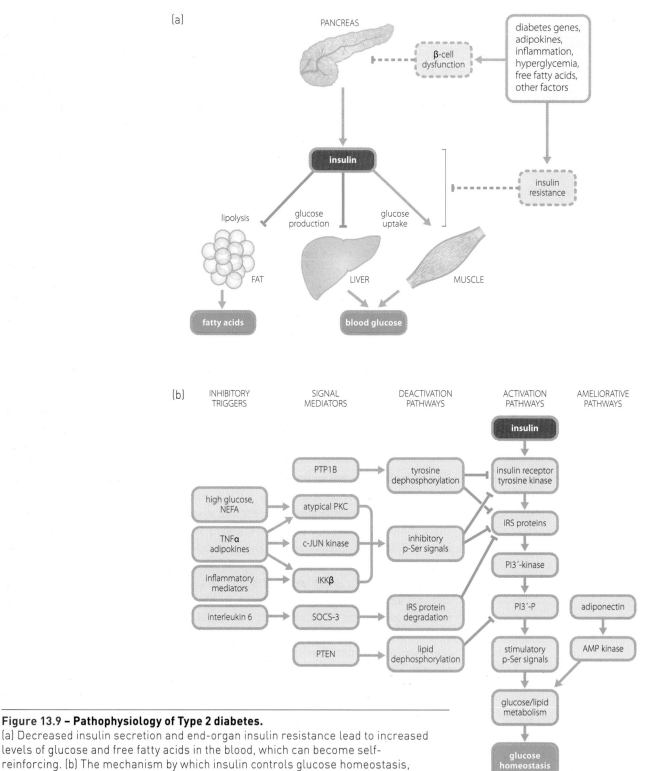

Figure 13.9 – Pathophysiology of Type 2 diabetes.
(a) Decreased insulin secretion and end-organ insulin resistance lead to increased levels of glucose and free fatty acids in the blood, which can become self-reinforcing. (b) The mechanism by which insulin controls glucose homeostasis, and factors influencing it. NEFA, non-esterified fatty acids; TNFα, tumour necrosis factor α; PTP1B, phosphotyrosine phosphatase 1B; PKC, protein kinase C; IKKβ, NFκB inhibitory unit kinase (an activator of NFκB); SOCS-3, suppressor of cytokine signaling-3; IRS, insulin receptor substrate; PI, phosphoinositol. Both figures reproduced from Stumvoll *et al.* (2005) with permission from Elsevier.

Overall, genetic research into adult onset T2D has been marked by massive investments of time and resources for very meager returns. Some people claim this is because the wrong hypothesis is being obstinately pursued, and that T2D is in fact a disorder of epigenetic programing, as described in *Chapter 7*. However, given the very large numbers of possible players in the pathogenesis (see *Figure 13.9*), it is entirely likely that the problem is extensive genetic heterogeneity with no gene variants having a major effect. The review by Florez *et al.* (2003) is recommended reading, not for the factual detail but because it gives a good picture of the extreme difficulty of reaching definitive conclusions in this field.

13.4. **Summary and extension**

The examples of Alzheimer disease and T2D are quite typical of the frustrating nature of research into the genetics of complex diseases. The whole area has proved very much more difficult than most people expected. When the genetics community embarked on ASP studies of common disease in the early 1990s, many people believed that most factors would be identifiable by testing a few hundred affected sib pairs. In the event, lod scores were generally weak and studies of every disease were plagued by inability to replicate positive findings.

Failure to replicate a finding does not necessarily mean it was wrong. An initial whole genome study will report any region that gives an interesting lod score. A replication study has to find a good score for that particular region – clearly a more demanding task. If there are a dozen or more susceptibility loci, but the studies are only marginally powerful enough to detect any effect of any of them, it is quite unlikely that one study will replicate the findings of another. Understandable though this may be, it doesn't help researchers trying to identify true linkages among a sea of not very significant results. Although the ASP method is robust, calculations by Risch and Merikangas (1996) showed that it is only able to detect highly potent susceptibility factors (*Table 13.7*). The conclusion from 15 years of effort is that susceptibility to most common diseases is the cumulative result of many weak factors rather than a few strong ones.

The Risch and Merikangas paper was hugely influential because it not only identified a problem but proposed a solution. They showed that association studies could detect far weaker susceptibility factors than linkage analysis, using feasible numbers of subjects. Their calculations helped to stimulate a major shift away from linkage and towards association studies. Usually these took the form of case–control studies of polymorphisms in candidate genes suggested by the known biochemistry or physiology of the disease in question. However, association studies face a number of problems.

Table 13.7 – **Numbers of affected sib pairs needed to detect a disease susceptibility factor**

Relative risk of disease due to this locus	5x	3x	2.5x	2x	1.5x
Probability of allele sharing by affected sibs	0.634	0.556	0.536	0.518	0.505
Number of affected sib pairs needed to detect effect	94	559	1366	5379	67805

Affected sib pairs are powerful for detecting factors that raise the risk by a factor of more than 3. The poor track record of affected sib pair analysis suggests that most risk factors have a smaller effect than this. Data from Risch and Merikangas (1996).

Problems with association studies

Multiple testing

Association studies have once again produced a flood of reported positive results, very few of which have been confirmed. The review by Florez *et al.* (2003) gives a good flavor of the data in one area. One problem is multiple testing. When a large number of SNPs are tested for association to a disease, it is necessary to think about the threshold for statistical significance. Consider the two possible thresholds:

- a 0.05 chance that *this particular SNP* would show a deviation this large from random expectation
- a 0.05 chance that *any one of 1000 SNPs tested* would show a deviation this large from random expectation

Clearly a result that is significant using the more stringent threshold is more believable. This is analogous to the linkage thresholds shown in *Box 13.3*. The most rigorous correction for multiple testing (**Bonferroni correction**) is to multiply the P value for each single question by the number of questions asked. So with 1000 SNP tests an individual P value of 0.00005 is needed to give an overall P value of 0.05. Naturally researchers are loathe not to report an association with a P value of 0.0001 if this is the best result from many months of hard work.

Replicating a positive finding

If there are 20 true associations with the disease, but only one is detected in a study, that one probably crossed the significance threshold by a lucky combination of genotypes in the particular samples used. A replication study will probably not find it, even if it is true, unless the replication study is statistically much more powerful than the original. One way of getting high statistical power is to limit the number of questions asked – but of course it is frustrating to go through all the work of collecting a replication sample and then just type for a few markers, when your lab is well equipped to do another whole genome trawl. However, a meta-analysis of association studies in several diseases (Lohmueller *et al.*, 2003) gave some grounds for cautious optimism. All reported association studies of T2D, bipolar disease and schizophrenia were considered, plus all studies of eight other randomly chosen reported associations. Altogether, all published studies of 25 reported associations of a particular genotype with a particular disease were analyzed. For eight of these 25, meta-analysis supported a true association, while for the other 17 it was inconclusive or negative. The risk ratios for the eight confirmed associations ranged from 1.07 to 2.28. The overall conclusion was that initially reported associations might quite often be true, but that confirming this would require much larger studies than usually conducted, and that the initially reported risk ratios were almost always too high, for the reason explained above.

Matching cases and controls

One difficult area in association studies is the matching of cases and controls. Sex and age matching should not be important – the frequency of a marker allele should not depend on either of those variables – but is it sufficient to use people from the same ethnic group and country as controls, or should they be from the same locality? Many populations do exhibit fine-scale structure, as expected since local people are more likely to be part of the same extended family. Strong associations should not be sensitive to small local variations in marker allele frequencies, but current large studies look for quite subtle effects and so need more careful matching of controls. One solution is to use internal controls, where the non-transmitted chromosome of a parent is used as a control (the Transmission Disequilibrium Test, TDT).

Transmission disequilibrium test: The TDT avoids any risk of a mismatch between cases and controls by using non-transmitted parental chromosomes as controls. The study sample consists of cases and their two parents. It is irrelevant whether or not the parents are affected. For testing association with a particular allele of a marker, only parents who are heterozygous for that allele are informative. The test simply compares how often the heterozygous parent transmitted the allele in question, rather than his other allele, to the affected case (*Figure 13.10*). Significance is assessed using a simple χ^2 test.

The TDT is well suited to childhood diseases but would be difficult in late-onset Alzheimer disease, since the parents of affected people would be long dead. Variants of the TDT use sibs to get round this problem.

Finding the real causative variant

If an association is replicated and the controls look satisfactory, the next question is the identity of the true susceptibility factor. As mentioned above, the true causative variant may not be the SNP used to establish the association, but something in linkage disequilibrium with it. In mendelian conditions, sequencing candidate genes will usually reveal convincing mutations. For complex diseases the susceptibility factors may be much less obvious variants, as in the case of persistence of intestinal lactase (*Box 8.4*). It will be necessary to sequence the whole ancestral chromosome segment in a large number of cases and controls to look for differences. But irrelevant variants that were present in the ancestral segment will tend to be found in all the present-day cases, and

A_1 A_2

b times

a times

N unrelated affected cases with a parent heterozygous for the allele being investigated. $N = a + b$

if allele A_1 is associated with susceptibility we would expect A_1 to be transmitted to the affected person more often than A_2

test statistic: $(a-b)^2/(a+b)$

Figure 13.10 – The Transmission Disequilibrium Test.
The test statistic has a χ^2 distribution.

so simple comparison of sequences in cases and controls may not pinpoint the relevant change. Some biological insight into the function is needed, and it is very hard to know why, for example, in the lactase case, a C/T polymorphism 14 kb upstream of the start codon should have any effect on expression of the lactase gene. Thus this final hurdle is a far more significant challenge than in mendelian diseases.

A resource for association studies: the HapMap project

Consider the pattern of normal variation across the human genome. Most nucleotides are more or less invariant, with just occasional rare variants, but about 1 in 300 is polymorphic with two variants common in many or all human populations. What could cause such a pattern? It is not that the variable nucleotides are in some way intrinsically more likely to vary than the surrounding nucleotides. Rather, the different variants mark different ancestral chromosome segments. The variable nucleotide mutated just once, by random chance, in a remote ancestor, and significant numbers of all living people have inherited the mutated version, while others have inherited the original version.

High density SNP genotyping reveals a fascinating picture. If there is one SNP every 300 bp, a 10 kb segment might contain 30 or so SNPs. If each has two alleles there are 2^{30} possible haplotypes. But in fact for most such segments in all human populations, only 4–6 different haplotypes are reasonably common. This must be evidence of shared ancestral segments. It means that for any particular segment, all humans have only 4–6 ancestors. This does not mean we are all descended from the same 4–6 cavemen. The next chromosomal segment will also be derived from only 4–6 ancestors, but they will be different ancestors from the previous ones.

The International HapMap project is aiming to define the conserved haplotype blocks across several ethnic groups (see www.hapmap.org/). Data so far from typing over 1 million SNPs confirm the picture of our chromosomes as a mosaic of ancestral blocks (*Figure 13.11*). Blocks are statistical entities, not unambiguously identifiable features of the genome. As the figure shows, the block structure is obvious, but the exact boundaries of blocks are not: the precise number, size and identity of blocks depends on the statistical criteria adopted. The blocks vary in size, but average around 5–15 kb. Some scattered regions of the genome have no readily identifiable block structure. These might be regions of extended high recombination, or regions where gene conversion has been frequent. Despite these reservations, identifying ancestral blocks is a key feature in the design of association studies.

Blocks can be defined by the genotype of maybe two or three selected SNPs ('tagging SNPs'). We can begin to imagine describing somebody's genome by using tagging SNPs to compile a list of which of the 4–6 alternative blocks is present at each chromosomal location. The relevance of this to mapping susceptibility factors is that if we compiled such a list from each of a number of people affected with our favorite disease, we might quite easily be able to spot which ancestral blocks they shared. Shared blocks would be strong candidates for containing the ancient common variants that conferred susceptibility to the disease. Whereas ASP mapping defines shared regions of 20–50 Mb, far too large to search for sequence variants, the shared haplotype blocks would be only a few kb long and readily searchable.

Figure 13.11 – An example of the haplotype block structure of the human genome as revealed by the HapMap project.
In the triangular plot, an ordered set of SNPs from a 500 kb region of chromosome 2q37 is listed along each of the sloping axes. Where there is complete linkage disequilibrium between any pair of SNPs, the cell at the intersection of their co-ordinates is coloured red. The result can be read along the horizontal axis as a map of haplotype blocks along that chromosomal region. The lower figure plots recombination frequencies across the region. Although the genome-wide average is 1 cM/Mb, almost all recombination occurs in a few hotspots, marked by the red triangles. Recombination hotspots generally correspond to boundaries of haplotype blocks. Adapted from The International HapMap Consortium (2005), with permission from Macmillan Publishers Ltd.

A risk in association studies: everything depends on the Common Disease – Common Variant hypothesis

The combination of data from the HapMap project and very high throughput genotyping technologies holds the promise of real progress in this difficult area of research. The same calculations by Risch and Merikangas that showed how poor ASP studies were at identifying weak susceptibility factors, demonstrated that association studies had far greater power with quite feasible sample sizes. However, there is one important difference between linkage and association. Linkage is a relationship between loci, while association is a relationship between alleles or phenotypes (see *Box 13.2*). As long as a collection of families have mutations in the same gene, they will show linkage to nearby markers. This is true even if the actual mutation is different in each family, provided the locus is the same. But the same collection of families would not tend to share the same allele at a nearby marker locus unless they all had the same ancestral mutation, carried on the same ancestral chromosome segment.

The **Common Disease – Common Variant hypothesis** holds that most common disease susceptibility factors will be ancient variants that are common polymorphisms in the present-day population. As we saw in *Chapters 5* and *6*, most mendelian diseases show great allelic heterogeneity. There are exceptions, but mostly they show a disparate collection of relatively recent mutations. If the same were true of common disease susceptibility factors, the whole approach described here would fail. It is argued that mutations causing mendelian disease will have a much higher turnover because natural selection is constantly removing them, and they are maintained by recurrent mutation. Susceptibility factors, it is argued, are not significantly affected by natural selection, so they persist in the population as ancient common variants. The argument is an extension of the argument made in *Chapter 10* about the slow turnover of mutations causing recessive diseases, compared to the rapid turnover of mutations causing dominant diseases. It is wholly plausible, but only further work will tell whether, or how far, it is correct.

If we can identify susceptibility factors, what then?

So far we have described a lot of hopefully interesting science – but what practical use is it? If the research is successful, how will identifying susceptibility factors make clinicians in 10 or 20 years' time manage their patients differently from now? And is there any other value to the research?

One hope is that, whether or not knowledge of susceptibility factors affects clinical practice, it should provide leads for pharmaceutical research. Identifying a novel susceptibility factor for diabetes identifies a novel part of the pathogenesis, which might be targeted by novel drugs. Twenty years ago the small number of known drug targets was seen as a limiting factor in drug development. Nowadays pharmaceutical companies are almost embarrassed by the large number of possible targets, and their ability to prioritize them has become a more important factor. The long lead times for drug development mean that it is too early yet to know whether genetic susceptibility studies will eventually lead to effective new drugs. One caution is that most company profits come from a very small number of 'blockbuster' drugs. Necessarily these are drugs that can be prescribed to large numbers of people. For a common disease like T2D the most promising targets must lie in final common pathways that are affected in every sufferer. But these are already well explored by research into the physiology of the disease. A susceptibility factor that is important for only 2% of sufferers is a much less attractive area for development.

Regarding possible effects on clinical practice, there is a great division of opinion. According to the optimists, medicine in the 21st century will move from a diagnose-and-treat model to a predict-and-prevent model. No longer will people wait until they become ill before consulting their physician. Instead, they will give a DNA sample which will be screened for a large number of disease susceptibility factors. The computer will identify which common diseases they are particularly at risk of, and the physician will advise them how to avoid the risk.

This view has the support of many of the most eminent human geneticists. *Box 13.4* shows an example of this vision. Others, equally eminent, are less optimistic about the leap from diagnosis to prediction to prevention. They use three main arguments:

- Most predictions will be relatively weak compared to those that can be made on the basis of diet, smoking, exercise, etc. If we know 20 genetic risk factors for a disease, then a person with all 20 high-risk or all 20 low-risk will get a strong prediction. But such people will be very rare. Most people will have some combination of high-risk and low-risk factors that will not lead to a strong prediction. Thus the optimists' view over-emphasizes genetic factors at the expense of known and more readily manipulable lifestyle factors (see the example of T2D).

- The lifestyle advice you would give would not depend on the prediction – for example, you would never tell a person who has low-risk factors for lung cancer that he can smoke as much as he likes without worrying. The limitations of 'lifestyle' genotyping were discussed in *Chapter 11*. Since the intervention does not depend on the test result, what benefit is there in doing the test? (The optimists would reply that you might advise more strongly or recommend more surveillance and maybe extra preventative measures for somebody at high risk, and that knowing he is at high risk might motivate a person to take more precautions.)

- Prediction does not automatically lead to prevention. Often there is no known means of prevention; even when there is, people are unlikely to follow advice unless the prediction is extremely strong and the prevention involves no inconvenience or expense. We have excellent predictors of lung cancer and of T2D, and highly effective preventive measures that are known to everybody and available at zero cost – yet these diseases remain major public health problems. Why should relatively weak genetic predictors be more successful?

We hope we have presented both sides of this major controversy here. Today's medical students will find out who is right.

A hypothetical case in 2010

The text that follows is taken from the 1999 Shattuck Lecture given by Francis Collins, head of the US National Human Genome Research Institute. It is reproduced here from Collins (1999) with permission. © 1999, Massachusetts Medical Society.

General visions of gene-based medicine in the future are useful, but many health care providers are probably still puzzled by how it will affect the daily practice of medicine in a primary care setting. A hypothetical clinical encounter in 2010 is described here.

John, a 23-year-old college graduate, is referred to his physician because a serum cholesterol level of 255 mg per deciliter was detected in the course of a medical examination required for employment. He is in good health but has smoked one pack of cigarettes per day for six years. Aided by an interactive computer program that takes John's family history, his physician notes that there is a strong paternal history of myocardial infarction and that John's father died at the age of 48 years.

Box 13.4

To obtain more precise information about his risks of contracting coronary artery disease and other illnesses in the future, John agrees to consider a battery of genetic tests that are available in 2010. After working through an interactive computer program that explains the benefits and risks of such tests, John agrees (and signs informed consent) to undergo 15 genetic tests that provide risk information for illnesses for which preventive strategies are available. He decides against an additional 10 tests involving disorders for which no clinically validated preventive interventions are yet available.

A cheek-swab DNA specimen is sent off for testing, and the results are returned in 1 week (*Table 1*). John's subsequent counseling session with the physician and a genetic nurse specialist focuses on the conditions for which his risk differs substantially (by a factor of more than two) from that of the general population. Like most patients, John is interested in both his relative risk and his absolute risk.

John is pleased to learn that genetic testing does not always give bad news – his risks of contracting prostate cancer and Alzheimer's disease are reduced, because he carries low-risk variants of the several genes known in 2010 to contribute to these illnesses. But John is sobered by the evidence of his increased risks of contracting coronary artery disease, colon cancer, and lung cancer. Confronted with the reality of his own genetic data, he arrives at that crucial 'teachable moment' when a lifelong change in health-related behavior, focused on reducing specific risks, is possible. And there is much to offer. By 2010, the field of pharmacogenomics has blossomed, and a prophylactic drug regimen based on the knowledge of John's personal genetic data can be precisely prescribed to reduce his cholesterol level and the risk of coronary artery disease to normal levels. His risk of colon cancer can be addressed by beginning a program of annual colonoscopy at the age of 45, which in his situation is a very cost-effective way to avoid colon cancer. His substantial risk of contracting lung cancer provides the key motivation for him to join a support group of persons at genetically high risk for serious complications of smoking, and he successfully kicks the habit.

This vision of genetically based, individualized preventive medicine is exciting, and it could make a profound contribution to human health. For this vision to be realized, however, protections against the misuse of genetic information will need to be firmly in place. And another critical challenge must be met: physicians, nurses, and other health care providers will need to become familiar with the emerging fields of genetic medicine. The need for medical genetic specialists who can sort out the most complex cases will be considerable, but there will not be enough of them to go around, and genetic medicine will be practiced for the most part by primary care providers. Numerous surveys have shown that we are not currently prepared for this – most practitioners in primary care have not had a single hour of instruction in genetics as part of their formal training.

To meet this urgent need for education, the National Human Genome Research Institute, the American Medical Association, and the American Nurses Association have recently banded together to form the National Coalition for Health Professional Education in Genetics (NCHPEG). NCHPEG (accessible at http://www.nchpeg.org) is a national effort to promote professional education and access to information about advances in human genetics. An interdisciplinary group, NCHPEG comprises the leaders of approximately 100 diverse health professional organizations, consumer and voluntary groups, government agencies, private industry, managed-care organizations, and professional genetics societies. By facilitating frequent and open communication, NCHPEG seeks to capitalize on the collective expertise and experience of its members and to reduce duplication of effort.

Box 13.4 – continued

Box 13.4 – continued

Table 1 – Results of genetic testing in a hypothetical patient in 2010

Condition	Genes involved*	Relative risk	Lifetime risk (%)
Reduced risk			
Prostate cancer	HPCI, HPC2, HPC3	0.4	7
Alzheimer's disease	APOE, FAD3, XAD	0.3	10
Elevated risk			
Coronary artery disease	APOB, CETP	2.5	70
Colon cancer	FCC4, APC	4	23
Lung cancer	NAT2	6	40

*HPC1, HPC2 and HPC3 are three genes for hereditary prostate cancer; APOE is the gene for apolipoprotein E; FAD3 and XAD are hypothetical genes for familial Alzheimer's dementia; APOB is the gene for apolipoprotein B; CETP is the gene for cholesteryl ester transferase protein; FCC4 is the hypothetical gene for familial colon cancer; APC is the gene for adenomatous polyposis coli; and NAT2 is the gene for N-acetyl transferase 2.

Disease box 13

Autism

Since the first description of early infantile autism in the 1940s the range of disorders included under the heading of 'autistic spectrum disorders' has widened. Estimates of the frequency vary widely but, for the severe and moderate types, it is around 1 in 1000. By definition, children with autism must manifest delays in 'social interaction, language as used in social communication, or symbolic or imaginative play' with 'onset prior to age 3 years', according to the Diagnostic and Statistical Manual of Mental Disorders. Children with classic autism, which can sometimes present with regressive features around 18 months of age, generally have impairment of:

- social interaction, including poor eye contact, failure to develop age-appropriate peer relationships and to seek to share activities
- communication development, including delay or total lack of spoken language or use of repetitive language and lack of imaginative or imitative play
- behavior manifested by inflexibility of routines, obsessions and repetitive and stereotypical patterns of activity

Whilst children with classic autism usually require special educational provision and remain dependent for all their lives, those individuals at the milder end of the spectrum are often diagnosed later in childhood or adult life and live relatively normal lives.

Autism illustrates many of the problems that beset genetic analysis of psychiatric and behavioral characters. While definitions such as that quoted above ensure that clinicians mean the same thing when they use the word 'autism', such definitions are essentially arbitrary and do not necessarily describe a biological entity. Classic autism shades through Asperger syndrome into 'normal' personality variants without any natural boundaries (see the figure). The sex ratio for classic autism in multiple studies has been around 4M : 1F – but we all accept that 'normal' boys are more likely than girls to spend hours obsessively playing solitary computer games and to be socially inept. There are numerous cytogenetic and monogenic disorders where autism or autistic features are frequent; these include Rett syndrome, Fragile X syndrome and duplications of chromosome 15q11–13. A few percent of children whose primary diagnosis is autism turn out to have one or other of these conditions, but the great majority do not. Evidently autism is a pattern of behavior that can have many different causes.

Autistic spectrum disorders merge into normal behavior with no natural boundaries.

No environmental factors have been identified as major causes of autism. Early reports of abnormal parenting, with 'refrigerator mothers' were not substantiated by more careful studies, and despite the publicity it has received, no serious study has implicated the MMR (measles – mumps – rubella) or any other vaccine. By contrast, many observations point to important genetic determinants. The sibling recurrence risk (after the birth of a child with classic autism) is 6–8%, so that λ_s is over 50, among the highest for any complex disease (compare with *Table 13.1*). For second degree relatives the risk is sharply lower, around 0.18%. Concordance is much higher among monozygotic than dizygotic twins (70–82% versus 0–10%, depending on the criteria). The fall-off between MZ and DZ twins, and between first and second degree relatives, is much sharper than in most complex diseases. This might be for either of two reasons:

- genetic susceptibility might depend on combinations of an unusually large number of genes, say, 20 or more
- susceptibility might be largely due to new mutations; these might be conventional sequence changes or epimutations.

It would be nice to know which of these explanations is correct, because they have diametrically opposite implications for genetic research into autism. The first explanation would mean that studies need to be done on an extremely large (and expensive) scale to detect associations. The second implies that the association approach will never work; the best approach would be sequencing (including bisulfite sequencing) of candidate genes in a panel of affected individuals.

Genetic investigation so far has followed the usual routes. Twelve whole genome scans were reported between 1998 and 2004. Using the Lander–Kruglyak criteria (*Box 13.3*) there were no highly significant lod scores, and just one significant score, 3.74 for chromosome 2q.

Disease box 13 – continued

Several other studies supported 2q with suggestive lods. Other locations are 7q, 16p and 17q, supported by several suggestive but no significant lods. Different studies have reported suggestive lods for loci scattered over most other chromosomes, but these have seldom been replicated, even by slightly raised lod scores. Candidate genes for association studies have been chosen for their chromosomal location and/or likely involvement in neurotransmission. Several associations have been reported, but replication studies have been inconsistent or negative. A few individuals have been found with mutations in one or another gene, but no polymorphism has yet shown consistent associations or been identified as a major factor in autism.

Research into psychiatric and behavioral phenotypes involves all the same problems as research into any complex disease, but with the added difficulty that diagnostic labels are arbitrary. Autism is typical: the word describes a type of behavior that may have all sorts of different causes in different individual cases. Researchers try to define 'endophenotypes' to target more homogeneous groups – that is, characters that are part of the overall phenotype but that may lie closer to the underlying gene action. The choice of possible endophenotypes is wide, making confirmation studies and meta-analysis more difficult. In the meanwhile it is important in individual cases to investigate the possibility of one of the known monogenic or cytogenetic causes, to draw a detailed family pedigree recording cases of autistic spectrum disorders, and to give recurrence risks based on empiric data.

For information on autism see http://www.nimh.nih.gov/publicat/autism.cfm. Websites of the UK and US support groups are http://www.nas.org.uk/ and http://www.autism-society.org.

13.5. **References**

American College of Medical Genetics/American Society of Human Genetics Working Group on APOE and Alzheimer disease (1995) Statement on use of apolipoprotein E testing for Alzheimer disease. *JAMA*, **274**: 1627–1629.

Bertram L and Tanzi RE (2004) The current state of Alzheimer's disease genetics: what do we tell the patients? *Pharmacol. Res.* **50**: 385–396.

Eckel RH, Grundy SM and Zimmet PZ (2005) The metabolic syndrome. *Lancet*, **365**: 1415–1428.

Florez JC, Hirshhorn J and Altshuler D (2003) The inherited basis of diabetes mellitus: implications for the genetic analysis of complex traits. *Annu. Rev. Genomics Hum. Genet.* **4**: 257–291.

Holzman NA (1999) Promoting safe and effective genetic tests in the United States: work of the task force on genetic testing. *Clin. Chem.* **45**: 732–738.

The International HapMap Consortium (2005) A haplotype map of the human genome. *Nature*, **437**: 1299–1320.

Lander E and Kruglyak L (1995) Genetic dissection of complex traits: guidelines for interpreting and reporting linkage results. *Nat. Genet.* **11**: 241–247.

Lohmueller KE, Pearce CL, Pike M, Lander ES and Hirschhorn JN (2003) Meta-analysis of genetic association studies supports a contribution of common variants to susceptibility to common disease. *Nat. Genet.* **33**: 177–182.

Risch N and Merikangas K (1996) The future of genetic studies of complex human diseases. *Science*, **273**: 1516–1517.

Stumvoll M, Goldstein BJ and van Haeften TW (2005) Type 2 diabetes: principles of pathogenesis and therapy. *Lancet*, **365**: 1333–1346.

Warren V (1999) *Report of Work Group on Genetic Tests and Future Need for Long-Term Care in the UK.* Continuing Care Conference, London.

13.6. **Self-assessment questions**

(1) Which of the following would provide the strongest evidence for involvement of genetic factors in susceptibility to heart attacks?
  (a) A raised incidence of heart attacks among sibs of index cases.
  (b) Increased concordance of like-sex compared to opposite-sex twin pairs.
  (c) For index cases who were adopted, an increased incidence among the biological, but not the adoptive, relatives.
  (d) The observation that children tend to resemble their parents in healthy or unhealthy eating habits.

(2) Two unrelated women each suffer from a complex disease where family, twin and adoption data suggest that genetic susceptibility is important. The disease is twice as common in men as in women. Anne is the only affected person in her family; Betty's brother and son are also affected. For each of the following four comparisons, decide whether the risk is:
  (a) higher
  (b) lower
  (c) the same
  (d) impossible to predict from these data

  (1) The risk of Anne's or Betty's next child being affected, compared to the risk to the offspring of an affected man.
  (2) The risk of a son of Anne being affected, compared to the risk to a daughter of hers.
  (3) The risk of a son of Betty being affected, compared to the risk to a daughter of hers.
  (4) The risk Anne's next baby will be affected compared to the risk to Betty's next baby.

(3) A mutation arises on a chromosome bearing a particular haplotype of markers. What would be the half-life (in generations) of the association between the mutations and a marker located, (a) 1 cM and (b) 5 cM away?

(4) In the 1950s the statistician Ronald Fisher argued that the known association between smoking and lung cancer did not mean that smoking caused lung cancer. He suggested that incipient lung cancer causes an irritation in the lungs that drives people to smoke; or alternatively that

SECTION **13.6**: SELF-ASSESSMENT QUESTIONS **361**

people with a certain nervous constitution have a tendency both to develop lung cancer and, independently, to take up smoking. How would you prove him wrong?

(5) Locus A has three alleles, A*1, A*2 and A*3 with gene frequencies 0.5, 0.4 and 0.1, respectively. The linked locus B has three alleles B*1, B*2 and B*3 with gene frequencies 0.6, 0.3 and 0.1 respectively. Which of the following would be evidence of linkage disequilibrium?
(a) The frequency of the haplotype A*1, B*1 is 0.30.
(b) The frequency of the haplotype A*2, B*2 is 0.14.
(c) The frequency of the haplotype A*3, B*3 is 0.03.
(d) The frequency of the haplotype A*3, B*2 is 0.01.

(6) Which of the following is evidence for linkage disequilibrium between cystic fibrosis and the linked *KM19* DNA polymorphism?
(a) In a comparison of ten populations, the one with the highest prevalence of CF also had the highest frequency of *KM19* allele 2.
(b) *KM19* allele 2 is found on 91% of chromosome 7s carrying CF but only 25% of those not carrying CF.
(c) The *CFTR* and *KM19* loci both map to chromosome 7q31.2.
(d) In family studies, the *CFTR* and *KM19* loci show close linkage.

(7) In a bean-bag containing a very large number of black beans, one bean in 100 is red. Eyes shut, you put in your hand and take out a bean. If you are given ten tries, what is the chance you will pick out at least one red bean? Now apply this argument to a search for susceptibility genes. You test 1000 markers, each with 4 alleles, for association with a disease you are studying. What *P* value for an association will be significant at the 5% level? Would the answer be the same if instead of testing for association, you tested 1000 markers distributed across the genome for linkage?

(8) Developments in high-throughput genotyping have made whole-genome association testing technically feasible. One million SNPs are tested in a panel of 500 affected people and 500 controls. SNP 629 380 has two alleles that are present at frequencies of 50% each in the controls. What is the threshold number of affected people who must have SNP allele 1 for this to show significant association with the disease?

(9) At a disease susceptibility locus the relative risk of disease for genotypes 1–1, 2–1 and 2–2 is 4:2:1. Calculate the expected proportion of affected sib pairs who are both 1–1, both 2–1 or one each 1–1 and 2–1 if the parents are:
(a) 1–1 × 2–2
(b) 1–1 × 2–1

Chapter 14

What can we do about genetic disease?

Learning points for this chapter

After working through this chapter you should be able to:

- Describe the value of diagnosis and counseling for patients and parents
- Estimate recurrence risks for mendelian and certain multifactorial conditions in affected families (in straightforward cases)
- Describe the main methods of prenatal diagnosis, their uses and problems
- Describe the use of dietary manipulation to treat genetic diseases
- Describe in outline the principles of gene-based therapies by gene augmentation, gene replacement, gene targeting and manipulation of alternative splicing, and their general status in current clinical practice
- Describe possible applications of stem cells for treating genetic disease

14.1. Case studies

There are no new cases for this chapter, which will instead draw on all the previous cases used throughout the book

14.2. Background

Medical care in clinical genetics, as in most medical specialties, rests on a precise diagnosis. The main interventions in clinical genetics involve counseling, testing and therapy.

Diagnosis

As the cases in the text illustrate, clinical observations and examinations are the first steps in establishing a diagnosis. Many clinicians and other healthcare staff are involved in diagnosis and counseling of individuals and families with genetic disorders. In countries with well-developed health services, specialist genetic centers have been established that bring together clinical geneticists, genetic counselors and genetic scientists. Genetic disorders can affect all age groups and all body systems, so specialists need to have broad skills, although sub-specialization means that clinical geneticists build up expertise in specific areas.

A diagnosis is established by taking a detailed medical, pregnancy and family history, followed by systems examinations and then appropriate investigations. For some syndromes (e.g. Williams syndrome, achondroplasia), the diagnosis is first suggested by recognition of a pattern of facial and other features such as heart defects or body proportions. For other conditions (e.g. neurological or metabolic disorders), diagnosis is suggested by clinical symptoms and examination of body systems. The differential diagnoses can then be investigated by specific tests, where these are possible. Many genetic conditions still rely solely on clinical diagnosis because genetic tests are not available.

A diagnosis facilitates clinical management, anticipation of complications and, for a few conditions, treatment. Precise genetic counseling also rests on a precise diagnosis; if a mendelian or cytogenetic cause is established then counseling is relatively straightforward, but for many situations, e.g. learning disability or syndromes of birth defects not conforming to a previously described pattern and where tests are negative, counseling is less precise and is based on studies of groups of similarly affected families.

Risk assessment and genetic counseling

Genetic counseling involves much more than giving out recurrence risks – but an indispensable start is to get the recurrence risks right. Those giving risks need to have enough understanding of the science and the methods for risk calculation, to be able to justify a quoted figure, even if they did not calculate it themselves.

- *For mendelian conditions* the increasing availability and success of mutation testing have made this part of counseling much easier over the past decade. Where risks are based just on the pedigree, the main difficulties come with serious dominant and X-linked conditions where new mutations are frequent. In these cases Bayesian methods are important tools (see *Box 14.1*). Counselors (including clinicians offering counseling) need to have enough understanding of Bayesian methods to be able to follow and justify a calculation, whether or not they themselves normally do the calculations.
- *For chromosomal conditions* such as trisomies, recurrence risks are empiric risks. Where a parent carries a balanced abnormality (as with Ellen Elliott in Case 5) cytogenetic colleagues should be consulted about the risks of the various unbalanced outcomes. Although each case is a one-off, cytogeneticists can give guidance based on the geometry of meiotic pairing, for example in the tetravalent in a carrier of a reciprocal translocation.
- *For complex diseases* risks are empiric. The most important point is to use data that are up to date (risks change with changing incidences) and relate to the appropriate ethnic group.

Genetic counseling is essentially an information-giving and communication process. The widely accepted definition of genetic counseling (American Society of Human Genetics, 1975) states that genetic counseling is:

"a communication process which deals with human problems associated with the occurrence, or the risk of occurrence, of a genetic disorder in a family. This process involves an attempt by one or more appropriately trained persons to help the individual or family to:

(1) comprehend the medical facts, including the diagnosis, probable course of the disorder, and the available management;

(2) appreciate the way heredity contributes to the disorder, and the risk of recurrence in specified relatives;

(3) understand the alternatives for dealing with the risk of recurrence;

(4) choose the course of action which seems to them appropriate in view of their risk, their family goals and their ethical and religious standards, and to act in accordance with that decision; and

(5) make the best possible adjustment to the disorder in an affected family member and/or the risk of recurrence of that disorder."

Box 14.1

An introduction to Bayesian calculations in genetics

This method of combining probabilities was invented in the 18th century by the Reverend Thomas Bayes. It has turned out to be very useful for calculating genetic risks. It starts with a **prior probability** – how likely is a hypothesis in the first place? It then allows you to bring in relevant evidence supporting or opposing the hypothesis (conditional likelihoods) and to combine these to obtain an overall or posterior probability.

To apply this method:

(1) Set out each possible mutually exclusive hypothesis that you are testing. Cover all possibilities, so that one or other of your alternatives must be true. Usually there are just two alternatives – individual X either is or is not a carrier of this disease – but sometimes there are more (you might want to calculate the probabilities that X is aa, Aa or AA).

(2) Assign a prior probability to each. In genetics these are usually the mendelian 1 in 2, 1 in 4, etc. probabilities. They must add up to 1.

(3) Considering your first additional piece of evidence, for each alternative outcome in turn, write down the likelihood of having made that observation *if that alternative were the true one*. These are the conditional likelihoods. They do not necessarily add up to 1.

(4) If there are other relevant observations that are completely independent of the first one, repeat step 3 for each such observation.

(5) When the list is complete, multiply the numbers down each column of the table. The results are called joint probabilities.

(6) Since the final probabilities for each of the possible hypotheses must add up to one (i.e. one of them must be true), you must scale the joint probabilities so that they sum to 1. Do this by dividing each one by the sum of all the joint probabilities. The result is the final probability of each hypothesis, in the light of the prior probability and all the additional observations.

To illustrate it, here is how to calculate the risk that the healthy sister of a child with cystic fibrosis is a carrier. The steps are color coded.

Box 14.1 – continued

Hypothesis – sister is:	AA	Aa	aa
Prior probability:	¼	½	¼
Conditional: she's unaffected:	1	1	0
Joint probability	¼	½	0
Final probability	¼ / (¼+½+0) = $\frac{1}{3}$	½ / (¼+½+0) = $\frac{2}{3}$	0

1. Set out the alternatives. As the child of two carrier parents she could be AA, Aa or aa.
2. The prior probability is just the mendelian 1:2:1 probability.
3. This is the tricky bit. Remember, each conditional likelihood is the likelihood of the observation, *given that the particular hypothesis is true*. If she is AA then she will definitely be unaffected (likelihood = 1). Similarly if she is Aa. If she is aa there is no chance she would be unaffected (obviously you could introduce variable penetrances here, which is a major use of the method).
4. Multiply down each column.
5. Divide each joint probability by the sum of all joint probabilities, to make them sum to 1.

The *Guidance* for this chapter's *Self-assessment questions* give some more examples and discussion of Bayesian calculations. Bayesian approaches to questions of probability are attractive because they correspond to the way we decide whether or not to believe something in everyday life. As mentioned in the guidance for *SAQ1* of *Chapter 9*, you may well believe your friend if he tells you that he missed a lecture because he overslept, but not if he tells you it was because he had been abducted by aliens. You assess the overall credibility of his story in the light of its prior probability. Thus Bayesian calculations are a form of quantitative common sense.

Testing

Like any other clinician, a clinical geneticist will call on a wide range of tests, many of which are not specifically genetic. Making a diagnosis can involve all the usual clinical skills and tests. Here we restrict ourselves specifically to genetic tests.

Diagnostic testing
This can involve chromosomal, biochemical and DNA analysis.

- *Chromosome analysis* is indicated in babies with multiple congenital malformations, in patients of any age with a combination of mental retardation and dysmorphism, and for otherwise unexplained infertility, recurrent miscarriages or intersexual states. The methods were described in *Chapter 2*.
- *Biochemical analysis* is indicated when certain symptoms and signs occur, such as enlarged liver and spleen, early onset seizures, neurological deterioration and coarsening of facial features.
- *Molecular testing* is useful when there is a strong suspicion, but not certainty, of a specific mendelian condition. As explained in *Section 5.4*,

testing must be targeted, ideally at a specific mutation, but at least at one or two specific genes.

In general, diagnostic testing does not raise the same ethical issues as predictive testing, but clinicians need to be sensitive to possible implications for other family members.

Carrier testing

This is used for autosomal and X-linked recessive conditions, and also for balanced chromosomal abnormalities. It would normally be carried out at the request of the patient, and for a reason beyond mere curiosity. Counseling should always be part of the process, though when testing is done as part of a population screening program, pre-test counseling is likely to be quite minimal. Children should not be tested unless there is an immediate benefit to the child.

Predictive testing

This is used for late-onset conditions such as Huntington disease and familial cancers. It needs to be done within the context of a full clinical genetics service and to follow detailed written protocols that define in advance the response to each possible outcome. *Box 14.2* shows a protocol for predictive testing for Huntington disease.

Prenatal testing

This can be carried out at several stages of pregnancy.

- *Chorion villus biopsy* is performed at 10–12 weeks of gestation under ultrasound guidance (*Figure 14.1*). Either a transabdominal or transcervical route may be used. The chorion is the outermost of the fetal membranes, and the sampling instrument should not penetrate the amniotic cavity. Once removed, the material needs expert dissection under the microscope to pick fetal material free of contaminating

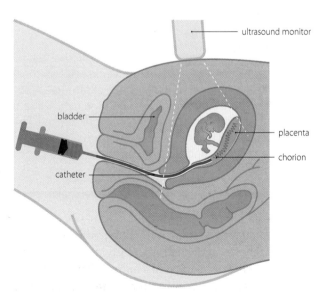

Figure 14.1 – Chorion villus biopsy.

Box 14.2

Protocol for predictive testing for Huntington disease

Various nationally agreed protocols differ in minor respects, but all require multiple counseling sessions. The following, reproduced from Tibben (2002) with permission from Oxford University Press, is typical. The patient is encouraged to bring a spouse, friend or supporter to each session.

Counseling session 1:
 Sociodemographic details
 Confirmation of family and clinical data
 Assessment of impact of Huntington disease and test results
 Assessment of knowledge of Huntington disease and of predictive testing
 Reasons for requesting prediction
 Neurological examination

Counseling session 2 (a month or more after session 1):
 Assessment of psychological, personality and social resources, using standardized
  instruments
 Further counseling and discussion of the disclosure session; agreement of the date of this
  session
 Nomination of professional support
 Signing of consent form
 Taking of blood sample

Laboratory work:
 The blood sample is split into two and sent to the laboratory on two different days, to
  minimize any risk of sample mix-up
 The laboratory uses PCR to estimate the CAG repeat sizes on both copies of chromosome 4,
  as in *Figure 4.18*

Counseling session 3 (within 2 weeks of session 2):
 Disclosure of test results

Follow-up 1:
 2 days – 1 week, normally by telephone

Follow-up 2:
 3 months

Follow-up 3:
 12 months

Only a small proportion of people at risk eventually take the predictive test. Follow-up support is important for people whose test result is negative, as well as those found to carry the disease allele. Genetics centers often maintain registers of families with Huntington disease (and other conditions where the risk extends beyond the nuclear family). These are administrative tools to provide a point of long-term contact for family members. In Manchester, for example, 1374 at-risk individuals in 514 extended Huntington disease families have volunteered to be included in the register, and they are each contacted once a year to check on any problems and advise them of any relevant new findings.

maternal tissue. Villi can be used for DNA extraction or for rapid cytogenetic analysis of dividing cells already present. Such short-term cultures need to be confirmed with longer term cultures. Mosaicism detected in villi is difficult to interpret: retrospectively it often turns out to have been confined to the placenta. For DNA testing, results should always be compared to a control sample of the mother's blood DNA, to ensure that the test result reflects the fetal genotype.

Chorion villus biopsy carries around a 2% risk of causing a miscarriage. There is a significant learning curve for the procedure, and it is always best to rely on an obstetrician who has already performed many such procedures.

- *Amniocentesis* is performed at 14–20 weeks of gestation (*Figure 14.2*). Amniotic fluid consists mainly of fetal urine and washings from the lungs. It can be analyzed biochemically, or fetal cells can be isolated from the fluid and cultured for cytogenetic or molecular analysis. Biochemical analyses include testing for AFP, a protein produced by the fetal liver: a high level indicates that the fetus has a hole, most likely an open neural tube defect, but possibly an abdominal wall defect. There is an extensive literature on the interpretation of biochemical findings. Culture of cells from amniotic fluid for cytogenetic analysis takes around 2 weeks to obtain good quality preparations. Amniotic fluid is a poorer source of DNA than chorionic villi, because there are fewer cells. Newer techniques that do not require cell culture, such as QF–PCR (quantitative PCR with fluorescence-labeled primers) to detect specific trisomies, are increasingly being introduced into practice.

Amniocentesis carries a 0.5–1.0% risk of causing a miscarriage.

(a)   (b)

Figure 14.2 – Amniocentesis.
(a) Diagram of procedure. (b) Withdrawing amniotic fluid.

- *Analysis of fetal cells or DNA in maternal blood* has often been suggested as a non-invasive method of prenatal diagnosis. Many reports have shown that fetal cells are often detectable in the maternal blood. Typically there is about one fetal cell per milliliter of maternal blood. These rare cells could in principle be used to screen for a long list of anomalies, but the tests are not reliable enough for routine clinical use. A large multi-center study (NIFTY study, Bianchi *et al.*, 2002) attempted to determine fetal sex and to check for aneuploidy by interphase FISH of fetal cells in 3502 maternal blood samples. Among women carrying a singleton male fetus, at least one cell showing an X and a Y FISH signal was found in 41%; the false positive rate was 11%. For aneuploidy the detection rate was 74% with 0.6–4.1% false positives.

  Because of these disappointing results, attention has moved to detecting free fetal DNA in the maternal circulation. Plasma from pregnant women contains free DNA, of which 3–6% is of fetal origin. The concentration of free DNA is much higher than the amount contained in the rare fetal cells. Fetal DNA is detectable from week 7, maybe earlier, and its concentration rises through pregnancy. The fetal DNA consists mainly of fragments <200 bp in length. Its origin is unknown, but is most likely to be placental (in which case confined placental mosaicism could be a problem, as with the chorion villus biopsy).

  Highly sensitive PCR protocols have been used to sex the fetal DNA or to check for paternally inherited mutations, Because of the large excess of maternal DNA, it is not possible to test for inheritance of maternal mutations. Many reports attest to the feasibility of fetal genotyping using this free fetal DNA (reviewed by Chiu and Lo, 2004). As usual with difficult new technologies, early reports tend to be from people who have got the method to work; those who tried and failed seldom report their experiences. It will take large controlled trials to discover how robust the method is for routine use in non-specialist centers or with samples sent from outlying hospitals – but clearly, the method has considerable promise.

- *Imaging* is discussed here because, when an anomaly is detected, it frequently leads on to a genetic test. It is the only thoroughly established non-invasive method for routine fetal testing. With each passing year imaging becomes more powerful and sophisticated. 3D and 4D imaging can now give really clear images of fetal structure and even facial features. A detailed fetal anomaly scan (different from the scans used to establish gestational age and check the number of sacs) is often done at around 18 weeks. A wide range of structural anomalies can be picked up and then investigated further, often by amniocentesis followed by cell culture and chromosome analysis, or by FISH analysis for specific disorders. For example, after detection of a heart defect, FISH analysis for 22q11 deletions may be performed. Imaging is also employed as a screening test to detect micro signs of Down syndrome; the most frequently sought sign is increased nuchal translucency, but other structural features such as absence of the nasal bone can increase the likelihood that a baby has Down syndrome.

Treatment

Here we will discuss the principles of the two great hopes for general progress in treating genetic diseases, gene therapy and cell therapy. Before getting into these, it is important to stress that, while the promise of these technologies lies in the future, there is already a lot that can be done here and now. The reputation of genetic disease for being untreatable is only very partially deserved. Genetic patients, just like any others, have problems and symptoms that can be alleviated even if no radical cure is possible. Specific treatments based on an understanding of the abnormal function are available for a range of diseases. A number of examples are given in *Section 14.3*, and *Table 14.2* at the end of this chapter lists others.

Gene therapy

The promise of gene therapy rests on the existence of well-established laboratory methods for getting genes into cells. It is surprisingly easy to get exogenous DNA into living cells in the laboratory, using any of a range of techniques (*Figure 14.3*). Broadly, these fall into physical methods and vector-dependent methods.

Physical methods include:

- *liposomes* – artificial membrane-bound vesicles that can fuse with cell membranes and release their contents into the cell;
- *receptor-mediated methods*, where the DNA is attached to the ligand for a cell-surface receptor which internalizes after binding the ligand;
- *electroporation*, where a short high-voltage pulse temporarily alters cell membranes such that they take up naked DNA from the medium.

Vector-based methods use engineered viruses that resemble the acute transforming retroviruses described in *Figure 12.4*. Compared to physical methods, these are often much more efficient at getting the foreign DNA into a good proportion of the target cells. Many different viruses have been used. Factors governing the choice include:

- *capacity*: how long a piece of genetic material they can hold;
- *tropism*: some viruses preferentially infect certain types of cell;
- *ability to infect non-dividing cells*: retroviruses can only infect dividing cells;
- *integrating or non-integrating vectors*: integrating vectors such as retroviruses integrate the transferred gene into a chromosome of the host cell, ensuring that all daughter cells will carry a copy. Non-integrating vectors such as adenoviruses remain as extrachromosomal **episomes**, which will eventually be diluted out during cell replication. As we will see in the case of the Portillo family (Case 16, immunodeficiency) there are advantages and disadvantages to integration.

Depending on the nature of the condition it is designed to treat, gene therapy can have any of three aims:

Gene supplementation or augmentation. This aims to put a working gene into a cell that currently lacks it. This would be the aim of gene therapy for any

Figure 14.3 – Methods of inserting an exogenous gene into a cell.

loss of function condition, which includes many of the conditions covered in our *Case studies* (see below). Additionally it could be used to introduce a novel gene into a cell, usually for the purpose of creating a vulnerability in cells that one wishes to eliminate. Cancer cells might be made to express a novel antigen that would trigger a cytotoxic attack by the immune system, or an intracellular enzyme that would convert a harmless pro-drug into a toxic metabolite.

Gene silencing aims to prevent expression of a resident gene. This type of gene therapy would be required for diseases caused by gain of function or dominant negative mechanisms. In most cases the silencing would need to be specific for the mutant allele, leaving expression of the normal allele unaltered. Gene silencing might also be used to prevent expression of viral genes in an infected cell.

Gene repair aims to correct a malfunction in an endogenous gene, rather than silence or replace it. Proposals for gene repair rely on highly targeted homologous recombination or mismatch repair to patch specific defects in a gene. Alternatively the repair might be at the expression level, for example, by manipulating splicing to cause skipping or retention of specific exons of a gene.

Any of these methods might be applied *ex vivo*, on cells taken from the patient which, after modification, will be returned, or *in vivo* by injecting or otherwise introducing the therapeutic construct into the patient's body. Equally, one could in principle treat either somatic or germ-line cells. Germ-line gene therapy has an appealing finality to it compared with somatic therapy – the problem is dealt with once and for all – but is generally regarded as ethically unacceptable. In truth, the technical obstacles to germ-line therapy are far greater than for somatic therapy, and it is quite hard to think of circumstances where germ-line therapy would be useful even if it could be done (*Figure 14.4*).

DOMINANT CONDITION
1 in 2 embryos OK

RECESSIVE CONDITION
3 in 4 embryos OK

Figure 14.4 – The limited usefulness of germ-line gene therapy.
The targets for germ-line therapy would most likely be embryos created by *in vitro* fertilization. Typically IVF might result in 5–10 embryos of which 1–2 are selected for implantation. A genetic test would identify which embryos would require the therapy. Depending on the mode of inheritance, either 1 in 2 or 3 in 4 embryos could be used without the need for any therapy.

Cell therapy

The obstacles to mending damaged tissues and organs by supplying new cells are the limited life and replicative potential of most cells, and the rejection of foreign cells. Although, of course, *organ* transplantation has been used successfully for decades, including for treating genetic diseases (e.g. kidney transplantation for polycystic kidney disease), *cell* transplantation usually relies on a small number of transplanted cells taking root and multiplying. This requires the use of **stem cells**.

It is believed that every tissue is maintained by a small number of stem cells. These cells have the potential to divide asymmetrically to produce another stem cell and a derivative cell that can go on to form the functioning cells of the tissue (*Figure 14.5*). Different stem cells differ in the range of cell types they can produce. **Embryonic stem cells** are totipotent. They can produce every cell type of the adult body. Perhaps when we understand much more about how to grow, maintain and differentiate them we will be able to grow organs and tissues to order from embryonic stem cells. Maybe this will be possible, maybe it will not. At present we don't know – but the potential is so alluring that laboratories throughout the world are devoting immense efforts to trying to find out.

Embryonic stem cells can only be obtained by destruction of a very early embryo (*Figure 14.6*). There is currently much debate about the potential of non-embryonic stem cells. The science is difficult and uncertain. Isolating and identifying stem cells requires an exceptional degree of laboratory skill, and experiments to explore their potential are often very hard to interpret. On top of the scientific difficulties, are political and religious agendas that promote certain interpretations of the experiments. It will be some years before the science is secure enough to force consensus on the facts. Of course, the science can never dictate the ethics, but we look forward to a time when all parties to the ethical arguments can at least start from an agreed base of facts.

Amid the uncertainty, one form of stem cell transplantation is already part of routine clinical practice. Cord blood contains stem cells that can reconstitute every type of blood and bone marrow cell (and maybe other types of cell too). It can be collected at every birth with no risk or pain to the mother or baby. Methods for extracting stem cells are well established. Banks of cord blood great majority of cloned animal blastocysts produced in this way fail to develop, and those few that come to term are usually abnormal. Even those animals that appear normal when young, like Dolly the sheep, usually die early. Embryonic stem cells, however, appear to have erased all previous epigenetic programming.

14.3. Investigations of patients

Rather than discuss each case separately, they are collected into groups for most of the discussion of what could be done.

Possibilities for prenatal diagnosis

Prenatal diagnosis could, in principle, be offered for almost all of the conditions described in the *Case studies*. The exceptions would be leukemia (an acquired condition), and Alzheimer disease and type 2 diabetes (complex diseases where genetic prediction is not possible). For most of the mendelian conditions it would only be possible if the causative mutation had been previously identified – as we saw in *Chapter 9*, this was a particular challenge in the case of hearing loss.

Several of the chromosome abnormalities occurred *de novo* (in Cases 7, 8, 9, 13, 17 and 18). In these cases the recurrence risk is very low and in general the parents would be reassured rather than offered prenatal diagnosis in future pregnancies. For the *de novo* structural rearrangements (Cases 7, 13 and 17) germ-line mosaicism can never be ruled out, so there is a finite though small recurrence risk. If the parents were particularly anxious it would be appropriate to offer prenatal testing, but to point out that the chance of detecting a recurrence is probably smaller than the risk of losing the pregnancy because of the procedure. Of course, the two risks are not necessarily equally important, and families will make their own judgement of the relative weights to put on them. In our cases, of those six families only Anne Howard (Case 8, Down syndrome) was tested in her next pregnancy. In her case she and her husband decided to have tests partly because of the small increase in risk associated with her age and partly because they felt they would not be able give Helen all the attention she needed if they had another baby with Down syndrome.

For the other conditions, decisions about prenatal diagnosis would be governed by several factors:

- the legal and ethical framework in the country – in some countries prenatal testing is legal only for a defined list of conditions; in others it is left to negotiation between parents and clinician
- the practical availability of testing, including whether somebody else – the state or an insurance company – will pay for it
- the severity of the condition – for example, many people would not regard hearing loss as an indication for termination of affected fetuses
- the availability and effectiveness of treatment – demand for prenatal diagnosis of cystic fibrosis, for example, depends on views about the current and future prospects for treatment

- the age of onset of the condition – many people do not see late-onset conditions such as Huntington disease as appropriate for prenatal diagnosis
- the situation of the individual family – how well could they cope, emotionally, physically and financially with the birth of an affected child?
- the moral principles or religious beliefs of the individuals concerned – some people would not countenance a termination, whereas others would see it as the least bad option.

Current possibilities for treatment

None of the conditions discussed is untreatable, although most are incurable at present. In *Table 14.1* they have been split into those where the current problem is the result of things that happened, or failed to happen, early in development, and those where the problem is largely due to things happening, or failing to happen, here and now. For the first group treatment is necessarily symptomatic, while for the second, in principle, a more fundamental treatment or cure might be possible.

Table 14.1 – Summary of the 26 *Case studies* used in this book

Case	Family	Conditions where the problem affected development, so that treatment is necessarily symptomatic	Case	Family	Conditions where the problem is a continuing malfunction, where therapy might, in principle, aim to rectify the malfunction
3	Choudhary	Hearing loss	1	Ashton	Huntington disease
5	Elliot	Chromosomal anomaly	2	Brown	Cystic fibrosis
7	Green	22q11 deletion	4	Davies	Duchenne muscular dystrophy
8	Howard	Down syndrome	6	Fletcher	Leber's optic neuropathy
9	Ingram	Turner syndrome	11	Kavanagh	Sickle cell disease
10	Johnson	Marfan syndrome	12	Lawton	Hemophilia
13	Murphy	Chromosomal anomaly	14	Nicolaides	Thalassemia
15	O'Reilly	Stickler syndrome	16	Portillo	X-linked severe combined immunodeficiency
17	Qian	Angelman syndrome	20	Tierney	Acute lymphocytic leukemia
18	Rogers	Prader–Willi syndrome	21	Ulmer	Tay–Sachs disease
19	Stott	Congenital adrenal hyperplasia	22	Vlasi	Phenylketonuria
			23	Wilson	Breast cancer
			24	Xenakis	Familial adenomatous polyposis
			25	Yamamoto	Alzheimer disease
			26	Zuabi	Type 2 diabetes

Phenylketonuria (Case 22 – Vlasi family) comes nearest to being curable at present. Once diagnosed, the baby is put on a low protein diet to minimize its intake of phenylalanine. Some protein is of course necessary, as is some phenylalanine. Phenylalanine is an essential amino acid, that is, one that humans cannot synthesize but have to obtain from dietary protein. Careful titration of the phenylalanine level is necessary. Too low a level of protein or phenylalanine will cause malnutrition, retarded growth, etc., while too high a level of phenylalanine will cause brain damage. Keeping a child on the diet is immensely demanding for the family, especially if there are unaffected siblings. Well-intentioned friends or neighbors may feel sorry for a child who seems to be being subjected to a crank diet, and may slip it surreptitious treats. Peer-group pressure to conform may be very hard for the child to resist. Special phenylalanine-reduced flour is available so that the child can have its own cakes and cookies.

Once the brain has stopped growing it is no longer so susceptible to the toxic action of high levels of phenylalanine, and so at some age between 8 and 14 years the child can move on to a normal diet. The transition may be marked by emotional disturbance. As mentioned in *Figure 11.4*, a phenylketonuric woman needs to go back on the diet during pregnancy, or else the high phenylalanine level in her blood will damage her baby's brain, even though genetically the baby is not phenylketonuric.

In *Table 11.3* and the final section of this chapter other examples are given of inborn errors of metabolism that can be treated by dietary manipulation.

Congenital adrenal hyperplasia (Case 19 – Stott family) is one of the few genetic conditions that can be treated *in utero*. As explained in *Chapter 8*, the virilization of baby girls is the result of a feedback loop that over-stimulates the adrenal glands. If a couple have previously had an affected child, in subsequent pregnancies the mother is given oral dexamethasone, a glucocorticoid that can cross the placenta, to damp down the adrenal hormone production. This is started at the earliest possible stage of the pregnancy. If a subsequent fetal sex test shows that the fetus is male the treatment can be discontinued. Children with CAH are treated with steroids to ensure normal growth and development.

Acute lymphoblastic leukemia (Case 20 – Tierney family) in children is nowadays quite successfully treated (the disease in adults has a much worse prognosis); 75–80% of children can expect to survive 5 years without any recurrence, and in the best centers true cure (long term disease free survival) rates are 80% or better. The response to therapy is partly a question of the genetics of the leukemia cells – a variety of chromosomal rearrangements produce different chimeric oncogenes that influence prognosis – and partly a question of genetic polymorphisms controlling the pharmacokinetics (absorption, metabolism and clearance) and pharmacodynamics (response of the target) of the drugs used. Treatment response is measured by the level of residual disease after induction of remission. PCR of the specific chimeric oncogene is used to check the number of remaining cells with the leukemic genotype. In favorable cases this is 0.01% or less of the original level. Stem-cell transplantation is also often used, especially in adult cases. The cells are derived from cord blood from unrelated infants (see above).

Jason Tierney (Case 20) had two prognostically favorable features, his *TEL–AML1* translocation, and his thiopurine methyltransferase deficiency. Although the latter caused initial problems, it also meant that his cells had received very high effective doses of the drug.

For the *late-onset conditions* in *Table 14.1* there is the hope of prevention. The risk of type 2 diabetes (Case 26 – Zuabi family) can certainly be greatly reduced by physical activity and weight control. People with familial adenomatous polyposis (Case 24 – Xenakis family) are strongly advised to have their colon removed; unfortunately there is still a risk of gastric and peri-ampullary tumors. An appropriate diet can reduce the risk of recurrence. Prophylactic mastectomy is one option for women who carry mutations in *BRCA2* (Case 23 – Wilson family); those with *BRCA1* mutations often also opt for oophorectomy. Regular enhanced surveillance is important for people at high risk of cancer. No interventions are currently known that reduce the risk of Huntington disease (Case 1 – Ashton family) or Alzheimer disease (Case 25 – Yamamoto family)

Treatment of most of the other conditions in *Table 14.1* is symptomatic.

Possibilities for gene therapy

In principle, gene therapy might be applicable to any of the conditions in the right-hand column of *Table 14.1* where the problem is a continuing genetic malfunction.

- For complex diseases (Alzheimer's, diabetes) any such therapy would not try to correct the initial genetic susceptibility because, as we have seen, the effect of any one gene is small. Possibly some point in a final common pathway of pathogenesis might present a suitable target, but in general gene therapy is an unlikely first line of attack with complex diseases.
- For the leukemia and cancers, any therapy would be directed at the neoplastic cells. Clinical trials have attempted to make neoplastic cells more immunogenic by expressing a foreign antigen on the cell surface.
- As a gain of function condition, Huntington disease would need a more sophisticated version of gene therapy than the remaining diseases in our list, all of which are caused by loss of function and might, in principle, be treatable by gene augmentation.
- As mentioned above, the easiest targets for gene augmentation are diseases where the exact level of expression of the introduced gene is not important, and a low level could be clinically useful. This makes cystic fibrosis, Duchenne muscular dystrophy, hemophilia and X-SCID the most appropriate targets.
- For Duchenne muscular dystrophy, the huge size of the gene and the difficulty of getting a foreign gene into a high proportion of muscle cells have so far frustrated attempts at gene therapy.

X-SCID is so far the one success story of gene therapy (Case 16 – Portillo family) In *Section 9.3* we mentioned that a second affected boy was born recently to a distant relative in the Portillo family. For this baby, the prospects are much brighter than for Pablo, who was born in 1989. There are two options:

- Bone marrow transplantation. As mentioned, provided this is done early the results are good. If a perfectly HLA-matched sib is not available, marrow can be used from a parent or a sib who shares one HLA haplotype with the affected baby, though the success rate is not as high. The marrow is first depleted of T cells to avoid graft-versus-host disease.
- Gene therapy. Pioneering work by Alain Fischer's group in Paris (Hacein-Bey-Abina *et al.*, 2002) successfully cured 9 of 11 babies with X-SCID (*Figure 14.8*). Other groups have now achieved similar results. However, high optimism turned to gloom when two of the treated babies, and later a third, developed T cell leukemia. In two of the cases this was shown to be due to integration of the retroviral vector close to an oncogene, *LMO2*. The strong promoter used to cause high expression of the therapeutic *IL2RG* gene had the effect of up-regulating expression of *LMO2*. This is similar to the way the 8;14 translocation in Burkitt's lymphoma up-regulates the *MYC* oncogene by placing it next to the highly expressed immunoglobulin heavy chain gene (*Chapter 12*).

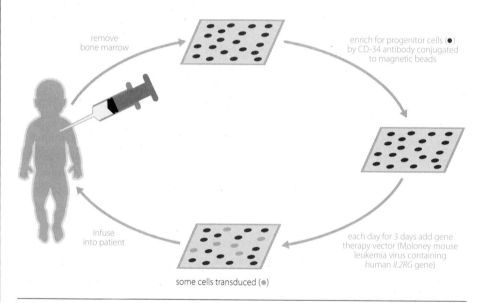

remove bone marrow

enrich for progenitor cells (●) by CD-34 antibody conjugated to magnetic beads

each day for 3 days add gene therapy vector (Moloney mouse leukemia virus containing human *IL2RG* gene)

some cells transduced (●)

infuse into patient

Figure 14.8 – Gene therapy protocol for severe combined immunodeficiency.
The disease is caused by loss of function mutations in the *IL2RG* cytokine receptor gene. A retroviral vector was used to integrate a working copy of the gene into chromosomes of hemopoietic precursor cells. This gave them a selective advantage when re-infused into the patient, and they were able eventually to reconstitute T cell and NK cell function in 9 of 11 babies treated. Similar treatment was not successful in older patients with a partial malfunction of the gene.

After the initial shock, when trials of retroviral gene therapy were halted worldwide, some measure of optimism returned. The leukemia was brought under control. Without gene therapy these babies would have died. Where there is no alternative, the risk seems worth taking. Possibly some modification of vector design or the treatment protocol may lessen the risk. It remains true that the risk of this sort of insertional activation has moved up the list of potential problems of gene therapy using integrating vectors.

Possibilities for cell therapy

Huntington disease and Alzheimer disease are high on the list of candidates for cell-based therapy. Regardless of the initial cause, in both cases it is loss of cells from specific brain regions that causes the clinical problems. The brain is an immunologically privileged site – that is, allografts (grafts from a different individual of the same species) are not usually rejected, although xenografts (grafts from a different species) often are. Animal studies have demonstrated the long-term survival of transplanted brain cells.

Preliminary trials have already been made of striatal cell transplantation in Huntington disease. A 6-year follow-up of one trial has recently been published (Bachoud-Levy *et al.*, 2006). Five Huntington disease patients received grafts into the striatum of fetal brain tissue. The tissue was obtained from the corresponding brain regions of 7.5–9 week aborted human fetuses – a developmental stage at which the brain contains suitable neuronal precursor cells. The results of this small trial showed real clinical improvement in some cases, and a temporary halt in the normal progression of the disease. By 6 years the normal decline was again evident. The transplanted cells can (sometimes) replace the lost cell population, but not halt the neurodegeneration in the rest of the affected brain regions. Other trials have also been reported, though with less intensive follow-up, and further trials are in progress.

These trials give real hope that cell-based therapy for Huntington disease can eventually be developed. The greatest present limitation is the source of cells. Quite apart from the ethical problems of using tissue from aborted fetuses, the tissue must be used fresh and it cannot be properly characterized or grown up in the laboratory. Real progress depends on identifying stem cells that can be preserved, grown in the laboratory when required, and induced to differentiate in the appropriate way.

14.4. **Summary and extension**

Most people's long term hopes for effective treatment for many genetic diseases rest on gene therapy or stem cell transplantation, although in fact treatments based on knowledge of the genetic and cellular mechanisms may prove to be equally effective and without so many associated risks.

Gene therapy

Hopes for gene therapy have followed a manic-depressive course over the past 20 years, with recurrent highs and lows. In the beginning many people thought it might be easy to transfer the techniques from the laboratory to the clinic. As early as 1990 it was claimed that a child with combined immunodeficiency (an autosomal recessive type due to deficiency of adenosine deaminase, not the X-linked type described in Case 16) had been cured by gene therapy. In fact it was enzyme replacement therapy, used simultaneously with the attempted gene therapy, that was probably responsible.

The continuing problem with gene therapy is obtaining reasonably long lasting and reasonably high level expression of the introduced gene.

- First, a sufficient proportion of cells in the target tissue must be transfected. Retroviral vectors give the highest efficiency, but they can be used only on dividing cells and, as we saw with X-SCID, integration is a mixed blessing. Adenoviruses seemed to be promising non-integrating vectors, but high doses can cause inflammatory responses that, in the case of Jesse Gelsinger (see http://www.uvm.edu/~cgep/Education/Expert.html) were fatal. None of the physical methods detailed in *Section 14.2* can target a useful proportion of cells under realistic clinical conditions. Novel viral vectors may have the most promise.

- Next, a sufficiently high level of expression must be achieved. Because this is difficult, most work has focused on conditions where even a low level of expression should be beneficial. Cystic fibrosis and hemophilia are examples of diseases where 10% of the normal expression level would bring real clinical benefits.

- If adequate expression could be achieved, the next problem would be to control it. The hemoglobinopathies should be good targets for therapy – the genes are small and exceptionally well understood, and the conditions are hugely important. The problem is that the expression level of an introduced globin gene would need accurate control. Over-expression of an introduced β-globin gene might convert a patient's β-thalassemia into α-thalassemia.

- Stable expression has proved extremely difficult to achieve. Cells commonly use epigenetic mechanisms to shut down expression of transgenes. Non-integrating vectors are especially likely to cease working after a short time. This has led many researchers to focus on situations where long-term expression is not needed – killing cancer cells or virally infected cells, for example.

Despite all these problems, there is a huge ferment of research and development in gene therapy. Many ingenious systems have been demonstrated in laboratory proof-of-principle experiments. Dozens of companies are pursuing novel approaches. Hundreds of phase I clinical trials have been run, particularly for cancer and infectious disease rather than for mendelian conditions. Despite the problems, X-SCID remains a real landmark success. Given the ever-growing number of methods we have for manipulating genes and their expression, it is hard to believe that nothing useful will be achieved over the next decade. Perhaps the main question is whether any achievement will be a generally applicable breakthrough, leading to gene therapy for a whole list of conditions, or whether it will be a series of disease- and cell-specific tricks that will be of great benefit to a few patients but leave the whole field little further forward.

Stem cell therapy

This has suffered from the same over-hype as spoiled the reputation of gene therapy in the 1990s. It is easy to paint a beguiling picture of tissues and organs grown to order in a brave new world – whether this will ever bear any relation to reality is quite another question. We still know very little about the real potential of embryonic stem cells or any other stem cells. The number of embryonic stem cell lines presently available is very small, which for such an intensively researched high profile subject illustrates just how difficult these techniques still are. Compared to the technical difficulties, legal obstacles will probably not be major factors impeding progress. Research will simply move to countries where it is not only permitted but strongly encouraged. If any of the promised clinical benefits are realized, pressure from patient groups to allow the technology will be politically irresistible. The supply of eggs may be a more significant factor.

While we wait for these new technologies to live up to the hype, it is too easy to overlook all that has already been achieved.

Diagnosis and counseling

These may be undramatic, but they can make a huge difference to the lives of families affected by genetic disease.

- A diagnosis is the cornerstone of clinical management. Without it clinical management is unfocused and complications not anticipated.
- When the diagnosis is of a lethal condition, e.g. trisomy 18, the most appropriate management is usually supportive care even if a structural malformation is present where surgery would normally be undertaken.
- Families will often consult many doctors and their child may be made to undergo multiple tests in search of a diagnosis. Getting to the right specialist is important.
- Establishing a diagnosis and providing information about a condition has real therapeutic value for many people even if there is no cure. Links can be made with support groups. The families have something to write on forms, and educational and social services are more readily provided.
- A diagnosis and counseling can help dispel the guilt and anger that can seriously impact the quality of life in families after the birth of a child with a malformation or disease. It is not enough simply to tell the parents that it wasn't caused by something one or other of them did. The professional skills of a counselor can help parents work through the natural reactions of shock, grief and anger.
- Counseling can relieve the burden of anxiety by dispeling exaggerated general estimates of recurrence risks and, especially in X-linked and recessive diseases, identifying family members who are at negligible risk. Contrary to popular belief, more people have good news and low risks given in genetic clinics than bad news and high risks.
- While counseling cannot abolish the real problems of living with an affected family member, it can help people focus on solutions rather than problems. Appropriate help can be given. Parents can be given a range of options for handling the recurrence risk.

Testing

Testing is a crucial part of the overall aim of allowing families affected by a genetic condition to live as normal lives as possible. This is well illustrated by a study by Modell *et al.* (1980) on families at risk of serious forms of thalassemia.

Before prenatal diagnosis was available, when the birth of an affected child made a couple aware of their 1 in 4 risk of having further affected children, they virtually ceased reproduction. Most subsequent pregnancies were accidental and they sought termination of 70% of them. Prenatal diagnosis for this condition became available in 1975. At-risk couples then resumed normal reproduction, with fewer than 30% of pregnancies being terminated for thalassemia. The effect of prenatal diagnosis was to reduce the number of terminations and to enable at-risk couples to have normal families.

The real example described below of a family with Duchenne muscular dystrophy further illustrates how the increasing accuracy of both carrier testing and prenatal testing can allow couples to avoid termination of wanted pregnancies. *Figure 14.9* shows how the distribution of carrier risks for Duchenne muscular dystrophy among families known to one large genetics center has changed as new knowledge allowed more precise genetic testing.

Figure 14.9 – Distribution of DMD carrier risks among women in families on the North West Genetic Register, Manchester.
Blue bars: risks based on pedigree and creatine kinase, before any molecular testing was available. Green bars: risk distribution in 1989 among women where the pedigree structure allowed gene tracking. Red bars: risks when direct mutation testing became available. The peaks at intermediate risks in the latter series are mostly from girls currently too young to test. Data courtesy of Dr Elizabeth Howard, St Mary's Hospital, Manchester.

Treatment

Treatment is available for a wide range of genetic diseases. Concentrating on the hopes for dramatic technologies such as gene and stem cell therapy distracts attention from the incremental but very real advances that have been made in treating a whole range of genetic diseases. We are indebted to an excellent brief article by Munnich (2006) for a list of some of these incremental advances; the article should be consulted for more details and references.

A central point made by Munnich is that patients do not suffer from their mutations, but from the functional consequences of those mutations. Often knowledge of the mutation or even the gene is irrelevant to treatment. We do not need to know whether a genetic patient's kidney failure is due to Alport syndrome, polycystic kidney disease or nephronophthisis to know that a kidney transplant will greatly improve his life. We do not need to know which of the 100 possible genes has caused a child's deafness before we can consider the possible benefits of a cochlear implant. Even with Huntington disease, a famously 'untreatable' condition, life for the patient and his carers can often be improved by drugs such as neuroleptics and antidepressants, and attention to diet and the home environment.

In other cases a closer knowledge of the gene function, though not necessarily of the gene itself, is the key to treatment. *Table 14.2* lists some examples and particularly interesting cases include the following.

- Type I tyrosinemia (OMIM 276700) is a severe inborn error of metabolism that is especially prevalent in the Saguenay-Lac Saint Jean region of Quebec because of a founder effect. Referring to the diagram of tyrosine catabolism (*Figure 8.4*), the defective enzyme is downstream of the final step shown. The block results in accumulation of maleylacetoacetic acid, and overflow reactions then produce succinyl acetone. This abnormal metabolite inhibits production of porphobilinogen in the heme biosynthesis pathway (see figure in *Disease box 8*). The result is a severe porphyria-like syndrome and death through liver failure or cancer. Type II tyrosinemia, by contrast, is a mild condition in which the first step in tyrosine catabolism is blocked (*Figure 8.4*). NTBC (2-(2-nitro-4-trifluoromethylbenzoyl)-1,3-cyclohexanedione) inhibits the enzyme, tyrosine transaminase, that is deficient in this mild form of tyrosinemia. It produces a **phenocopy** of Type II disease. Because of this block, there is no production of maleylacetoacetic acid, and the patient's disease is converted from the fatal Type I to the mild Type II disease.
- In carbohydrate-deficient glycoprotein disease type Ib (OMIM 602579) the underlying defect is an inability to isomerize fructose to mannose (deficiency of mannose phosphate isomerase). The symptoms of profuse diarrhea and severe liver disease are entirely due to lack of mannose. They can be completely rectified by oral mannose.
- Cystinosis (OMIM 219800) is an atypical lysosomal storage disease. The defect is not in a lysosomal enzyme, but in a lysosomal membrane transporter protein. Non-functioning of the transporter means that cystine is unable to get out of lysosomes. The accumulation produces symptoms including renal failure, pancreatic insufficiency, corneal erosions, central nervous system involvement and severe myopathy. Oral cysteamine is an effective treatment. Cystine consists of two molecules of cysteine linked by an S–S bridge (*Figure 14.10*). Cysteamine, given orally, enters lysosomes using a specific transporter. There it can displace one cysteine molecule from cystine to form a mixed cysteamine–cysteine disulfide, which is able to exit the lysosome, apparently using a lysine transporter. Once outside the lysosome, the mixed disulfide may be reduced, freeing the cysteamine to ferry another cysteine molecule out of the lysosome.

In other cases interventions are targeted more specifically at changing gene expression. Such treatments are mostly still experimental, for example:

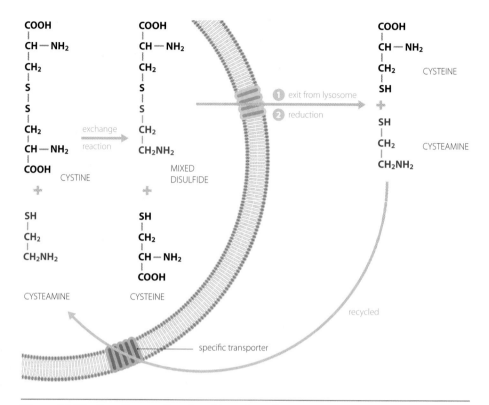

Figure 14.10 – Treating cystinosis with cysteamine.
Cysteamine and the mixed disulfide are able to cross the lysosomal membrane, but cystinosis patients lack the specific transporter protein that in normal people allows cystine to exit lysosomes. Their symptoms are caused by accumulation of cystine in lysosomes.

- Symptoms of deficiency or abnormality of β-globin in sickle cell disease or β-thalassemia are milder in patients who continue to express some fetal hemoglobin during adult life (hereditary persistence of fetal hemoglobin, HPFH). Patients in whom production of the fetal γ-globin has been shut down as part of normal development may be stimulated to re-express the gene by treatment with hydroxyurea.
- The antibiotic gentamycin can induce mis-reading of mRNA by ribosomes, such that the ribosome occasionally ignores a stop codon. Gentamycin has been used to improve symptoms in cystic fibrosis patients who have a nonsense mutation. Clearly it would be catastrophic to cause ribosomes to ignore a high percentage of stop codons, but even a very small degree of read-through may allow significant clinical improvement in cystic fibrosis.
- The anti-epileptic drug valproate affects intron–exon splicing. Preliminary trials in spinal muscular atrophy (OMIM 253300, see *Section 6.2*) suggest valproate may prolong the life of affected infants. More targeted ways to modify splicing have been attempted in the dystrophin gene. The aim is to induce specific exon skipping so as to make frameshifting deletions frame-neutral and thus convert Duchenne muscular dystrophy into the milder Becker form (see *Section 6.2*).

Table 14.2 – Examples of genetic diseases where symptoms can be ameliorated or sometimes abolished by treatments based on a knowledge of the malfunction, but not necessarily of the DNA sequence

Strategy	Example	Disease
Supply missing molecule		
	Insulin	Diabetes
	Growth hormone	Pituitary dwarfism
	Factor VIII	Hemophilia A
Replace defective enzyme		
	Acid beta-glucosidase	Gaucher disease
	Alpha-galactosidase	Fabry disease
	Alpha-glucosidase	Pompe disease
Dietary supplementation		
	High carbohydrate diet	Glycogen storage diseases
	Cholesterol	Smith–Lemli–Opitz syndrome
	Mannose	Carbohydrate-deficient glycoprotein syndrome 1b
	Biotin	Biotin-responsive carboxylase deficiency
	Pyridoxine	Pyridoxine-responsive homocystinuria
	Cobalamin	Cobalamin-responsive organic aciduria
	Alpha-tocopherol	Pseudo-Friedreich ataxia
	Creatine	Creatine synthesis deficiency
Dietary restriction		
	Low phenylalanine diet	Phenylketonuria
	Low protein diet	Maple syrup urine disease
	Low fat diet	Hypercholesterolemia
	Avoid phytanic acid	Refsum disease
Enhance residual enzyme activity		
	Fibrates	Fatty acid oxidation disorders
Remove a toxic product		
	Bleed regularly	Hemochromatosis
	Cysteamine	Cystinosis
Block a pathogenic process		
	NTBC	Tyrosinemia Type I
	Bisphosphonates	Osteogenesis imperfecta

Data from Munnich (2006).

Oligonucleotides are custom-designed to match the relevant exon–intron junction. This approach falls more into the realm of gene therapy, with the usual problems of securing effective delivery and expression of the oligonucleotide.

The true story of one Manchester family (note that only the names have been changed) affected by Duchenne muscular dystrophy shows how the advances in genetics over the past three decades have improved their lives, even though a cure or effective treatment for the disease remains elusive.

- In 1977, a 3-year old boy Alan was diagnosed as having DMD, on the basis of clinical examination (problems running and climbing stairs, pseudohypertrophy of his calves), elevated serum creatine kinase and muscle histology.
- His mother Betty was referred to the genetics service. When the pedigree was taken (*Figure 14.11*, grey part), it showed that Betty had two affected brothers, both now wheelchair-bound in their early 20s. Thus Betty and her mother Christine are obligate carriers. Betty had two sisters, Delia and Elly. Through Betty, Delia and Elly were invited to attend the genetic clinic and were counseled about their 50% risk of being carriers. Blood was taken for creatine kinase testing, but the results on Delia and Elly were not either high or low enough to significantly modify their carrier risks.
- In 1982 Delia, now married, was pregnant. She requested fetal sexing. Amniocentesis was carried out at 16 weeks. It took 2 weeks to get enough dividing cells for cytogenetic analysis. This showed the fetus was male. This wanted pregnancy was terminated by induced delivery at 18 weeks.
- In 1984 Delia was pregnant again, but miscarried at 10 weeks before any testing. Elly was now married but, having watched the traumas of her two sisters, was not willing to risk having children.
- By this time DNA markers had been defined that were linked to the *DMD* locus. Gene tracking (see *Chapter 9*) was used to estimate Delia's and Elly's carrier risks. Because all markers showed at least 5% recombination with the disease, two markers were used, one mapping proximal and the other distal to the disease locus. If a meiosis was non-recombinant for the two markers, there was only a very small risk that it would nevertheless be recombinant between the markers and the disease – only double recombinants would produce that result. If a meiosis showed recombination between the two markers, then no prediction could be made, but at least a false prediction would have been avoided. The result of the analysis (magenta lines in *Figure 14.11*) suggested that Delia had a >99% risk of being a carrier, while Elly's risk was very low, conservatively reported as 2%. Retrospectively, the risk that the fetus terminated in Delia's first pregnancy would have been affected was increased from 25% to 50%, which made Delia feel more confident that she had done the right thing. Elly now felt able to start a family.
- In 1985 Delia was pregnant for the third time. By now chorion villus biopsy was available (green lines in *Figure 14.11*). This was performed at 10 weeks. Rapid cytogenetic analysis showed the fetus was male. The pregnancy was terminated surgically at 11 weeks.

- In 1988 chorion villus biopsy in Delia's fourth pregnancy showed the fetus was female. She went on to deliver a normal healthy girl.
- In 1993 Delia was pregnant for the fifth time. By now the dystrophin gene had been cloned (blue lines in *Figure 14.11*). Testing Alan's DNA identified the family mutation, a frame-shifting deletion of exon 45 (see *Table 6.2*). Chorion villus biopsy was performed. Cytogenetic analysis showed a male fetus. Molecular testing for Y-specific sequences confirmed that the fetus was male, but exon 45 of the dystrophin gene could be PCR-amplified from the fetal DNA, showing it had not inherited the mutation. The pregnancy continued and Delia delivered a normal boy.

This family story illustrates several aspects of genetic services. First, how rapidly scientific advances can be delivered into clinical service; secondly, how options for individual family members can change even when the disease remains incurable, and thirdly, the importance of long-term follow up of families. Delia's daughter will soon wish to know her carrier status and options.

Figure 14.11 – How advances in genetics affected a family with Duchenne muscular dystrophy.
This is a real family; only the names have been changed. The colors show how the pedigree evolved over time. The black rules represent the results of gene tracking using two DNA polymorphisms, A and B that map either side of the disease locus. Allele numbers are arbitrary; + signifies the normal allele at the *DMD* locus. TOP, termination of pregnancy.

Finally we should perhaps consider some of the objections that have been raised against continuing progress in clinical genetics.

- *Helping people with genetic disease to live normal lives allows them to pass on their genes and shows an irresponsible lack of concern for future generations.* We dealt with this in relation to mendelian diseases in *Chapter 10*. In relation to complex diseases, this is really an objection to the whole of medicine – indeed to the whole of civilization. What is a civilized society but a collective attempt to prevent the operation of natural selection?

- *Offering prenatal diagnosis for a genetic condition devalues people with that condition.* Understandably, people living with spina bifida, achondroplasia or Down syndrome are highly sensitive to the suggestion that they should never have been born. The desire of parents for healthy children does indeed conflict with the need to respect the lives of people with disabilities. Each of us probably has our own point at which we would draw the line. The only general solutions to the conflict (allowing no choice or unfettered choice) are unacceptable to a majority of people in most countries. Perhaps the wisest course is to try as far as possible to circumvent the conflict by insisting that, whatever indications we may accept for termination of pregnancy, when an affected child is born we must value it as much as we would any other person and provide appropriate support and services to the family.

- *Curing certain conditions is another way of devaluing people with that condition.* This has particularly surfaced in relation to cochlear implants for deaf children. If these are done on a very young child they can be quite successful in terms of enabling the child to understand speech. Most hearing people would not question the benefit of enabling a deaf child to hear, but many people in the Deaf Community see it otherwise. They contend that attempting to cure deafness is tantamount to trying to undermine their culture.

  This is similar to the question whether people in small linguistic isolates should be educated in their own minority language or in the national language of their country. For an individual, learning the national language widens his opportunities, but it threatens the minority culture with extinction in two or three generations. Perhaps the best aim in cochlear implantation is to make the child bilingual, in signing and in spoken language. This is the policy in Sweden but in few other places. It is worth pointing out that most children with profound congenital hearing loss are born into hearing families and are not part of the Deaf Community in their formative years. The Swedish solution leaves them free to make their own decisions about where they belong when they are old enough to do so.

- *Advances in genetic testing and reproductive choice put us on a slippery slope.* The 'designer baby' catchphrase, so beloved of journalists, usually surfaces early in this discussion. It has been repeatedly used in connection with 'savior siblings'. These are babies born after *in vitro* fertilization, where embryos were selected to be HLA-compatible with an older child who has a serious disease that could be cured by a transplant of HLA-compatible cord blood stem cells. Allowing this selection, say the critics, opens the door to much more extensive selection of embryos for non-medical reasons.

  The absurdity of this objection can be seen by looking at *Figure 14.4*. Suppose Mr and Mrs Frank N. Stein decide they want a tall blue-eyed blonde boy with an IQ of 150. They go through the trauma and expense of IVF and end up with eight embryos in a dish. Four are female and are discarded. Blue eyes and pale hair are not simple mendelian characters, but they are usually recessive. Photographs of the parents do not show us blue-eyed blonde people, so we must assume they are at best heterozygous for these attributes. Thus only 1 in 4 of their embryos will fit their pigmentary aspirations. Out go three, leaving them with just one. What a pity it happens to grow into a man 160 cm tall with an IQ of 95!

The 'designer baby' example just quoted shows that there is very little mileage in embryo selection. However, if the gene therapy technique of *Figure 14–8* were applied to the embryos of *Figure 14–4*, the story might be very different. Suppose that one day in the future all the limitations of gene manipulation had been overcome, so that any desired genetic alteration could be achieved safely and with high efficiency. Perhaps babies really could be designed to order. Maybe ambitious parents could browse a catalog of desirable human characters and place their order. Moving further into science fiction territory, why stop at existing human characters? Like every new technology, this would bring risks as well as benefits. The ethical problems would be mind-boggling. But it is important to remind ourselves that this is science fiction and not everything in science fiction ever gets developed in reality – for example, we already know that time travel, as imagined by Hollywood, will never be developed. Unless every gene transfer into an embryo worked with 100% efficiency and 100% safety, attempts at multiple manipulation would run into the same problem of diminishing returns as embryo selection. And unless every one of the 100–150 cells in the inner cell mass of a blastocyst could be manipulated, the resulting baby might just be a low-level mosaic for the designed genotype. In short, while we must remain alert to new possibilities, moral panic about genetics is misplaced. For the foreseeable future, clinical genetics services will remain a small but important part of normal medicine, bringing great and ever-increasing benefits to those families needing them, while genetic science will increasingly become the foundation of much broader medical practice.

14.5. **References**

American Society of Human Genetics (1975) Genetic counseling. *Am. J. Hum. Genet.* **27**: 240–242.

Bachoud-Lévi A-C, Gaura V, Brugieies P *et al.* (2006) Effect of fetal neural transplants in patients with Huntington's disease 6 years after surgery: a long-term follow-up study. *Lancet Neurol.* **5**: 303–309.

Bianchi DW, Simpson JL, Jackson LG, *et al.* (2002) Fetal gender and aneuploidy detection using fetal cells in maternal blood: analysis of NIFTY I data. *Prenat. Diag.* **22**: 609–615.

Chiu RWK and Lo YMD (2004) The biology and diagnostic applications of fetal DNA and RNA in maternal plasma. *Curr. Topics Dev. Biol.* **61**: 81–111.

Hacein-Bey-Abina S, Le Deist F, Carlier F *et al.* (2002) Sustained correction of X-linked severe combined immunodeficiency by *ex vivo* gene therapy. *New Engl. J. Med.* **346**: 1185–1193.

Modell B, Ward RH and Fairweather DV (1980) Effect of introducing antenatal diagnosis on reproductive behaviour of families at risk for thalassaemia major. *Br. Med. J.* **280**: 1347–1350.

Munnich A (2006) Advances in genetics: what are the results for patients? *J. Med. Genet.* **43**: 555–556.

Tibben A (2002) Genetic counseling and presymptomatic testing. In: *Huntington Disease*, 3rd edition, eds Bates G, Harper PS and Jones L. Oxford University Press, Oxford.

14.6. **Self-assessment questions**

(1) A woman has a son with Duchenne muscular dystrophy. There are no previous cases in the family, there are no other children and the mother is an only child. She might be a carrier, or the boy might be a new mutation. Calculate the chance that she is a carrier. (See the *Guidance* for two ways of doing this important calculation.)

(2) This calculation uses the carrier risk, 2/3, calculated in the previous question. The woman has another child, a girl. Calculate the risk the girl is a carrier.

(3) The woman in *SAQ2* has two more children, both unaffected boys. Does this alter your estimate of her carrier risk? If so, use a Bayesian calculation to calculate her revised risk.

(4) A man comes from a large family in which an autosomal dominant condition is segregating. His mother is affected but he is healthy. The condition is 90% penetrant, so he might either not have inherited the disease allele or he might be a non-penetrant case. He marries. Calculate the risk that his first child will be clinically affected by the disease.

(5) Generalize the result of *SAQ4* for a condition with penetrance x, and calculate the maximum risk that such a person would have an affected child, if x could have any value.

(6) Your mother has Huntington disease. You are healthy at age 45. If half of people who have inherited the disease gene show symptoms by age 45, what is the chance that you have inherited the disease gene?

(7) Score each of the following statements as true or false:
    (a) Empiric risks are used in counseling for non-mendelian diseases
    (b) Empiric risks are based on mathematical simplifications
    (c) Empiric risks embody no assumptions about genetic mechanisms
    (d) Empiric risks are valid only for a particular population and time

(8) Outline proposals to develop gene therapy for (a) cystic fibrosis, (b) Duchenne muscular dystrophy, and (c) a rapidly growing brain tumor. In each case, consider the advantages and disadvantages of this condition as a target for gene therapy, the gene(s) and constructs you would use, which tissue or cells you would target and how.

Guidance on self-assessment questions

Chapter 1

SAQ 1, 2 and 3. Following the two questions as suggested in the text should lead you to a convincing answer. We are told that each disease is rare, so the chance of an unrelated person who marries into the family being a carrier (if the disease is recessive) is small.

Pedigree 3. Unlike every other pedigree in this book, this pedigree shows a real family. The disease is hemophilia A (OMIM 306700) and the family is Queen Victoria's. Queen Victoria is 1–2. The affected people are Leopold (II-1), Frederick (II-8), Leopold and Maurice Mountbatten (III-18, III-19), Rupert (IV-2), Alexis, Tsarevitch of Russia, murdered with his four sisters by the Bolsheviks in 1918 (IV-8), Waldemar and Henry of Prussia (IV-9, IV-11) and Alfonso and Gonzalo of Spain (IV-14, IV-19). V-1 is the present Queen Elizabeth II of Britain.

SAQ 4. This pedigree is ambiguous (you shouldn't be given one like this in an exam). Try each possible mode of inheritance. Don't be misled by the affected female, and don't jump to the conclusion that there is male to male transmission. An affected man has an affected son – but are you sure the son inherited his disease gene from his father? The risk for a child of IV-3 may depend on which mode of inheritance is correct.

Chapter 2

SAQ 1a. Consider events in oogenesis that could result in a missing X (egg fertilized by an X-bearing sperm) and events in spermatogenesis that could result in a sperm with either a missing X or a missing Y. Note that in reality, Turner syndrome is usually the result of anaphase lag rather than non-disjunction (see *Section 2.3*).

SAQ 2a. Use *Figure 2.8* to check whether the breakpoints are proximal (near the centromere) or distal (towards the telomere) on the chromosome arm. 2q22 is about one-quarter of the way down the long arm on chromosome 2 and 4q32 is about three-quarters of the way down the long arm of chromosome 4. Draw out the cross-shaped tetravalent formed when the two translocated chromosomes pair with their two normal counterparts. Draw it very roughly to scale, using different colors for the chromosome 2 and chromosome 4 sequences. Check that you are always pairing segments of matching color. Then draw out possible gametes. You could consider 3:1 segregation patterns as well as the 2:2 patterns shown in *Figure 2.17*.

Chapter 3

SAQ 2   CTCAAAAGCACGCTCCAGTTCCTCCAGCTG
CAGCUGCAGGAACUGGAGCGUGCUUUUGAG

Remember that strands are anti-parallel but are always written in the 5′->3′ direction.

SAQ 3. Transcription starts at the start of exon 1. The first codon is the AUG initiation codon. Intron 1 starts at the end of exon 1.

SAQ 4. You could use a word processor to interleave and align the two sequences, or just compare them manually. Sequences present in the genomic DNA but absent in the mRNA are introns.

Chapter 4

SAQ 1a. First ask yourself, to get a 50 bp product, will the primers flank the underlined 50 nt sequence or will they lie inside it? Write in the complementary strand for the regions where your primers will anneal. Then put in all the 5′ and 3′ directions and remember that the primers will extend from their 3′ ends.

SAQ 4. Imagine you had one copy of each possible sequence n nucleotides long. There are 4^n such sequences, so the total length of all these would be $4^n \times n$. Look for a value of n such that this total $> 3\,000\,000\,000$. Of course, this exercise ignores the fact that the human genome is not a random sequence, and contains many repeated sequences – but it shows that a sequence does not need to be very long to be *potentially* unique within the human genome.

Chapter 5

SAQ 2. Hybridization is a property of single-stranded DNA. Double-stranded DNA doesn't hybridize to anything else.

SAQ 3. Remember that sequences must be read 5′ -> 3′. CTTAAG is not an *Eco*RI site. If you write in the complementary strand, you will notice that GAATTC, like most restriction sites, is palindromic – that is, it reads the same on both strands.

Chapter 6

SAQ 1. Ask whether each change would specifically cause a failure to transport chloride ions across apical cell membranes.

SAQ 2. Two of the changes are deletions of one or a few nucleotides. One change affects a splice site.

SAQ 3. A laboratory might report the last sequence variant as p.V29M but in fact it might very well affect splicing – it replaces the last nucleotide in exon 1, and a G at this position is part of the normal consensus splice site sequence.

SAQ 4. c.216C>G is a mis-sense mutation, p.172M – it creates an internal methionine codon. This is not an initiator codon: translation initiates at the first suitable AUG in the mRNA, and once initiated, further AUGs are just read as normal methionine codons.

Chapter 7

SAQ 1. Here is one possible pedigree. The condition is autosomal dominant and so it affects both sexes and the mutant gene can be transmitted by both sexes – but it is always non-penetrant when it is inherited from the mother.

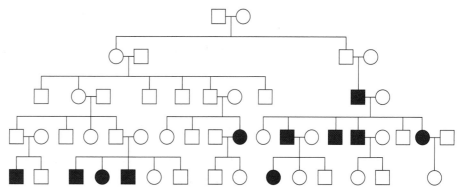

SAQ 6. This is the sequence recognized by the primer giving the 313 bp product in *Figure 7.14*. You can see all the sequences in the paper by Zeschnigk *et al.* (1997).

SAQ 7. There is an obligate crossover in every male meiosis between the Xp and Yp copies of the pseudoautosomal region. The crossover point might be proximal or distal to the location of the marker. You could try assuming that 50% of the crossovers are located between the centromere and the marker locus. In female meiosis crossovers within this region are quite uncommon.

Chapter 8

SAQ 2. Consider possible blocks in a multi-step pathway, or a block in post-translational processing (see *Section 8.4*).

SAQ 5. Eliza is homozygous for HLA-B27 and for HLA-DR4. You need to use the latter fact to work out the DR allele in each haplotype.

Chapter 9

SAQ 1. Although every meiosis may be recombinant or non-recombinant, only the meioses in the mother of the third generation are informative about this. The χ^2 result (3.6, 1 d.f.) is almost significant at the 5% level, while the lod score is well below the threshold for significance [L1 = $(\frac{1}{2})^{10}$; L2 = $(1-\theta)^8.(\theta)^2$; maximum lod score = 0.83 at θ = 0.2]. The reason is that the lod score, but not the χ^2 test, takes into account the low prior probability of linkage. That is, given two loci picked at random, the chance they would show linkage is of the order of only 1 in 50 – they would probably be on different chromosomes, and even if they were on the same chromosome they might well be sufficiently far apart not to show linkage. Common sense tells us that we need to take the prior probability into account when deciding whether or not to believe something. For example, you may well believe your friend if he tells you that he missed a lecture because he overslept, but not if he tells you it was because he had been abducted by aliens. See Strachan and Read *Human Molecular Genetics* (Chapter 11 in the 2nd edn, available on the Internet, Chapter 13 in the 3rd edn.) for a brief explanation of how the lod score threshold includes the prior probability, or Ott, *Analysis of Human Genetic Linkage* for full details.

SAQ 2. Work out the haplotypes, starting with generation 2. The marker alleles have been chosen in this example to allow unambiguous haplotypes to be assigned to each individual. You can then identify which haplotype in individual II-1 is linked to the disease locus (remember we have been told that the disease is linked to this chromosomal region). When you examine the paternal haplotypes in generation III you can see that individuals III-3 and III-5 have inherited recombinant paternal disease-carrying haplotypes. The positions of crossovers show that the disease locus must map below marker A (from III-3) but above marker C (from III-5). III-6 has a recombinant maternal haplotype. The crossover might be anywhere between markers A and D. This recombinant does not provide any data for mapping the disease locus.

SAQ 4. The combination of deafness and diabetes is known sometimes to be caused by mutations in the mitochondrial DNA. NB Although it is sensible to attempt this sort of prioritization, when the causative gene is finally found, often it is not one of the more obvious candidates.

Chapter 10

SAQ 2. Remember that only people who are homozygous at one or other locus are affected; people who are heterozygous at two or more loci are unaffected. In reality, as explained, it would be unwise to rely on Hardy-Weinberg figures for such a rare recessive condition.

SAQ 3. You could try solving this by saying $p^2 + 2pq = 0.64$; substitute (1-p) for q, and you get a quadratic equation to solve for p. It can be done – but it is a lot easier to start by noting that $q^2 = 0.36$

SAQ 4. Treat the first part as a 3-allele Hardy–Weinberg problem, as in *Box 10.1*, with non-functioning, low functioning and normal alleles.

SAQ 5. Remember the difference between obligate carriers and possible carriers.

SAQ 6. Genetic counseling is non-directive.

Chapter 11

SAQ 4. Estimate the relative numbers by counting squares under the appropriate part of each curve. The curves have been drawn having equal total areas, but remember that the curve for NTD should really have 1/100 the area of the normal curve.

SAQ 5. The risk before any screening that a couple are both carriers is $1/40 \times 1/40 = 1/1600$. We need to calculate the sensitivity of a test such that when the partner tests negative, there is only a 1 in 1600 chance that this is a false negative. You can see from *Table 11.1* that this is not readily achievable.

Chapter 12

SAQ 1. In regard to Statement 8, although it is generally true that mutations in oncogenes are somatic and not inherited, there are a few exceptions. Inherited mutations in the *RET* oncogene are found in familial thyroid cancer. If a gene product has more than one function it may be simplistic to talk simply of loss or gain of function. Equally, the classification of genes into oncogenes and tumor suppressor genes is a very useful tool for thinking about the molecular pathology of cancer, but it has its limitations.

SAQ 3. If the chance of a mutation in one cell is μ and there are n cells, the chance that no cell will suffer a mutation is $(1-\mu)^n$. Since μ is very small, this approximates closely to $1-n\mu$, and is equal to the chance of non-penetrance in a familial case. It is interesting that in order to get a combination of a realistic penetrance and a realistic frequency of sporadic cases with this simple calculation, it is necessary to postulate an unrealistically high mutation rate. Maybe a single somatic mutation affects the target cells in such a way as to make a second mutation more likely.

SAQ 4. Using the scoring system of *Table 12.4*, simply adding up points across each pedigree gives a 12% chance of a *BRCA1* mutation in family A and a 14% chance in family B. But all 12 points in family A come from the paternal side, while in family B the paternal side has 9 points and the maternal side has 5. If there is a *BRCA* mutation, it is most likely to come from the father, but the likelihood is only 9%. This is of course a rather contrived example.

Chapter 13

SAQ 1. The familial eating habits might be learned or genetic. Opposite sex twins are all dizygotic, while like-sex twins may be either monozygotic or dizygotic. The first three observations all suggest genetic factors. The adoption data give the cleanest separation of genetic from environmental effects, though the Barker hypothesis (see *Chapter 7*) would sound a caution against drawing dogmatic conclusions.

SAQ 2. Because the disease is commoner in men than in women, the risk is always higher for a son than a daughter of a given person. The logic of *Box 13.1* dictates that the risk is higher for a child of an affected woman than for a child of the same sex of an affected man. Because Betty has two affected male first-degree relatives she is likely to have a higher susceptibility than Anne, so the risk for her child is greater.

SAQ 3. If the recombination fraction is θ, after n generation a proportion $(1-\theta)^n$ remain associated.

SAQ 7. This is the multiple testing problem and a Bonferroni correction is appropriate. Sometimes it is hard to decide how many questions were asked. If a marker has n alleles, and you check each for association, is that one question, or n or $n-1$? The Bonferroni correction is over-rigorous if the questions are not fully independent. If you look not only for associations with individual marker alleles but also with multi-marker haplotypes, are those extra independent questions? If you use linkage analysis and you know that there are susceptibility loci somewhere in the genome, each negative result reduces the area of the genome where the susceptibility factor(s) must be hiding – so are tests of the few remaining areas independent? In short, the multiple testing problem is severe in complex disease studies and requires expert statistical insight.

SAQ 9. For the $2-1 \times 1-1$ parents the mendelian proportions among the sibs must be modified by the fact that you have selected pairs that were both affected. This is most easily done by a Bayesian calculation, with the mendelian proportions as the prior probability and the fact that both sibs are affected as a conditional:

Genotypes of sibs:	(1–1, 1–1)		(1–1, 2–1)		(2–1, 2–1)
Prior probability	¼		½		¼
Conditional likelihood (both affected):	16	:	8	:	4
Joint likelihood	4	:	4	:	1
Final probability:	4/9		4/9		1/9

For an explanation of this method see *Box 14.1*.

Chapter 14

SAQ 1. This is an important basic calculation in genetic risk estimation so we show it in detail. There are two ways of arriving at the answer, which applies to any X-linked recessive condition where affected males never reproduce.

(a) If the population contains equal numbers of males, who each have one X chromosome, and females who each have two, then one-third of all X chromosomes are in males. Equally, one-third of all DMD X chromosomes are in males. Any DMD X chromosome that is in a male will not be transmitted to the next generation, thus one-third of all DMD X chromosomes are lost each generation. If the disease frequency remains constant over the generations, this must be balanced by new mutations. Thus one-third of cases are new mutations, so the chance that the mother of an isolated case is a carrier is 2/3.

(b) An alternative method starts by calculating the probability that any woman, picked completely at random, is a carrier of DMD. Call this probability P. Suppose she has a daughter. The probability that the daughter is a carrier is made of three parts:

- She might be a carrier because her mother is a carrier and she has inherited her mother's mutated X. The probability of this is $P/2$.
- She might be a carrier because although her mother was not a carrier, the X she received from her carried a new DMD mutation. Call the mutation probability μ.
- She might be a carrier because the X she received from her father carries a new DMD mutation. Again the probability of this is μ.

The daughter's overall carrier risk is $P/2 + 2\mu$. But our original woman was selected completely at random; exactly the same logic could have been applied to her and her mother. The carrier risk of the mother and daughter must actually be the same (if it weren't, by repeating the exercise over enough generations, you could get the risk to either 0 or 100%, which would be absurd). Therefore $P = P/2 + 2\mu$, from which we see that $P = 4\mu$.

Now we have worked out the prior probability that a woman is a DMD carrier, we can return to the original question and do a Bayesian calculation of the carrier risk of the woman who has a son with DMD. Either she is a carrier or she is not. The calculation goes as follows:

Woman is:	a carrier	not a carrier
Prior probability:	4μ	$1-4\mu \approx 1$
Conditional: affected boy	½	μ
Joint probability:	2μ	μ
Final probability	$2\mu/3\mu = 2/3$	$\mu/3\mu = 1/3$

SAQ 2. The daughter's risk is half the mother's risk – there is a 1 in 2 chance she will inherit her mother's 'risk' X rather than the other one.

SAQ 3.

- *Method 1*: repeat the calculation of SAQ1, adding in an extra line of conditionals for the two unaffected boys. Given that she is a carrier, the chance of having two unaffected boys is 1 in 4. Given that she is not a carrier, it is 1–2μ, which is effectively 1.
- *Method 2*: start with her 2/3 carrier risk as your prior probability. In that case, this has already used the information that she has an affected boy, so the only conditional likelihoods are for the unaffected boys.

   This illustrates the fact that it doesn't matter which pieces of information you put as prior probabilities and which as conditionals, just as long as you use each piece of information once and only once.

SAQ 4. First you need to calculate the chance that the man is a non-penetrant carrier. Use a Bayesian calculation. The prior probability is his mendelian 1 in 2 risk, the conditional is the fact that he is clinically unaffected. Having got his risk, the risk his son has inherited the disease gene is half the risk the father carries it. Then remember that even if the child inherits the gene there is only a 90% chance he will be clinically affected.

SAQ 5. The formula is $\frac{1}{2} \times \frac{(1-x)}{(2-x)}$. The answer, 8.6% risk for 59% penetrance, is surprisingly and reassuringly low. If a condition has low penetrance, this increases the risk the unaffected father may carry the disease gene, but at the same time it reduces the risk the child will be clinically affected if it does inherit the gene.

SAQ 6. The 'obvious' answer, 1 in 4, is wrong. Use Bayes to get the correct answer.

Glossary

3′ untranslated sequence – in a messenger RNA, the part downstream of the stop codon.

5′ untranslated sequence – in a messenger RNA, the part upstream of the translation initiation (AUG) codon.

Acrocentric – of a chromosome, having the centromere close to (but not at) one end. In humans, chromosomes 13, 14, 15, 21 and 22.

Acute transforming retrovirus – a small RNA virus, part of whose genome has been replaced by an activated oncogene (see *Figure 12.4b*).

Affected sib pair (ASP) method – a model-free method of linkage analysis that seeks chromosomal segments which pairs of brothers or sisters who have the same disease share more often than by chance (see *Table 13.3*).

Alleles – alternative forms of a gene.

Allelic heterogeneity – the situation where a clinical condition can be caused by any of several (often very many) different mutations within a certain gene. Characteristic of loss of function conditions (cf. **locus heterogeneity**).

Alternative splicing – alternative choices of which segments of an RNA primary transcript are retained in the mature messenger RNA (see *Figure 3.11*).

Amniotic fluid – the fluid surrounding a fetus, contained by the amnion.

Analytical validity – of a test, the extent to which it measures that which it claims to measure.

Anaphase – the phase of cell division (mitosis or meiosis) in which chromosomes or chromatids separate and are pulled to opposite poles of the cell.

Aneuploid – of a cell, not **euploid**; having missing or extra chromosomes.

Anneal – of complementary single strands of nucleic acid, to hybridize forming a base-paired double helix.

Anticipation – the tendency of a disease to become more severe, more frequent, or to start at an earlier age, in successive generations. Often an artifact of biased ascertainment.

Apoptosis – a specific mechanism by which a cell kills itself.

Association – the statistical tendency of two things to go together more often or less often than by random chance. The combination occurs at a frequency that is not equal to the product of the individual frequencies.

Assortative mating – choosing a mate who is genetically similar to oneself. Can be based either on having a similar phenotype or on being related.

Autosome – any chromosome that is not the X or Y sex chromosome.

Autozygosity mapping – mapping a recessive condition in inbred kindreds by finding a shared ancestral chromosome segment that is homozygous in all the affected people (see *Figure 9.8*).

Balanced – of a chromosomal constitution, having nothing extra or missing. Also used loosely of Robertsonian translocations, even though these lack part of the short arms of the acrocentric chromosomes involved.

Bias of ascertainment – collecting a sample that is statistically unrepresentative of the larger population.

Bisulfite sequencing – a method of identifying unmethylated cytosines in DNA; after treatment with sodium bisulfite they are converted to uracil, which is scored as thymine on sequencing (see *Figure 7.10*).

Bonferroni correction – a rigorous statistical correction for multiple testing, consisting of multiplying the *P* value for an observation by the number of different questions asked.

cDNA – complementary DNA; a DNA copy of messenger RNA made using reverse transcriptase. Human cDNAs represent only 1–3% of the genomic DNA but contain most (but not all) of the clinically relevant sequences. Unlike genomic DNA, cDNAs are tissue-specific.

Cascade screening – ascertaining gene carriers by systematic testing of the extended family of an affected person (see *Disease box 11*).

Cell cycle checkpoint – a regulatory interaction that prevents a cell progressing through the cell cycle unless certain conditions are met (see *Figure 12.8*).

Centromere – the point at which the sister chromatids of a replicated chromosome are joined, and the location of the kinetochore, to which spindle fibers attach during cell division. Marked by heterochromatin containing a special histone H3 variant, CENP-A protein.

Chimera – of a person, having cells derived from two different zygotes – a rare condition, the opposite of twinning. Of a gene, made by a chromosomal rearrangement that brings together exons of two different genes to form a novel gene. A common occurrence in cancer (see *Box 12.3*).

Chorionic villi – outgrowths of fetal origin on the external surface of the chorion, the outermost of the fetal membranes.

Chromatid – a single DNA double helix packaged into a chromosome. Chromosomes normally exist as a single chromatid, but when they are seen during cell division they consist of two sister chromatids joined at the centromere.

Chromatin – a general term for the DNA–protein complex of which chromosomes consist.

Chromatin disease – a disease caused by faulty regulation of chromatin structure (see *Disease box 2*).

Chromosomal instability – accumulation of structural and/or numerical chromosome abnormalities in abnormal (e.g. cancer) cells.

Coefficient of inbreeding – the probability that a person is homozygous at any given locus because of the inbreeding of his parents. Equal to half the coefficient of relationship of the parents.

Coefficient of relationship – the proportion of their genes that two people share by virtue of having identifiable common ancestors (see *Section 10.2*).

Common disease–common variant hypothesis – the hypothesis that most genetic susceptibility factors for common complex diseases are ancient variants that are common in the general population. The hypothesis underlying attempts to identify susceptibility alleles by association studies. The contrary hypothesis is that susceptibility is due to a heterogeneous collection of recent mutations.

Comparative genomic hybridization – (CGH) – a technique for detecting sequences anywhere in the genome that are present in an abnormal number of copies (see *Figures 4.7* and *4.8*).

Compound heterozygote – a person with a recessive condition who has two different mutant versions of the relevant gene.

Congenital – present at birth; not necessarily genetic.

Consensus sequence – of a family of related sequences, the sequence having the most common nucleotide at each position (which may or may not be the most common actual whole sequence).

Conserved sequences – sequences that are unchanged or little changed in related species.

Cousin – in genetics, used specifically to mean first cousin (q.v.).

CpG dinucleotide – a cytosine immediately upstream of a guanine in a DNA sequence. The target of DNA methylating enzymes, and hotspots for CpG→TpG mutations.

CpG islands – short chromosomal regions (typically less than 1 kb) where the usual genome-wide depletion of CpG dinucleotides has not taken place. See *Section 7.4* for their significance.

Cryptic splice site – a sequence in an exon or an intron that resembles a splice site but not sufficiently to be used as one; a mutation may change it so that it does get used as a splice site ('activating a cryptic splice site').

Denaturing – separating the two strands of a double helix by heat or high pH; also called melting.

Denaturing high performance liquid chromatography (dHPLC) – a method of testing a PCR product or other double-stranded DNA fragment for changes, compared to a reference fragment, by checking the speed with which it passes through a column.

Diagnostic test – a test that establishes the diagnosis in a patient affected by a disease (cf. a **predictive test**, a **screening test**).

Dichotomous character – a character such as a disease, that some people have and others do not (cf. **quantitative** or **continuous characters**, that everybody has).

Dideoxynucleotide (ddNTP) – a chemically modified nucleotide used in DNA sequencing to terminate growing DNA chains (see *Figure 5.2*).

Diploid – of a cell or organism, having two genomes. The normal condition of human somatic cells.

Dominant – a character is dominant if it is manifest in a heterozygote. Dominance and recessiveness are properties of characters, not of genes or alleles.

Dominant negative – a mutation where the product of the mutant allele interferes with the function of the normal product in a heterozygote.

Dosage-sensitive – of a gene, where different non-zero copy numbers have an effect on the phenotype.

Dot blotting – a hybridization test in which either the test DNA or the probe is spotted on to a solid support to immobilize it.

Downstream – on a nucleic acid strand, in the 3′ direction (of the sense strand in a gene).

Embryonic stem cell (ES cell) – a totipotent stem cell obtained from the inner cell mass of a blastocyst (see *Figure 14.6*).

Empiric risks – risks defined by survey data, as distinct from risks worked out by applying genetic theory.

ENCODE Project – an international collaborative project (Encyclopedia of DNA Elements, http://www.genome.gov/10005107) that aims to identify all functions of human DNA (see *Section 6.2*).

Epigenetic – making heritable (from cell to daughter cell, or sometimes from generation to generation) changes in gene expression without changing the nucleotide sequence. Effected by DNA methylation and/or changing chromatin structure.

Epimutation – a mutation that causes an epigenetic change but not a DNA sequence change.

Episome – an extrachromsomal genetic element.

Euchromatin – chromatin with a relatively open structure in which genes can be active if suitable transcription factors and co-activators are present; the opposite of **heterochromatin**.

Euploid – of a cell, containing some number of complete chromosome sets, without any extra or missing chromosomes. The opposite of aneuploid.

Exon – a segment of genomic DNA that corresponds to sequence in a mature mRNA. Exons include the 5′ and 3′ untranslated regions of a gene as well as the coding sequence.

Expression array – a microarray of oligonucleotides or cDNAs that will hybridize to individual mRNAs or cDNAs. When hybridized to bulk cDNA from a cell or tissue the pattern of hybridization reflects the repertoire of mRNAs in the source material (see *Sections 4.4* and *12.4*).

Familial – tending to run in families; not necessarily genetic.

Fetal exclusion test – a linkage-based method of telling whether or not a fetus is at risk of inheriting a late-onset dominant disease present in a grandparent, without doing a predictive test on the parent (see *Figure 9.10*).

First cousins – Jack and Jill are first cousins if one of Jack's parents is the sib of one of Jill's parents.

Fluorescence *in situ* hybridization (FISH) – *in situ* hybridization using a fluorescently labeled DNA or RNA probe (see *Figures 4.6, 4.14* and *4.15*).

Founder effects – an unusually high frequency of a particular allele or haplotype in a population that is descended from a small number of founders, one or more of whom happened to carry that sequence.

Fragile site – in a chromosome preparation, a region that appears relatively uncoiled and extended. Usually only seen under specific culture conditions, e.g. after treatment with bromodeoxyuridine or aphidicolin. Most fragile sites exist as non-pathogenic polymorphic variants. The FRAXA and FRAXE fragile sites (see *Disease box 4*) are unusual in being pathogenic.

Frame-shift mutation – a mutation that alters the reading frame of a coding sequence (see *Box 3.3* and *Section 6.2*).

Functional genomics – studying the functions of all the genes in a genome or all the genes expressed in a cell or tissue.

G-banding – a standard procedure in which chromosomes are treated so that they stain in a characteristic and reproducible pattern of dark and pale bands, as shown in *Figure 2.5*.

Gene conversion – a process in which a short stretch (typically 100 bp) of DNA sequence in a gene is replaced with similar but not identical sequence from another allele or gene. A recombination-like process but non-reciprocal – the donor gene is unchanged (see *Box 8.2*).

Gene frequency – the gene frequency of allele A_n is the proportion of all alleles of the A gene in a certain population that are A_n.

Gene pool – the totality of alleles at a particular locus in a certain population.

Gene tracking – using linked polymorphic markers to follow the segregation of a chromosomal segment through a pedigree. Used to follow a pathogenic mutation when, for any reason, it is not possible to check for the mutation directly by sequencing (see *Figure 9.9*).

Genetic drift – a change in gene frequencies between generations because of chance differences between the gene frequencies in one generation and the genes in the gametes that go to make the next generation. Only happens if the number of gametes is small, i.e. the breeding population is very small.

Genome – the totality of genetic material of an organism.

Genomic – of DNA, the DNA as it occurs in the cell nucleus, in contrast to cDNA.

Germ-line – the lineage of cells that are potentially transmissible to the next generation. In humans and other animals the germ-line separates from somatic cells very early in embryogenesis.

Germinal mosaic – a person who, owing to a mutation that occurred after they were conceived, has a mutant cell population in their germ-line, so that they can produce recurrent mutant gametes. A major pitfall in pedigree interpretation and risk estimation.

Haploid – of a cell or organism, having only a single genome (i.e. 23 chromosomes in humans).

Haplo-insufficiency – the condition in which a single functional copy of a gene is not sufficient to produce a normal phenotype, so that loss of function mutations in the gene produce a dominant character.

Haplotype – a set of closely linked alleles on a chromosome that is normally inherited as a block.

HapMap project – an international collaborative project that aims to catalog all the conserved ancestral chromosome segments in several different human populations (see *Section 13.4* and http://www.hapmap.org).

Hardy–Weinberg distribution – the mathematical relationship between gene frequencies and genotype frequencies seen when no distorting factors are present. Seldom applies in humans to rare recessive conditions where many cases are due to consanguinity (see *Box 10.1*).

Heritability – the extent to which differences between people with respect to a character (in a particular population at a particular time) are due to the genetic differences between them. Heritabilities are correlation coefficients, symbolized as h^2 and taking values between 0 (no genetic influence) and 1 (wholly determined by genetic differences) (see *Section 13.2*).

Heterochromatin – chromatin that is highly condensed and genetically inactive. Found mainly at centromeres.

Heteroduplex – a DNA double helix containing mismatches (see *Figure 5.7a*).

Heteroplasmy – of a person, having two or more genetically different types of mitochondria.

Homologous chromosomes – the two No. 1 chromosomes, etc. in a person. Homologous chromosomes contain the same array of loci but, unlike sister chromatids, they are not copies of each other. They may differ in small ways (minor DNA sequence differences) or sometimes in large ways (because of translocations, etc.).

Hybridize – of complementary single strands of nucleic acid, to anneal forming a base-paired double helix.

Informative meiosis – in linkage analysis, a meiosis where the genotypes allow it to be scored as recombinant or non-recombinant.

Intron – a segment of a gene that is part of the primary transcript but is excised by the splicing machinery and is not included in the mature mRNA.

Inversion – a structural abnormality in which part of a chromosome is in the wrong orientation compared to the rest (see *Figures 2.19* and *4.12*).

Karyogram – the correct term for a display of somebody's chromosomes, like in *Figure 2.9*. Usually loosely called a karyotype.

Karyotype – a person's chromosome constitution – also used loosely to describe a display of a person's chromosomes, as in *Figure 2.9*, etc.

Lepore – Lepore-type genes are chimeric genes produced by non-homologous recombination. Named after the hemoglobin β–δ chimeric gene that produces Hb–Lepore.

Library – in molecular genetics, a random collection of cloned fragments of a complex starting material (DNA or mRNA). The main types are genomic libraries and cDNA libraries (see *Box 4.5*).

Linkage – the phenomenon whereby loci that are close together on a chromosome tend to segregate together in families. The extent of the tendency (between random segregation and invariable co-segregation) measures the genetic distance in centiMorgans (between 0 and 50 cM) between the loci.

Linkage disequilibrium – a population association of particular alleles at two or more loci. Seen when the loci are closely linked and the alleles are features of a shared ancestral chromosome segment.

Locus – the position of a gene on a chromosome; a type of gene (as distinct from alleles, which are variant forms of the same type of gene).

Locus control region – a DNA sequence located many kilobases away from the transcription start site of a gene that controls the expression of a gene or group of genes (see *Section 3.4*).

Locus heterogeneity – the situation where a clinical phenotype can be caused by mutations at any one of several different loci, cf. **allelic heterogeneity**.

Lod score – the statistical measure of the significance of evidence for or against linkage. Equals the logarithm (base 10) of the odds that the loci are linked, with a given recombination fraction, rather than not linked (see *Section 9.2*).

Loss of heterozygosity – in cancer research, the observation that tumor DNA is apparently homozygous for a DNA polymorphism for which the normal DNA of the same patient is heterozygous. Usually the result of loss of a chromosome. If seen repeatedly, implies that the chromosome in question carries a tumor suppressor gene (see *Figure 12.7*).

Lyonization – X-inactivation (see *Figure 7.4*).

Lysosomal storage disease – an inborn error of metabolism where lysosomes are unable to degrade a certain type of material. As a result the material accumulates in lysosomes, leading to pathological effects.

Manifesting heterozygote – with an X-linked recessive condition, a female carrier who shows some clinical signs of the condition, most likely because by chance she has inactivated her good X in most cells of the affected tissue.

Meta-analysis – analysis of the combined data from a number of separate studies.

Metacentric – a chromosome that has its centromere in the middle (e.g. numbers 3 and 20).

Metaphase – the stage of mitosis or meiosis immediately before anaphase, when chromosomes are maximally contracted and aligned on the equatorial plane (metaphase plate) of the cell.

Methylation – attaching methyl (CH_3) groups to any molecule, but particularly used for converting cytosine in a CpG dinucleotide to 5-methyl cytosine as part of gene regulation (see *Figure 7.8*).

Methylation-sensitive restriction enzyme – a restriction enzyme such as *Hpa*II that will only cut unmethylated recognition sites (see *Section 7.2*).

Microarray – a solid support divided into a large number of cells in each of which a specific test sample or reagent has been anchored, allowing a large number of tests to be carried out in parallel. Microarrays of oligonucleotides, cDNAs, antibodies or tumor samples are widely used in genetic research.

Microdeletion – a chromosomal deletion that is too small (< 3–5 Mb) to be seen on a standard chromosome preparation; Detected by **fluorescence *in situ* hybridization, comparative genomic hybridization,** or **multiplex ligation-dependent probe amplification.**

Microsatellites – short tandem DNA repeats where the repeat unit is 1–6 nucleotides (tandem repeats with longer repeat units are called mini-satellites). Polymorphic microsatellites are one of the main types of DNA marker for linkage analysis.

Microsatellite instability – a property of tumors that are deficient in repair of DNA mismatches caused by replication errors. Compared to the normal DNA of the patient, tumor DNA contains new alleles of many microsatellites from all across the genome.

Mismatch repair – a protein complex, including the MSH2 and MLH1 proteins, checks newly replicated DNA for wrongly incorporated nucleotides, cuts them out and re-synthesizes that stretch of the DNA.

Modifier gene – a gene that modifies the phenotype of a mendelian condition whose primary cause is a different gene.

Monosomy – having one copy of one particular chromosome, but two of all the others (i.e. 45 in total for an autosomal monosomy).

Mosaic – having two or more genetically different cell lines. A person can be mosaic for a chromosomal variant or a single-gene change.

Multifactorial – a catch-all term to describe a character that is determined by many factors including several genes and environmental factors.

Multiplex ligation-dependent probe amplification (MLPA) – a method for simultaneously checking a large number (30–50) of short DNA sequences for copy number variations. Used especially for checking multi-exon genes for any whole-exon deletion (see *Figures 5.8* and *5.9*).

Non-parametric linkage analysis – linkage analysis that is based on the extent to which affected relatives share chromosomal segments, but does not depend on a specific genetic model for the cause of the phenotype (see *Section 13.2*).

Nonsense-mediated decay – a mechanism in cells that breaks down most mRNA molecules which contain a stop codon located more than 50 nucleotides upstream of the 3′-most splice site. Probably evolved to protect cells against dominant negative effects of truncated proteins (see *Figure 6.3*).

Nonsense mutation – a mutation that converts a codon for an amino acid into a stop codon (UAA, UAG or UGA in mRNA; TAA, TAG or TGA in the DNA).

Northern blotting – analyzing RNA by gel electrophoresis, transferring to a membrane and hybridizing to a labeled probe.

Nucleosome – the basic unit of chromatin, comprising 146 bp of DNA wrapped round a core consisting of two molecules each of histones H2A, H2B, H3 and H4.

Nucleoside – a combination of a base and a sugar.

Nucleotide – a combination of a base, a sugar and a phosphate.

Oligonucleotide ('*oligo*') – a short piece of single-stranded DNA or RNA.

Obligate carrier – a person whose pedigree shows that they must be a carrier of a recessive (autosomal or X-linked) condition. For X-linked conditions where new mutations are frequent, an obligate carrier must have affected or carrier relatives both in her own or a previous generation, and among her children or grandchildren. Having more than one affected child does not make a woman an obligate carrier because she might be a germinal mosaic.

Okazaki fragments – intermediates in DNA replication. As a replication fork moves along a double helix, one new strand growing in the 5′→3′ direction can grow continuously in the same direction as the movement of the fork, but the other is synthesized as a set of short (100–200 nucleotide) fragments that are later ligated together (see *Figure 12.3a*).

Oncogene – a gene that suffers gain of function mutations in cancer. Strictly applies only to the mutated version; the normal version is strictly called a **proto-oncogene**, but this distinction is often ignored.

One gene–one enzyme hypothesis – the hypothesis (defined by Beadle and Tatum in the 1940s) that the function of each gene is to direct synthesis of one specific enzyme. Now seen as only part of the story.

Penetrance – the probability of a character being manifest, given a certain genotype. Penetrance is a property of a character or phenotype, not a gene or allele.

Pharmacogenetics – the study of single gene effects on the metabolism or action of a drug.

Pharmacogenomics – the genome-wide study of drug targets or drug effects.

Phenocopy – a phenotype that resembles a genetic phenotype, but is produced by non-genetic means.

Phenotype – the observable characteristic of a person (including the result of tests).

Pleiotropic – of a mutation, having effects on many systems.

Polygene – an unfortunate term sometimes used to describe the genes responsible for a polygenic character. Polygenes are not a different type of gene, they are ordinary genes that have variants which have a minor effect on some particular character. The same genes may have major effects on a different character.

Polygenic – in mathematical theory a polygenic character is determined by the combined action of an infinite number of genes, each of which has an infinitesimally small effect. In reality, polygenic effects can be due to just a handful of genes.

Population attributable risk (population attributable fraction) – of a cause of disease, the extent to which that particular cause is responsible for the overall incidence of the disease in the population.

Positional candidate – in identifying disease genes, a gene located in a chromosomal region identified by linkage as containing a disease gene.

Positional cloning – identifying a disease gene through linkage analysis followed by testing positional candidates for mutations; as compared to identifying the disease gene through investigation of the pathogenesis.

Positive predictive value – of a test result, the proportion of cases positive on the test that actually have the condition being sought (see *Box 11.1*).

Predictive test – a test that shows whether a currently healthy person is likely subsequently to develop a late-onset disease.

Pre-mutation – in diseases caused by expanded nucleotide repeats, an expansion that is not long enough to cause the disease, but is long enough to destabilize the repeat, so that later generations are affected (see *Disease box 4*).

Primary transcript – the initial RNA product of transcribing a gene. Contains all the exons and introns of the gene. The introns are cut out when the primary transcript is processed to form the mature mRNA.

Primer – in DNA synthesis, a short (10–40 nt) oligonucleotide that hybridizes to a single strand of DNA and that is then extended by DNA polymerase adding nucleotides to its 3′ end.

Prior probability – in Bayesian risk estimation, the initial estimate of how plausible each alternative hypothesis is.

Probe – a piece of single-stranded DNA labeled, for example, with ^{32}P or a fluorescent dye, that is used in a hybridization assay to test for the presence of a complementary sequence.

Promoter – the DNA region immediately upstream of a gene on which the RNA polymerase complex is assembled to enable transcription of the gene.

Prophase – the first stage of mitosis or meiosis when the chromosomes are gradually condensing and becoming visible. Ends with the dissolution of the nuclear membrane.

Prometaphase – late prophase of cell division. Cytogeneticists normally karyotype mitotic cells in prometaphase because the chromosomes are more extended than at metaphase and show the banding better.

Proteome – the complete set of proteins in a cell or tissue.

Proto-oncogene – the normal, unactivated version of an **oncogene**.

Pseudoautosomal region – the regions at the tips of the X and Y chromosome short arms that contain 2.6 Mb of homologous DNA and recombine in meiosis. Genes in this region show an autosomal pattern of inheritance. There is another short pseudoautosomal region at the tips of the long arms (see *Figure 7.5*).

Pseudogene – a non-functional copy of a gene. Pseudogenes are very common in the human genome.

Quantitative trait locus (QTL) – a locus that contributes to the phenotype of a quantitative character.

Quantitative character – a character like blood pressure that everybody has, but with varying magnitude. Sometimes called a continuous character, cf. **dichotomous character.**

Random mating – a choice of mate unrelated to genotype; the opposite of **assortative mating.**

Real-time PCR – various methods by which the accumulation of a PCR product can be followed as the reaction proceeds. The basis of most quantitative PCR assays.

Recessive – a character is recessive if it is not manifest in a heterozygote. Recessiveness and dominance are properties of characters, not of genes or alleles.

Recombinant – a gamete produced by a person is recombinant for two loci if the two alleles that it carries came from different parents of the person.

Recombinant DNA – DNA produced by ligating together sequences derived from different sources – typically a human sequence of interest ligated into a vector.

Relative risk – the risk of a disease for a person with a specific genotype, or a specific relationship to an affected person, compared to the risk in the general population. Note that relative risks are quite distinct from absolute risks. A relative risk of 10 may be of no clinical significance if it only raises the absolute risk from 1 in 10000 to 1 in 1000.

Reproductive cloning – a procedure that aims to produce a cloned baby (see *Section 14.4*).

Restriction endonuclease – an enzyme that cuts double-stranded DNA at a specific sequence, usually a 4- or 6-nucleotide palindrome.

Restriction fragment length polymorphism (RFLP) – a DNA polymorphism due to a nucleotide change that creates or abolishes the recognition site for a restriction enzyme (see for example, *Figure 5.14*).

Reverse dot blot – a **dot blot** where the probe rather than the test DNA is immobilized on the solid support. DNA **microarrays** are massively parallel reverse dot blots.

Robertsonian translocation – a special type of translocation in which two acrocentric chromosomes are joined close to their centromeres (see *Figure 2.20*).

RT–PCR – reverse transcriptase – polymerase chain reaction; a technique for making many DNA copies of an RNA. A common method for studying messenger RNA.

Screening test – a test used to select people at high risk from a population. Normally followed by a **diagnostic test** (see *Section 11.2*).

Second cousins – two people are second cousins if their parents are first cousins.

Sense strand – in a gene the strand of the double helix whose sequence corresponds to the sequence of the messenger RNA (the opposite of the template strand).

Sensitivity of a test – the proportion of people with the disease, etc. that is being sought, that the test picks up (see *Box 11.1*).

Sex-limited – a character that is seen in only one sex for anatomical or physiological reasons.

Sibs – brothers or sisters.

Signal peptide – the N-terminal dozen or so amino acid residues of a nascent protein that determine where it will be transported. Signal peptides are cleaved off once they have performed their function.

Single nucleotide polymorphism (SNP) – any polymorphic variation at a single nucleotide.

Single strand conformation polymorphism (SSCP) – a quick but fallible method for scanning a DNA fragment (up to 300 nt) for mutations (see *Figure 5.7b*).

Sister chromatids – the two chromatids of a chromosome as seen in a dividing cell. Sister chromatids are copies of each other, made during the preceding round of DNA replication.

Slipped-strand mis-pairing – a mistake in replication of a tandemly repeated sequence that results in the newly synthesized strand having extra or missing repeat units compared to the template.

Somatic mutation – a mutation in a cell of the body that will not be transmitted to offspring.

Southern blotting – analyzing DNA by restriction digestion, gel electrophoresis, transfer to a membrane and hybridizing to a labeled probe (see *Figure 4.5*).

Splice isoforms – alternative forms of a protein produced by alternative splicing of exons.

Stem cell – a cell that is capable both of self-replication and of giving rise to a variety of differentiated cell lineages (see *Figure 14.5*).

Stop codon – in a messenger RNA, a UAG, UGA or UAA codon that signals the ribosome to dissociate and cease extending the polypeptide chain; the corresponding sequence in a gene.

Submetacentric – of a chromosome, having a long arm and a short arm, e.g. most human chromosomes (the others are metacentric or acrocentric).

Tandem repeat – direct DNA sequence repeats that are adjacent to each other. Other types of repeats are inverted repeats (or palindromes) and dispersed repeats.

Telomerase – a ribonucleoprotein that can add TTAGGG units to the telomeres of chromosomes.

Telomere – the special structure that stabilizes the ends of chromosomes, comprising specific proteins complexed to tandemly repeated TTAGGG DNA sequences.

Template strand – in a gene, the strand of the double helix that base-pairs with the nascent RNA during transcription.

Therapeutic cloning – a procedure that aims to produce embryonic stem cells genetically matched to a patient, in order to obtain cells or tissues for transplantation (see *Figure 14.7*).

Trans-acting – of a genetic regulatory element, regulating a gene or genes that lie elsewhere in the genome (normally by making a diffusible regulatory product).

Transcription factor – a protein whose action is to facilitate transcription of a gene or genes by helping bring the RNA polymerase to the promoter.

Translocation – a structural abnormality in which two chromosomes swap non-homologous segments (see, for example, *Figure 2.14*).

Transmission disequilibrium test (TDT) – a test for association in the presence of linkage. Used in identifying disease susceptibility factors (see *Figure 13.9*).

Transposon – a 'jumping gene': a mobile genetic element that can move from one chromosomal location to another, either via excision or by making a mobile copy. They can be seen as a sort of intracellular virus. Transposons can be recognized by certain sequence features. About 50% of the human genome consists of transposons, but the great majority have accumulated mutations that destroy their ability to transpose.

Triploid – a cell or organism having three copies of the genome (in humans, 69 chromosomes). Normally lethal in animals including humans.

Trisomy – having three copies of one particular chromosome, but two of all the others, i.e. 47 in total. (see for example, *Figure 2.11*).

Trisomy rescue - the main mechanism producing uniparental disomy. A chance mitotic non-disjunction in a trisomic early embryo produces one cell with the correct chromosomal number, from which the whole baby develops (see *Figure 7.16*).

Tumor suppressor gene – a gene that suffers loss of function mutations in cancers.

Unbalanced – of a chromosomal abnormality, having extra or missing material, rather than just the correct material rearranged.

Uniparental disomy – having both copies of one chromosome pair inherited from the same parent. In isodisomy the two are copies of the same parental chromosome, in heterodisomy both chromosomes of that parent are present.

Unrelated – everybody is related if you go back far enough. In genetics, people are usually described as unrelated if they do not share any common great-grandparent.

Upstream – on a nucleic acid strand, in the 5′ direction (of the sense strand in a gene).

Vector – a DNA sequence into which a piece of DNA of interest can be ligated, allowing it to be introduced into cells and manipulated. Most vectors are engineered versions of natural plasmids or bacteriophages (see *Box 4.5*).

X-inactivation – the mechanism whereby in each cell of a person, genes on all but one of the X chromosomes are switched off, so that only one gene copy is active regardless of the number of X chromosomes present (see *Figure 7.4*).

Index

b after a page number means entry is in a box, f in a figure, g in the glossary, t in a table; bold pages are principal entries. References to diseases have as far as possible been listed under the heading 'Syndrome'.